Interferon Treatment of Neurologic Disorders

Interferon Treatment of Neurologic Disorders

edited by

RICHARD ALAN SMITH

Center for Neurologic Study
San Diego, California

MARCEL DEKKER, INC. New York and Basel

Library of Congress Cataloging-in-Publication Data

Interferon treatment of neurologic disorders.

   Includes bibliographies and index.
   1. Interferon--Therapeutic use. 2. Nervous
system--Diseases--Chemotherapy. 3. Nervous system--
Infections--Chemotherapy. I. Smith, Richard Alan,
         [DNLM: 1. Interferons--therapeutic use.
2. Nervous System Diseases--therapy. WL 100 I595]
RC350.I45I58 1988   616.8'0461   88-11816
ISBN 0-8247-7935-5

COPYRIGHT © 1988 by MARCEL DEKKER, INC. ALL RIGHTS RESERVED

Neither this book nor any part may be reproduced or transmitted in any form or by any means, electronic or mechanical, including photocopying, microfilming, and recording, or by any information storage and retrieval system, without permission in writing from the publisher.

MARCEL DEKKER, INC.
270 Madison Avenue, New York, New York 10016

Current printing (last digit):
10 9 8 7 6 5 4 3 2 1

PRINTED IN THE UNITED STATES OF AMERICA

Foreword

There are many books about interferons, but to my knowledge, this is the first one that focuses on the interferon therapy of neurologic diseases. Is there a need for a book like this? I think so and believe that the contents of this book represent just the beginning of a long series of investigations in a field which will become increasingly important in the future.

The clinical applications of interferons started slowly. During the first 25 years of interferon research there was a continual shortage of interferons. In the 1970s, almost all clinical work with interferons was carried out with natural human leukocyte interferon-a. In the 1980s, lymphoblastoid interferon-a, recombinant interferon-a_2 and recombinant interferons-γ have become abundantly available. But at present very little solid information is available about the clinical usefulness of interferons. In my opinion, interferon is today applicable for the routine treatment of two diseases only—dendritic keratitis and hairy cell leukemia. It is my belief that there will be other diseases in which interferon will be the treatment of choice.

As the contents of this book show, our information about the value of interferons in the treatment of neurologic diseases is still very preliminary and fragmentary. Some promising hints, however, encourage further work. It seems clear to me that, for optimum results, interferons will have to be combined with other treatment modalities, especially with other biologic response modifiers. Such studies will take decades.

I find the "neurotoxicity" of interferons intriguing. Do the effects of interferons on memory, mood, and behavior suggest that interferons or related molecules may have physiologic functions in the brain? Can we use these molecules as our tools to unravel some of the infinitely complex mechanisms of the brain functions? Finally, a thought that has been nagging me for years: Could interferons have beneficial effects on psychiatric diseases such as schizophrenia?

Kari Cantell

Preface

With the advent of biotechnology clinicians have seen new opportunities to undertake the treatment of presently incurable diseases. This is particularly the case for some neurologic disorders in which treatment has not changed appreciably in spite of a general advance in medical and scientific progress. As recently as 1980, interferons were in short supply and laboratories were gearing up to identify and produce other lymphokines including interleukin, tumor necrosis factor, and so forth. Most, if not all, of the biotechnical milestones of the decade pertain to interferon, which was the first human gene to be sequenced, the first human protein to be cloned, and the first recombinant-derived biological to be approved for human use. The people who have made this happen are some of the most remarkable personalities of contemporary science. In these heady times of biotechnology it is worth recalling the effort and commitment that was needed to isolate and purify a protein in the recent past.

Following the discovery of interferon in the 1950s, interest in interferons remained relatively dormant; in fact, this area of inquiry was accorded very little respect. Most observers credit Kari Cantell, a Finnish physician, with bringing interferon to center stage. Over the course of 10 years Dr. Cantell painstakingly developed the procedures for purifying interferon from human leukocytes. Subsequently, the Finnish Red Cross became the major supplier of interferon-α, allowing investigators to study the pharmacology and pharmacokinetic properties of the drug and initiate clinical trials. At this point—in the early 1980s—a number of factors brought interferon to public attention. An anxious populace, spurred on by the media, saw in interferon the possibility of a miracle drug that would eradicate cancer and other scourges of humankind. The biotechnological industry, then in its infancy, was understandably eager to bring to market a product with the reputed potential of interferon. A breakthrough drug also fit the needs of foundations, which look to the public to support their various causes, including cancer and multiple sclerosis.

This volume, assembled over the course of several years, provides a balanced view of interferon as it relates to the nervous system. The authors represent a spectrum of persons working in the field. The majority are at academic institutions, small institutes or corporations. While most are North Americans, I was fortunate to be able to enlist the support of authors from Europe and Asia. Contact throughout the world has been facilitated by frequent meetings, which have given the interferon community a sense of camaraderie. In very few fields has international collaboration attained such success.

Although the clinical results with interferons, particularly as they relate to neurologic disorders, have been modest, even the casual reader will be impressed with the knowledge that has accumulated on the subject. The tools available to researchers in an era of molecular biology have permitted elaborate investigation into the mechanisms of action of interferons. Although the story continues to unfold, investigators have uncovered a great deal about the inner workings of interferons on cells. Acting in the manner of a hormone, interferons induce a cascade of intracellular events which prepare host defenses against viral attack. As each of these pathways has been elucidated, our understanding of viral-host interactions has been enhanced. It is likely that this information will lead to novel means for interfering with viral replication and controlling cell growth. Seen from this perspective, interferons can be viewed as probes that provide insight into the workings of cells and into the mechanisms they employ to preserve their integrity.

The clinical studies reported in this volume suggest that the course of several diseases, most notably multiple sclerosis, can be modified with administration of interferon. This has encouraged investigators to proceed with additional trials. Second-generation studies will employ highly purified, recombinant-derived interferons. As a result there are few constraints on the dose or the number of patients to be enrolled. Although it may be hazardous to predict the outcome of an individual trial, it seems safe to predict that interferons will ultimately prove to have a role in the treatment of a number of presently incurable neurologic diseases. It may take years to realize this prediction. Dramatic, immediate results would have been preferred, but nature does not always make the physician's task easy.

As the century comes to a close, it is clear that our human capabilities are expanding at an unprecedented pace. In this environment patients increasingly look to society to address their hopes for a better life. This expectation may seem unreasonable to some, but from the patient's perspective medicine and science represent society's commitment to its less fortunate members. Although it is an imperfect world, I do believe that patients and their families sense through interferon the worth of those who take science or medicine as their calling.

Although the idea to explore the usefulness of interferon for the treatment of neurologic diseases was mine, George F. Thagard, Jr., and Kari Cantell, M.D., made it possible for me to do so. This book is dedicated to them and to supporters Arlene and George Hecht, Toby and Leon Gold, Al Herzog, Betty and Cindy Bordner, Alese and Jack Shapiro, Joan Thagard, Dee Norris, and Charles Taubman; family Lucie, Tania, and Daryl Smith, Alfred and Norma Cohen, and Herbert Smith; colleagues Charles Bakst, Shen Wang, J. Lakshmanan, James Nelson, Dee Silver, Ed Chapman, Brian Copeland, and Forbes Norris; and patients Charles Bordner, Rosalie Mills, James Waldal, Fred Clark, Arthur Levien, Ida Harvey, and Frank Parodi.

Richard Alan Smith

Contributors

Samuel Baron Department of Microbiology, University of Texas Medical Branch, Galveston, Texas

Ernest C. Borden Department of Human Oncology, University of Wisconsin Clinical Cancer Center, Madison, Wisconsin

Ferdinando Dianzani Institute of Virology, University of Rome Medical School, Rome, Italy

Markus Färkkilä Department of Neurology, University Hospital of Helsinki, Helsinki, Finland

W. Robert Fleischmann, Jr. Department of Microbiology, University of Texas Medical Branch, Galveston, Texas

David Goldstein Department of Human Oncology, University of Wisconsin Clinical Cancer Center, Madison, Wisconsin

Jean-Claude Guillon Department of Experimental Physiopathology, Oncology Unit, Pasteur Institute, Paris, France

Robert M. Herndon Department of Neurology, University of Rochester School of Medicine and Dentistry, Rochester, New York

Ara G. Hovanessian Department of Virology, Pasteur Institute, Paris, France

Lawrence Jacobs Baird Multiple Sclerosis Center, Dent Neurologic Institute, Millard Fillmore Hospital, and Department of Neurology, State University of New York School of Medicine at Buffalo, Buffalo, New York

Kenneth P. Johnson Department of Neurology, University of Maryland School of Medicine and Veterans Administration Medical Center, Baltimore, Maryland

Rugimar Markovistz Department of Virology, Pasteur Institute, Paris, France

Jean E. Merrill Department of Neurology, Reed Neurological Research Center, University of California-Los Angeles School of Medicine, Los Angeles, California

Osamu Nakamura* Department of Neurosurgery, University of Tokyo Hospital, Tokyo, Japan

Forbes H. Norris ALS Research Center, Pacific Presbyterian Medical Center, San Francisco, California

Hillel S. Panitch Department of Neurology, University of Maryland School of Medicine and Veterans Administration Medical Center, Baltimore, Maryland

George J. Pazin Department of Infectious Diseases, School of Medicine and Graduate School of Public Health, University of Pittsburgh, Pittsburgh, Pennsylvania

---

Present affiliation:
*Department of Neurosurgery, Tokyo Metropolitan Komagome Hospital, Tokyo, Japan.

CONTRIBUTORS

V. Ramamurthy* Department of Microbiology, University of Texas Medical Branch, Galveston, Texas

Peter Reese Department of Biomathematics, Roswell Park Memorial Institute, Buffalo, New York

Yves Rivière Department of Virology, Pasteur Institute, Paris, France

Ama Z. S. Rohatiner Department of Medical Oncology, St. Bartholomew's Hospital, London, England

Andres Salazar Department of Clinical Investigation, Walter Reed Army Medical Center and Uniformed Services University of Health Sciences, Bethesda, Maryland

Richard Alan Smith Center for Neurologic Study, San Diego, California

G. John Stanton Department of Microbiology, University of Texas Medical Branch, Galveston, Texas

Kintomo Takakura Department of Neurosurgery, University of Tokyo Hospital, Tokyo, Japan

Stephan R. Targan Department of Medicine, University of California-Los Angeles School of Medicine, Los Angeles, California

Henri Tsiang Rabies Unit, Department of Virology, Pasteur Institute, Paris, France

Bryan R. G. Williams Department of Pediatrics and Medical Genetics, Research Institute, Hospital for Sick Children, Toronto, Ontario, Canada

Present affiliation:
*Department of Biochemistry, Baylor College of Medicine, Houston, Texas.

Robert J. Wills Department of Drug Metabolism, Hoffmann-La Roche Inc., Nutley, New Jersey

Allan J. Yates Division of Neuropathology, Department of Pathology, College of Medicine, The Ohio State University, Columbus, Ohio

Contents

Foreword (Kari Cantell)		*iii*
Preface		*v*
Contributors		*ix*
1.	**Interferon: Mode of Action and Clinical Applications**	1
	W. Robert Fleischmann, Jr., V. Ramamurthy, G. John Stanton, Samuel Baron, and Ferdinando Dianzani	
	I. Introduction and Overview	1
	II. Historical Perspective	5
	III. Production and Properties of Interferons	7
	IV. Large-Scale Production by Recombinant DNA Techniques	8
	V. Assay Techniques	9
	VI. Interferon Activation of Responding Cells	12
	VII. Biologic Activities of Interferons	15
	VIII. Interferon in Disease States	21
	IX. Therapeutic Application of Interferon	22
	X. Future Prospects	25
	References	27

2. **Molecular Mechanisms of Interferon Action** 43
   Bryan R. G. Williams
   - I. Interferon-Receptor Interactions 44
   - II. Genes Regulated by Interferons 46
   - III. Interferon-Induced Changes in Intracellular Functions 48
   - IV. The 2-5A System 50
   - V. The Protein Kinase 54
   - VI. Regulation of Oncogene Expression by Interferon 56
   - References 57

3. **The Immunologic Basis for the Use of Interferons** 65
   Jean E. Merrill and Stephan R. Targan
   - I. Classes of Interferons and Leukocytes that Produce Them 65
   - II. General Biologic Effects of IFN 67
   - III. Induction and Suppression of IFN by Immunoregulatory Mechanisms 68
   - IV. IFN Effects on Cell Growth and Proliferation 70
   - V. Effects of IFN on Differentiation 71
   - VI. Production and Response to IFN in Patients with Multiple Sclerosis 79
   - VII. Conclusions 82
   - References 83

4. **Pharmacokinetics of Interferons** 103
   Robert J. Wills and Richard Alan Smith
   - I. Introduction 103
   - II. Pharmacokinetic Concepts 104
   - III. Interferon Pharmacokinetics 108
   - IV. Conclusion 125
   - References 126

5. **Neurotoxicity of Interferon Therapy** 135
   Ama Z. S. Rohatiner and Markus Färkkilä
   - I. Introduction 135
   - II. Clinical Toxicity 135
   - III. Neuropsychiatric Manifestations 137
   - IV. EEG Changes 138
   - V. Conclusion 140
   - References 140

6. Interferon Treatment of Herpes Simplex and Varicella-Zoster Virus Infections of the Nervous System   145
George J. Pazin
   I.   Introduction   145
   II. Laboratory and Animal Studies: Herpes Simplex Virus Infections   146
   III. Clinical Herpes Simplex Virus Studies   146
   IV. Clinical Varicella-Zoster Virus Studies   152
   V.   Summary   154
        References   154

7. Production and Action of Interferon in Rabies Virus Infection   157
Ara G. Hovanessian, Rugimar Marcovistz, Yves Rivière, Jean-Claude Guillon, and Henri Tsiang
   I.   Introduction   157
   II. Effect of Interferon on Rabies Infection of Animals   158
   III. Production and Action of Interferon During Rabies Virus Infection in Mice   161
   IV. Action of Exogenous Interferon on the Prophylaxis of Rabies Infection in Mice   168
   V.   Conclusions   176
        References   179

8. Treatment of Subacute Sclerosing Panencephalitis with Interferon   187
Hillel S. Panitch
   I.   Introduction   187
   II. Etiology and Pathogenesis   188
   III. Changing Clinical Course of SSPE   190
   IV. Treatment of SSPE   191
   V.   Directions for Future Therapeutic Trials in SSPE   198
        References   200

9. Treatment of Multiple Sclerosis by Systemic Administration of Interferon   209
Hillel S. Panitch and Kenneth P. Johnson
   I.   Introduction   209
   II. Clinical Trials of Systemic Interferons in Multiple Sclerosis   214
   III. Treatment of MS with an Interferon Inducer   226

	IV.	Studies in Progress	227
	V.	Complications of Study Designs	228
	VI.	Conclusions	231
		References	232

10. **Intrathecal Interferon in the Treatment of Multiple Sclerosis**   241
    Lawrence Jacobs, Andres Salazar, Robert M. Herndon, and Peter Reese

	I.	Introduction	241
	II.	Patients and Methods	242
	III.	Results	248
	IV.	Discussion	255
	V.	Addendum	259
		References	262

11. **Treatment of Amyotrophic Lateral Sclerosis with Interferon**   265
    Richard Alan Smith and Forbes H. Norris

	I.	Introduction	265
	II.	Viral Studies	266
	III.	Treatment Trials	268
	IV.	Methodology	269
	V.	Results	271
	VI.	Conclusions	272
		References	274

12. **Effects of Interferons on Malignant Brain Tumors**   277
    Kintomo Takakura, Osamu Nakamura, and Allan J. Yates

	I.	Introduction	277
	II.	In Vivo Studies	278
	III.	In Vitro Studies	298
	IV.	Summary	312
		References	313

13. **Interferons and Neurologic Disease: Epilogue**   321
    David Goldstein and Ernest C. Borden
    References   327

Index   *333*

Interferon Treatment of Neurologic Disorders

1
Interferon: Mode of Action and Clinical Applications

W. ROBERT FLEISCHMANN, JR., V. RAMAMURTHY,*
G. JOHN STANTON, and SAMUEL BARON

University of Texas Medical Branch, Galveston, Texas

FERDINANDO DIANZANI

Institute of Virology, University of Rome Medical School, Rome, Italy

I. INTRODUCTION AND OVERVIEW

In 1957, Isaacs and Lindenmann discovered an activity in cell supernatant fluids and animals that had the capability of blocking virus replication. They named this activity "interferon" (1). The possibilities for understanding natural defenses and for the therapeutic application of interferon were immediately recognized.

In the almost 30 years since interferon's discovery, the field of interferon research has progressed tremendously. We now know that the interferon of Isaacs and Lindenmann is really a family of molecules that can be divided into three species: IFN-α, IFN-β, and IFN-γ (Fig. 1). The interferons differ according to the agent

---

*Present affiliation: Baylor College of Medicine, Houston, Texas.

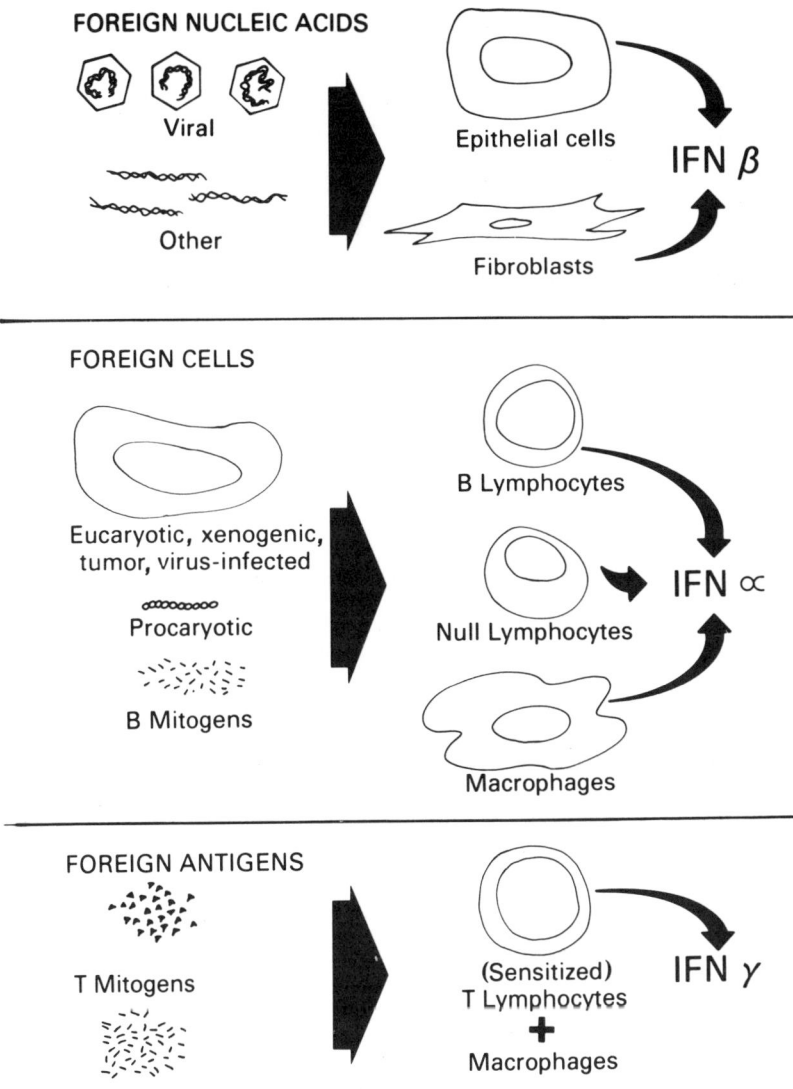

Figure 1 Induction of fibroblast interferon (IFN-β), leukocyte interferon (IFN-α), or immune interferon (IFN-γ) by foreign nucleic acids, foreign cells, or foreign antigens, respectively. [Reproduced with permission from Baron, S., Dianzani, F., and Stanton, G. J. *Texas Rep. Biol. Med.* 41:1-12 (1982).]

Table 1 Biological Activities of Interferon

Antiviral activity

Antiproliferative activity on dividing cells

Direct lytic effect on some cells

Immunoregulatory activity

Activation of macrophages

Enhancement of natural killer cell cytotoxicity

Enhancement of lymphocyte cytotoxicity

Hormonelike activity

---

that induces them and the cell type that produces them. The interferon proteins have been purified, and the interferon genes have also been cloned in bacteria. A wide variety of interferon activities, including antiviral effects, antiproliferative effects, immunomodulatory effects, and hormonal effects, have been described and partially characterized (Table 1).

To induce these activities, interferon must activate cells to produce effector proteins (Fig. 2). Briefly, the interaction of an interferon inducer with a cell causes the induction of the mRNA for the interferon. The mRNA for the interferon is translated, and the interferon protein is then released from the producing cell. Once outside the producing cell, it interacts with specific receptors on the cell membranes of the producing cell and on those of surrounding cells. This interaction of interferon with its receptor somehow triggers the synthesis of new mRNA and new proteins. These proteins establish a virus-resistant state in the responding cells and are called antiviral proteins. A considerable amount is known about some of the interferon-induced cellular proteins. It has been noted that responding cells can also stimulate neighboring cells to achieve a virus-resistant state by a still unknown mechanism (2).

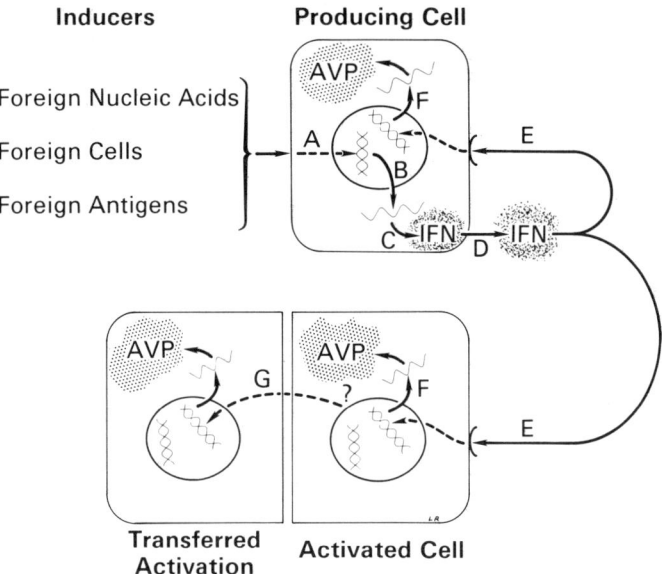

Figure 2 Cellular events of the induction, production, and action of interferon. Inducers of interferon (IFN) react with cells to derepress the IFN gene(s) (A). This leads to the production of mRNA for IFN (B). The mRNA is translated into the IFN protein (C) that is secreted into the extracellular fluid (D), where it reacts with the membrane receptors of cells (E). The IFN-stimulated cells derepress genes (F) for effector cell proteins (AVP) that establish antiviral resistance and other cell changes. The activated cells also stimulate contacted cells (G) by a still unknown mechanism to produce AVP. [Reproduced with permission from Baron, S., Dianzani, F., and Stanton, G. J. *Texas Rep. Biol. Med. 41*:1-12 (1982).]

It is well established that interferon is a natural body defense against many viral infections. Interferons may also play a role in the destruction of spontaneously arising tumors in animals and humans. Indeed, interferon has been used with some success in the clinic for the experimental treatment of viral diseases and malignancies. These experimental uses of interferon also include neurologically relevant diseases, such as Guillain-Barré syndrome, Reye's syndrome, and multiple sclerosis. Unfortunately, interferon treatment is not without side effects, including neurologic effects.

Interferon has now been approved for use in some malignancies and viral diseases. However, a better understanding of interferon's action may be required before interferon will completely fulfill its initial promise as a therapeutic agent.

II. HISTORICAL PERSPECTIVE

In 1957, Isaacs and Lindenmann (1) observed that pieces of chick chorioallantoic membrane infected with heat-inactivated influenza virus released a substance into the surrounding medium that could make other pieces of chick membrane resistant to virus infection. They named this substance interferon. Chick interferon was shown to be a protein (3). Comparative studies with chick and calf interferons demonstrated that the interferons exhibited "species specificity," with chick interferon having no activity on calf cells and vice versa (4). More recently, some cross-species activity has been noted (5-7). Indeed, two subtypes of human IFN-α have been shown to have higher antiviral activity on bovine cells than on human cells (8).

The cellular origin of interferon was established by biologic and biochemical studies. The properties of a given interferon were shown to be dependent on the cell of origin rather than on the virus that induced it (9, 10). Further, interferon was shown to be distinct from the virus by its resistance to inactivation by antisera prepared against viral proteins (11). Also, actinomycin D, which effectively blocks host mRNA synthesis but has no effect on the replication of most RNA viruses, was shown to block the induction of interferon (12). Finally, interferon genes have been mapped to specific chromosomes in the cell (13).

Interferons do not directly inactivate viruses. A prolonged exposure of metabolically active cells to interferon is required to establish an antiviral state. Interferons bind to specific receptor proteins and activate cells through a process that requires cell mRNA and protein synthesis (14–17). A number of interferon-induced proteins have been identified and are described here (15, 16).

Although interferons were first recognized for their antiviral properties, they have since been shown to have growth regulatory (18), immunoregulatory (19, 20), and hormonelike activities (21). The growth regulatory and immunoregulatory properties of interferon have suggested the potential use of interferon as an antitumor agent. Studies evaluating the efficacy of interferon as a therapeutic agent were limited by two difficulties: (1) interferon was produced in very small quantities, and (2) interferon was very difficult to purify.

The demonstration by Cantell and his colleagues (22) that interferon could be produced in relatively large quantity and partially purified from the supernatant fluid of leukocytes exposed to Sendai virus provided impetus for the clinical application of interferon. Indeed, Strander et al. (23) employed Cantell's interferon in the treatment of osteosarcoma to provide the first evidence to suggest that interferon may have antitumor activity. Even so, early clinical trials were hampered by the relative scarcity of human interferon.

This scarcity of human interferon has been largely alleviated by the production of interferon by recombinant DNA techniques, as described in Section III. The Extraction of active interferon mRNA from induced cells and the demonstration of its in vitro activity by its translation in *Xenopus* oocytes (24) were key initial steps that led to the application of recombinant DNA techniques to the production of human interferons in bacteria. In rapid order, the interferon protein was synthesized in very large quantity by the bacteria and was purified from the bacterial cultures.

With the large-scale production of interferon by recombinant DNA methodology, clinical trials have focused on the potential therapeutic effects of interferon on viral and neoplastic diseases as described in the following sections.

III. PRODUCTION AND PROPERTIES OF INTERFERONS

A. Biologic Properties

Early in the development of interferon research, before interferon was purified and monoclonal antibodies were available, a set of essential properties of interferons was identified (25). Briefly, to be considered as an interferon, a molecule had to be a protein that had no direct effect on the stability of viruses but exerted an antiviral effect against a broad and characteristic range of viruses through the activation of mRNA and protein synthesis in responding cells. A number of molecules have been identified that meet these criteria. They have been divided into three families of interferons: IFN-α, IFN-β, and IFN-γ (26). The assignment of interferon molecules to the three families has been on the basis of the cell type that produces them, the agent that induces them, and their antigenic and molecular relatedness (Fig. 1).

B. Interferon Inducers

IFN-α is produced by lymphocytes and macrophages that have been induced with viruses, foreign nucleic acids, and a variety of other synthetic polymers, bacteria and bacterial components, tumor cells, or heterologous cells (Fig. 1). Genetic sequences for at least 17 different IFN-α subtypes are encoded in human DNA. At least 8 are naturally expressed (27–29). The genes for IFN-α are all located in one region of human chromosome 9 (13). IFN-α molecules are composed of 166 amino acids (27–29).

IFN-β is produced by fibroblast and epithelial cells that have been induced with foreign nucleic acids, including those in viruses (Fig. 1). Genetic sequences for at least two IFN-β subtypes are encoded in human DNA (30, 31). Both are expressed naturally. The gene for one of the IFN-β subtypes has been mapped (13). It is located in close proximity to the IFN-α genes on human chromosome 9. IFN-β molecules are composed of 166 amino acids (30).

IFN-γ is produced by T lymphocytes that have been stimulated with foreign antigens to which they have previously been sensitized or with mitogens that simulate this induction (Fig. 1). The interaction of these IFN-γ inducers with T lymphocytes may involve a galactose residue on the lymphocyte membrane, since IFN-γ can also be induced by galactose oxidase (32). Only one genetic sequence for IFN-γ has been identified in human DNA (33, 34). It is located on human chromosome 12 (35). IFN-γ molecules are composed of 146 amino acids (33, 34).

C. Relatedness of the Interferon Types

IFN-α and IFN-β share considerable homology at the nucleotide and amino acid levels (36, 37). They interact with the same receptor molecule on the surface of responding cells (see below) (38). They appear to exert their biologic effects by identical mechanisms. Thus, these interferons have probably been generated by divergent evolution from a common ancestral interferon gene (39).

IFN-γ does not share significant homology with IFN-α or IFN-β at either the nucleotide or the amino acid level (33, 34). IFN-γ interacts with its own unique receptor molecule to activate responding cells (38). Further, there is some evidence to suggest that IFN-γ exerts its antiviral activity via a different mechanism than IFN-α and IFN-β (40).

However, IFN-γ does show some similarity with IFN-α and IFN-β in its secondary structure (41). Further, all three interferon types appear to share at least some common epitopes that are involved in the induction of the antiviral state (42). The data suggest that although IFN-γ may be unrelated to IFN-α and IFN-β, IFN-γ may be representative of convergent evolution.

IV. LARGE-SCALE PRODUCTION BY RECOMBINANT DNA TECHNIQUES

Interferons are currently being produced in large scale by recombinant DNA techniques. The procedure has been described in a recent general review (43) and is illustrated in Figure 3. Briefly, mRNA molecules from induced cells are extracted and purified. Complementary DNA copies of the mRNAs (cDNAs) are made using the retrovirus reverse transcriptase enzyme. Each cDNA copy is inserted into a suitable expression vector (often a bacterial plasmid) that contains a selectable marker, such as a gene for antibiotic resistance. The expression vector is then introduced into a bacterium, such as *Escherichia coli*. The bacteria are cloned in the presence of the appropriate selective agent (antibiotic), which selects for the bacteria that have taken up the expression vector. The clones that produce interferon are then identified. The remainder of the clones are discarded. The interferon-producing clones of *E. coli* carry the cDNA for the interferon gene and are cultured in large batches. The interferon is collected from the bacterial cultures and purified by a variety of techniques that may include specific binding on affinity columns made with monoclonal antibodies.

V. ASSAY TECHNIQUES

Interferon titers are generally expressed as antiviral units per milliliter (U/ml). A number of different assay systems are employed to quantitate the amount of interferon activity. Recently these assay systems have been extensively reviewed (44).

The plaque reduction assay is perhaps the most widely used assay system (45). Lindenmann et al. (3) demonstrated that, to be effective, interferon must be placed on the cells for some time before viral challenge. Thus, cell monolayers are exposed to serial dilutions of interferon for an overnight incubation. The cell monolayers are then challenged with an appropriate virus (often vesicular stomatitis virus). Following a period for virus absorption, the monolayers are overlaid with medium containing a stiffening agent, such as starch, agar, or methyl cellulose, which prevents the diffusion of progeny viruses. Plaques that develop in 24–48 hr are visualized by staining the monolayers with a dye, such as crystal violet, methylene blue, or neutral red. The number of plaques are expressed as the percentage of control plaques. A unit of interferon is defined as the reciprocal of the

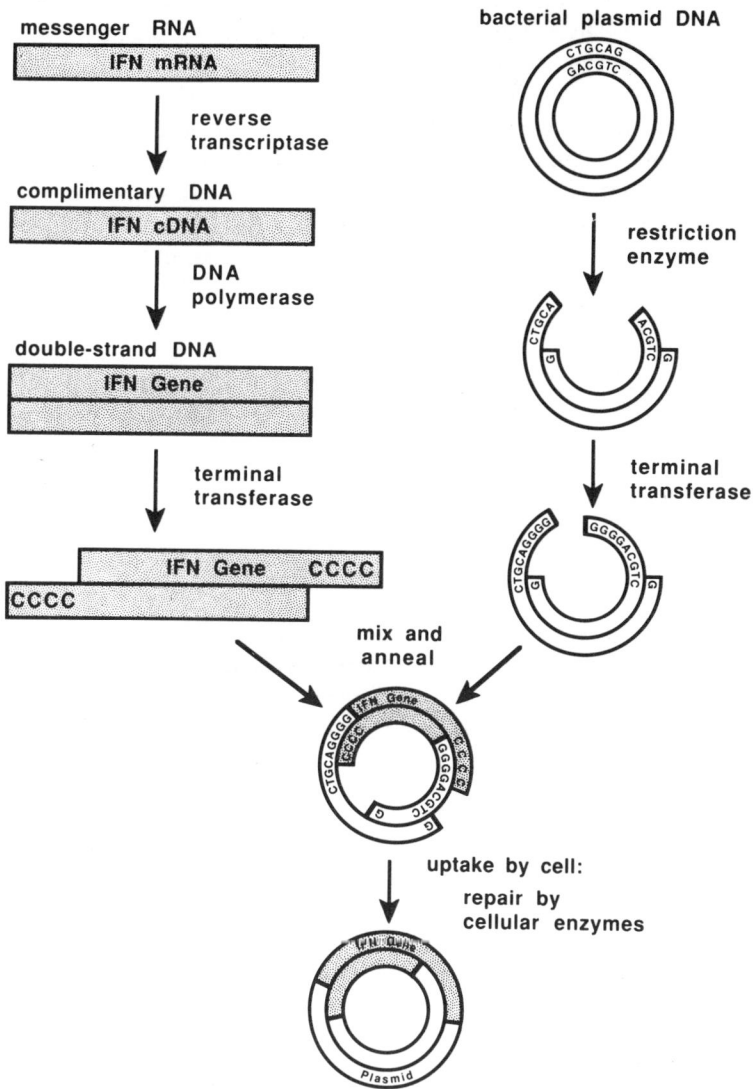

Figure 3 Production and isolation of an interferon-producing *Escherichia coli* clone by recombinant DNA techniques.

dilution that causes a 50% reduction in the control number of plaques.

The cytopathic effect (CPE) reduction assay is another frequently used assay system (46–48). This system measures the cytopathic effect of virus replication in the presence of interferon. The CPE reduction assay is performed as described for the plaque reduction assay except that, following virus absorption, the monolayers are overlaid with medium without a stiffening agent. Progeny virus are free to diffuse and infect distant cells. The monolayers are incubated until all of the control cells are infected and the CPE of control wells (no interferon treatment) is complete. The interferon-treated monolayers are then graded. Grading of the monolayers may be based on a visual examination through a microscope (46, 47) or on a spectroscopic quantitation of dye uptake by cells (48). A unit of interferon is defined as the reciprocal of the dilution that causes a 50% reduction in the CPE.

With the advent of monoclonal antibodies and recombinant DNA-derived interferons, radioimmunoassays (RIA) and enzyme-linked immunosorbent assays (ELISA) have also been employed. The RIA technique involves the immobilization of a monoclonal antibody to an interferon on polystyrene beads (49). Serial dilutions of the interferon are added to the beads and allowed to interact. The beads are spun down and then resuspended. A second, radiolabeled monoclonal antibody that recognizes a different epitope on the interferon is then added. The radiolabeled second monoclonal antibody binds to the polystyrene bead-first monoclonal antibody-interferon complex. The complex is spun down, and the amount of precipitated radiolabel is quantitated.

The ELISA technique (50) is similar to the RIA technique, except that the first antibody is immobilized on a microtiter plate and the second antibody is linked to an enzyme that can catalyze a colorimetric reaction. The amount of colorimetric change that has occurred is quantitated using a spectrophotometer. The RIA and ELISA techniques permit the very rapid quantitation of interferon molecules. However, these techniques are less sensitive than the biologic assays already described, and they do not distinguish between active and inactive interferon molecules in the preparations.

VI. INTERFERON ACTIVATION OF RESPONDING CELLS

Interferons interact with specific high-affinity receptors on the surface of responding cells to activate the cells by inducing the synthesis of new mRNA molecules, which are then translated into new proteins. IFN-α and IFN-β induce 12 new proteins (51, 52). IFN-γ induces these same 12 new proteins plus 12 more (52).

A. Interferon-Receptor Interactions

Interferon has a very high affinity for its receptor (log Ka = 10-11) (38). This affinity is of the same order of magnitude as the affinity of polypeptide hormones for their receptors.

The interaction of interferon with its high-affinity receptor is essential for the induction of the new mRNA synthesis in responding cells. Interferon-producing cells incubated in the presence of antisera to interferon fail to give an interferon response (53). Similarly, microinjection of interferon into sensitive cells failed to activate the cells (54). These results indicate that the intracellular production or administration of interferon is not sufficient to activate an interferon response.

The degree of interferon activation of a cell is dependent both on the external interferon concentration and on the receptor gene dosage level. For example, the receptor for IFN-α and IFN-β is located on human chromosome 21. Cells that are trisomic for human chromosome 21 are much more sensitive to a given concentration of these interferons than normal diploid cells (55).

B. Induction of New mRNAs

Considerable attention has focused on the possible generation of second messengers, such as cAMP or cGMP, that may provide a link between receptor and interferon binding and the induction of new mRNA synthesis (56). However, to date there is no clear and convincing evidence to support a particular molecule as the second messenger.

Recently, a possible intracellular role for the receptor-interferon complex or some derivative has been suggested but not yet established (57).

C. Production of New Proteins

As indicated, IFN-α and IFN-β induce the production of 12 new proteins in responding cells (51, 52). IFN-γ induces these same proteins and an additional 12 new proteins (52). Some of these proteins have now been identified; however, the precise mechanisms by which these proteins express interferon's varied activities are as yet unknown. Of the best studied proteins, three are described below.

1. 2′, 5′-Oliogoadenylate Synthetase

Interferon has been shown to induce the production of a novel RNA polymerizing enzyme that synthesizes adenylate oligomers with a unique 2′,5′-phosphodiester linkage between the ribose residues (53–61). This enzyme has been designated 2′,5′-oligoadenylate synthetase. It is specifically induced by the interferons, and it functions in the presence of double-stranded RNA.

The production of 2′,5′-oligoadenylates by the synthetase activates a constitutively produced ribonuclease, RNase L. Activation of RNase L leads to the breakdown of single-stranded RNA of both viral and host cell origin. The 2′5′-oligoadenylates have a short half-life: they are broken down by a constitutively produced endonuclease that preferentially cleaves 2′,5′-phosphodiester bonds (62, 63).

It has been proposed that activation of the 2′,5′-oligoadenylate synthetase occurs only at the immediate site of double-stranded RNA synthesis, thus restricting the destructive activity of RNase L to localized areas within the cell (64).

It is interesting to note that interferons are not the only inducers of 2′, 5′-oligoadenylate synthetase. Glucocorticoid treatment of human lymphoblastoid cells induced the synthetase (65). Also, chick oviduct cells, which have a low level of the synthetase during treatment with dithylstilbestrol, have a greatly enhanced level of the synthetase after withdrawal of the hormone (66).

2. Protein Kinase

Interferon has been shown to specifically induce the production of a protein kinase that functions in the presence of double-stranded RNA (67–69). The principal substrates for this protein kinase are itself and the smallest subunit of initiation factor eIF-2 (70–72). Phosphorylation of eIF-2 results in the inhibition of an initiation step in protein synthesis (the formation of the 40S initiation complex is inhibited).

Regulation of the protein kinase system is provided through the activity of a phosphoprotein in phosphatase that dephosphorylates the phosphorylated eIF-2 (73, 74).

It is interesting to note that interferon treatment is not the only mechanism by which the phosphorylation of eIF-2 occurs. Hemin-deficient reticulocytes, which down-regulate their synthesis of hemoglobin proteins, have also been shown to have phosphorylated eIF-2 that blocks the formation of the 40S initiation complex (75). The phosphorylation of eIF-2 in hemin-deficient reticulocytes is at the same site as in eIF-2 extracted from interferon-treated cells and activated with double-stranded RNA (72).

Thus, the interferon-induced protein kinase-mediated phosphorylation of eIF-2 may represent a mechanism for the regulation of cellular protein synthesis.

3. The Mx Protein

Interferon has been shown to induce the synthesis of a protein called Mx that blocks influenza virus replication (76). Interferon-treated cells lacking the ability to produce the Mx protein develop much less resistance to influenza virus replication than interferon-treated cells that do produce Mx.

The mechanism by which Mx exerts its antiviral activity has been well studied. Influenza virus replicates in the nucleus of infected cells, and the nuclear Mx protein inhibits the synthesis of the influenza virus mRNA (77).

VII. BIOLOGIC ACTIVITIES OF INTERFERONS

Interferons were first identified by their ability to block viral replication. However, very shortly, interferons were seen to possess antiproliferative activities, immunomodulatory activities, and hormonelike activities (Table 1).

A. Antiviral Activity

Viruses infect cells at the local site of implantation and within a very few hours release hundreds or thousands of progeny viruses. These progeny viruses infect surrounding cells to initiate new cycles of virus replication. Lytic viruses can be shown to have a frighteningly efficient, devastating effect in tissue culture, destroying entire monolayers of cells. However, in the host animal, virus replication is usually dampened. Most often virus infections are controlled before symptoms of virus infection develop. Only rarely do viral infections lead to fatal consequences.

Interferons have been shown to play an important role in the recovery of the host from virus infection. A summary of the types of evidence that support this claim is presented in Table 2. They include time and place correlations; sufficiency of quantity to account for the biologic effect; reproducibility in a wide range of organisms; and deletions and transfer experiments.

Figure 2 schematically presents the presumed mechanism by which the interferon system functions in the host animal. Virus infection results in the induction and release of interferon from an infected cell and from cells of the reticuloendothelial system which come into contact with viruses, virus-infected cells, or viral subunits. In the case of lytic viruses, the infected, interferon-producing cell will die. However, the interferon that is produced and released by the dying cell comes into contact with the surrounding cells and activates those cells to synthesize new mRNAs and new proteins. These new interferon-induced proteins are called the antiviral proteins. It should be noted that, unlike antibody, which can directly inactivate viruses, interferons have no direct antiviral

Table 2 Evidence for Interferon's Defensive Role in Virus Infections

Type of evidence	Example
Time correlation	Interferon produced rapidly after virus infection, reaching maximal titers just before and during termination of virus replication
Place correlation	Interferon produced at the site of viral replication
Sufficient quantity correlation	Concentrations of interferon achieved naturally in vivo have been shown experimentally in vitro and in vivo to be sufficient to account for its antiviral action
Reproducibility	The effectiveness of interferon has been shown for humans and for many other animals
Deletion	Deletion of interferon in vitro and in vivo increases the severity of virus infections
Transfer	Exogenous administration of interferon blocks or reduces severity of virus infections

activities and exert their antiviral effects only through the activation of cells (14-17, 78).

It can be noted that the antiviral effect induced by interferon can be transferred by responding cells to neighboring cells not yet exposed to interferon (2, 79). This process may have significance under physiological conditions to accelerate and/or amplify the interferon effect.

Viruses that infect cells that have been activated by interferon are blocked in their replication. A wide variety of viruses can be blocked by interferon, although each virus type is inhibited to a unique extent (80). The precise molecular mechanisms by which inhibition occurs are not completely understood (see above). However, it is known that interferon can induce the inhibition of transcription of viral mRNA (particularly of influenza virus) (77), translation of viral mRNA (81), and glycosylation of viral proteins (82). At low interferon levels, these activities result in the delayed and decreased synthesis of progeny virus (83, 84). At high interferon levels, they block virus replication. Thus, the viral infection is eliminated and the host animal recovers.

B. Antitumor Activity

A number of animal studies have shown that interferons can have pronounced effects on the growth of malignant and normal cells in vivo as well as in vitro. Interferons inhibit the multiplication of many malignant and normal cells with an efficacy comparable to that of antineoplastic chemotherapeutics (85, 86). This antitumor effect of interferon has been shown in animals against numerous spontaneous neoplasms, virally induced neoplasms, and transplantable tumors (85, 87). The results of these animal tumor model studies have formed the basis for the use of interferon in the clinical treatment of neoplastic disease. It should be noted, however, that not all cells respond to the antiproliferative action of interferon (88). The following are a few examples of such studies.

1. Spontaneous Tumors

The majority of AKR mice spontaneously develop lymphomas 6 months after birth. Interferon treatment before the development of the lymphoma reduces this frequency to 65% (89). Interferon treatment after development of lymphomas increases the survival by twofold (90). Similar results have been seen with spontaneous murine mammary carcinoma (91).

2. Virally Induced Tumors

A number of virally induced tumors have been studied in animal systems. Tumors initially studied that showed sensitivity to interferon include those induced by polyoma (92), Rous sarcoma (93), and Shope fibroma (94).

3. Transplantable Tumors

A wide variety of transplantable tumors have been shown to be inhibited by interferon treatment. They include animal tumors and human tumors grown in nude mice (reviewed in Ref. 86).

Interferons cause their antitumor effect by a variety of mechanisms (Fig. 4). These mechanisms include a direct antiproliferative effect on the tumor as well as indirect effects mediated by cytotoxic effector cells, such as natural killer (NK) cells, cytotoxic T cells, and activated macrophages.

C. Direct Antiproliferative Activity

Several studies have suggested that interferons exert their direct antiproliferative activities by prolonging the time of passage

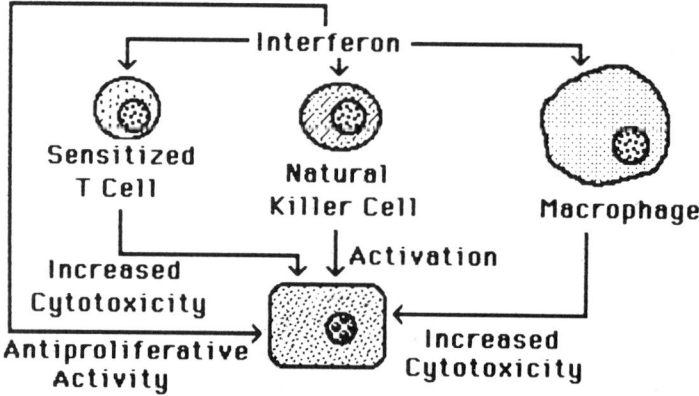

Figure 4 Possible factors involved in the antitumor activity of interferon.

through various parts of the cell cycle. However, the results have not pointed convincingly to a specific effect. Various investigators have documented a prolonged duration of G_1 and $S + G_2$ phases (95, 96), a block of the cell cycle at G_2 or S phase (97, 98), and a block that was independent of the cell cycle (99). Whatever the mechanism, interferon treatment can have a profound effect on the rate of cell proliferation of responding cells.

It should be noted that the antiproliferative activity of interferon can be transferred from one cell to a neighboring cell (100). It is believed that this transfer is analogous to the transfer of antiviral activity from a responding cell to a neighboring cell (2).

IFN-γ and IFN-β have been shown to cause the direct lysis of tumor cells (101, 102). However, IFN-γ appears to be more broadly active than IFN-β in its ability to cause direct lysis. The cell-lytic effects of individual interferons were observed only at relatively high interferon concentrations and low cell concentrations. However, combinations of IFN-γ and IFN-α or IFN-β have a potent lytic effect even at low interferon concentrations (103).

Thus, the antiproliferative activities of interferons can be highly potent. However, cells vary widely in their sensitivity to interferons, some being very sensitive and others being resistant (88).

D. Immunomodulatory Effects

Interferons play regulatory roles in modulating several aspects of the immune system, including the expression of the antibody response, the function of cytotoxic effector cells, and the expression of cell surface antigens. These indirect interferon effects on tumor cells have been shown to play an important role in interferon's antitumor activity. It was found that interferon treatment of mice inoculated with interferon-resistant L1210R cells (which are resistant to the direct antiproliferative effects of IFN-α and IFN-β) provided a significant antitumor effect when compared with untreated mice (104).

1. Modulation of Antibody Production

Interferon's main effect on the antibody response is inhibition. However, treatment of mice with low doses of interferon and careful timing of interferon treatment following antigen administration can cause enhancement (105). For example, an inhibitory effect is observed when lymphocytes are exposed to interferon at the time of antigen stimulation (106). However, interferon treatment 48-72 hrs after antigen stimulation results in an enhanced secretion of immunoglobulin (107). Thus, interferon treatment appears to block the differentiation of immature B lymphocytes to immunoglobulin-secreting plasma cells while enhancing the function of the differentiated cells.

2. Activation of Cytotoxic Cells

Macrophages. Macrophages are phagocytic cells that can directly kill foreign, virally infected, or tumor cells. They can also participate in antibody-dependent cell-mediated lysis (ADCC) of target cells. Interferons have been shown to activate macrophages. Mouse peritoneal macrophages treated with interferons have been shown to undergo morphologic changes, such as vacuolization and spreading (108). Interferon treatment has been shown to enhance the phagocytosis of colloidal carbon or latex particles (109) and *E. coli* (110). Further, interferon treatment increases Fc receptor expression, which leads to an enhanced level of immunoglobulin-mediated phagocytosis (ADCC) (111, 112). Indeed, more recent studies with recombinant DNA-derived interferons have shown that IFN-γ may be the major component of macrophage activating factor produced by T lymphocytes (113).

Cytotoxic T Lymphocytes. Cytotoxic T lymphocytes may be sensitized by exposure to specific cellular antigens to lyse cells that bear those antigens. The antigens may be present on foreign, virally infected, or tumor cells. Interferon treatment of sensitized T lymphocytes has been shown to enhance their specific cytotoxicity (114-116).

Natural Killer Cells. Natural killer cells are large granular lymphocytes that are distinct from cytotoxic T lymphocytes. They can kill a wide variety of foreign, virally infected, or tumor cells. Interferon treatment can enhance the cytotoxicity of natural killer cells (117-120). In addition to these in vitro studies, patients receiving interferon have been shown to have enhanced levels of natural killer activity (121). Unfortunately, interferon treatment can also protect target cells from natural killer activity (122), so the role of interferon in the activation of natural killer activity may still be an open question.

E. Protozoan and Bacterial Infections

Interferons may play an important role in the host's defense against a number of parasitic diseases. Much of the antiparasitic activity appears to be mediated by interferon enhancement of the activity of cytotoxic effector cells (see above) (123). However, interferon has also been shown to play a more direct role. IFN-γ treatment has been shown to deplete the intracellular pool of tryptophan in the target cell, resulting in the inhibition of trypanasome replication (124). Also, treatment of trypanosomes with IFN-β has been shown to cause a decrease in the efficiency of trypanosome uptake by target cells (125). In another study, interferon treatment of the target cells appeared to alter the cell membrane of the responding cells in such a way as to prevent penetration by *Salmonella* (126). A similar mechanism may be implicated in the interferon-mediated prevention of cell penetration by the invasive bacterium *Shigella* (127).

VIII. INTERFERON IN DISEASE STATES

The ability to produce and respond to interferon may have an effect on the general health of an animal or individual, but definitive studies remain to be done. For example, it has been recently reported that a pool of patients who were suffering from severe, fulminating viral diseases had a deficiency in their ability to produce IFN-α and IFN-γ (128). Similarly, the inability of natural killer cells to respond to interferon has been suggested as a contributing factor in such diseases as subacute sclerosing panencephalitis and multiple sclerosis (129, 130). Immunosuppression in Down's syndrome individuals may be due to their heightened sensitivity to interferon because their chromosome 21 trisomy causes an increased number of receptors to IFN-α and IFN-β (131).

High levels of circulating IFN-α have been associated with

several autoimmune diseases, including systemic lupus erythematosus (132), rheumatoid arthritis (132), and acquired immunodeficiency syndrome (133). Interestingly, the interferon detected in these patients is an unusal pH 2 labile form of IFN-a (134). Evidence suggests that IFN-γ causes the abberant expression of class II MHC antigens on thyroid epithelial cells, which in turn may trigger an autoimmune response leading to Grave's disease (135-137).

IX. THERAPEUTIC APPLICATION OF INTERFERON

As sufficient quantities of interferons have become available, interferons have been employed in clinical trials to determine their efficacy against malignancies and viral infections. It should be pointed out that, although interferon is effective against certain viral diseases and tumors, it is not yet as broadly active in people as it is in experimental animal systems. Some of the clinical data are summarized below.

A. Viral Infections

IFN-a has been found to be effective in preventing coryza due to influenza and rhinovirus infections (138, 139).

A therapeutic effect of IFN-a or IFN-β has been seen for ocular infections, such as herpes keratitis (140, 141) and adenovirus conjunctivitis (142). IFN-a has also been shown to have a modest effect on infections caused by various members of the herpesvirus group (Epstein-Barr virus, cytomegalovirus, varicella zoster, and herpes simplex virus-1) but the eradication of latent infections has not been demonstrated (143). However, it has been reported that interferon treatment causes a marked reduction in the frequency of reactivation of herpes labialis following neurosurgery (144).

IFN-a treatment has been shown to decrease viremia during chronic hepatitis B infections; however, it is not clear whether recovery is affected (145).

Finally, IFN-a has been effective against several tumors that are believed to have a viral origin, such as warts and condyloma acuminatum, juvenile laryngeal papillomatosis, and hairy cell leukemia (see below).

B. Neoplastic Disease

The antitumor potential of interferons has been shown in a number of studies against a variety of tumors (Table 3). For some tumor types, interferon does appear to have efficacy. Unfortunately, the demonstrated therapeutic potential of the interferon ranges widely from tumor type to tumor type. Also, for any given type of tumor, some patients may show a complete response (total regression of the tumor) but others may have no response.

Perhaps the best examples of interferon's potency are found in patients with hairy cell leukemia (146), warts and condyloma acuminatum (147-149), and juvenile laryngeal papillomatosis (150-152). These patients have response rates that are quite high, approaching 90%. Although long-term studies with hairy cell leukemia and condyloma acuminatum are not complete, long-term studies of patients with juvenile laryngeal papillomatosis suggest

Table 3 Malignancies and Other Tumors Evaluated for Interferon Antitumor Activity

Malignant melanoma	Ovarian carcinoma
Glioblastoma	Breast carcinoma
Malignant Glioma	Multiple myeloma
Bladder carcinoma	Non-Hodgkin's lymphoma
Kaposi's Sarcoma	Adult T-cell leukemia
Juvenile laryngeal papillomatosis	Hairy cell leukemia
Condyloma acuminata	Lymphocytic leukemia
Renal cell carcinoma	Granulocytic leukemia

that the interferon effect represents tumor management, not cure, since recurrence of the tumor occurs following withdrawal of the interferon therapy. Further, some findings indicate that the antipapilloma effect was often not sustained even with the continued administration of interferon (152).

C. Nervous System Disorders

Nervous system disorders of viral or suspected viral etiology have also been targets for interferon therapy.

Interferon administration in patients with systemic herpes zoster infections has been reported to modestly limit cutaneous and visceral spread of the virus (153). A somewhat decreased incidence of postherpetic neuralgia was also noted. This mild effect is consistent with the relative interferon resistance of the herpesviruses (154, 155).

Several studies have evaluated the efficacy of interferon therapy for multiple sclerosis. Intrathecal administration of IFN-β was reported to be effective for multiple sclerosis patients (156). The beneficial effects that were reported included decreased rates of exacerbation and improved neurologic status. A study employing systemic administration of 5 million U of IFN-α daily also showed some ability to decrease rates of exacerbation (157). A study employing systemic administration of IFN-γ did not show beneficial effects (158). Thus, interferon therapy, particularly intrathecally administered IFN-β, may be of some efficacy in reducing the frequency of exacerbations in multiple sclerosis patients.

Interferon inducers have also been employed with encouraging results in patients suffering from Reye's syndrome (159), multiple sclerosis (160), and polyneuropathy (Guillain-Barré's syndrome) (160).

D. Side Effects

A number of side effects have been associated with interferon therapy. They include fever, bone marrow suppression, malaise, fatigue, nausea, and anorexia, as well as some neurologic effects.

Originally, it was thought that these side effects were the result of contaminating proteins present in the impure interferon preparations that were first used in clinical trials. The persistence of these side effects with the use of recombinant DNA-derived interferons indicates that they are the result of the interferon molecules themselves. All the effects are reversible upon cessation of interferon therapy.

Fever is one of the more important side effects. Temperatures up to 39.5°C occur in a high proportion of patients when more than 1 million U of interferon are administered (162, 163). The fever occurs irrespective of the route of interferon administration, although it is accelerated and can be accompanied by major changes in blood pressure when interferon is given intravenously (164, 165).

Bone marrow suppression is another important side effect of interferon therapy (166-170). The bone marrow suppression results in decreased levels of circulating leukocytes, platelets, and reticulocytes.

Neurologic side effects are also important. When very high interferon doses (100-200 million U/day) were given to patients with amyotropic lateral sclerosis, the patients showed reduced tendon reflexes and reduced muscle force (171). In addition, significant slowing of electroencephalograph activity, auditory and visually evoked potentials, psychomotor retardation, and conditioning times were observed (172-176). Long-term interferon treatment has been shown to cause transient behavioral and cognitive changes. Some patients have been reported to exhibit severe lethargy and somnolence (sleeping up to 20 hr/day) with very high interferon doses (177, 178). Thus, interferon therapy can cause profound neurologic side effects.

X. FUTURE PROSPECTS

Improved efficacy of interferon is likely to come from improved delivery and a better understanding of the various mechanisms of the interferons. For example, we have much to learn before we know the best administration route, the best dosage level, and the best dosage schedule.

Other exciting prospects for enhancing the efficacy of interferons are currently under study. These involve the use of different types of interferons together, the use of interferons with other tumor therapies, and the use of interferons with other biologic response modifiers.

First, in vivo mouse studies and in vitro studies with mouse and human cells have shown that combination interferon therapy of IFN-γ with either IFN-α or IFN-β causes a synergistic enhancement of interferon's antiviral and antitumor activities (179-182). Combination interferon therapy is under evaluation in several clinical trials currently underway; however, no data are yet available.

Second, mouse studies have suggested that interferon therapy can be combined with chemotherapy to enhance the antitumor effect (183-185). These studies have since been extended to human cells in vitro (186-188) and to human tumors in a nude mouse model system (188).

Third, in vitro studies with human tumor cells have suggested that interferon therapy can be combined with γ irradiation to enhance the antitumor effect (188).

Fourth, animal studies have shown that combinations of tumor necrosis factor and IFN-γ produce a highly potent antitumor effect (189). Clinical trials to evaluate this combination of biologic response modifiers are currently underway.

Fifth, it may be possible to combine interferon therapy with the administration of bone marrow stimulatory substances to reverse interferon's bone marrow suppression and to provide increased numbers of cytotoxic cells. For example, colony stimulating factor-1 has been shown to block interferon-mediated myelosuppression (190, 191).

Thus, interferons have been shown to have some potential as antitumor and antiviral agents. However, much more work is required before the promise can be fulfilled, and increasing the efficacy of interferon therapy will be an important challenge for the future.

REFERENCES

1. Isaacs, A., and Lindenmann, J. Virus interference. I. The interferon. *Proc. R. Soc. Lond. (Biol.) 147*:258-267 (1957).

2. Blalock, J. E., and Baron, S. Interferon-induced transfer of viral resistance. *Nature 269*:422-425 (1977).

3. Lindenmann, J., Isaacs, A., and Burke, D. C., Studies on the production, mode of action, and properties of interferon. *Br. J. Exp. Pathol. 38*: 551-562 (1957).

4. Tyrell, D. A. J. Interferon produced by cultures of calf kidney cells. *Nature 184*:452-453 (1959).

5. Sutton, R. N. P., and Tyrell, D. A. J. Some observations on interferon prepared in tissue culture. *J. Exp. Pathol. 42*:99-105 (1961).

6. Buckler, C. F., and Baron, S. Antiviral action of mouse interferon in heterologous cells. *J. Bacteriol. 91*:231-235 (1966).

7. Moehring, J. M., and Stinebring, W. R. Examination of "species specificity" of avian interferons. *Nature 226*:360-361 (1970).

8. Rubinstein, M., Levy, W. P., Moschera, J. A., Lai, C.-Y., Hershberg, R. D., Bartlett, R. T., and Pestka, S. Human leukocyte interferon: Isolation and characterization of several molecular forms. *Arch. Biochem. Biophys. 210*:307-318 (1981).

9. Boxaca, M., and Paucker, K. Neutralization of different murine interferons by antibody. *J. Immunol. 98*:1130-1135 (1967).

10. Merigan, T. C. Purified interferons: Physical properties and species specificity. *Science 145*:811-813 (1964).

11. Isaacs, A. Interferon. *Adv. Virus Res. 10*:1-38 (1963).

12. Heller, E. Enhancement of Chickungunya virus replication and inhibition of interferon production by actinomycin D. *Virology 21*:652-656 (1963).

13. Owerbach, D., Rutter, W. J., Shows, B., et al. Leukocyte and fibroblast interferon genes are located on human chromosome 9. *Proc. Natl Acad. Sci. USA 78*:3123-3127 (1981).

14. Taylor, J. Inhibition of interferon action by actinomycin D. *Biochem. Biophys. Res. Commun. 14*:447-451 (1964).

15. Lockart, R. Z., Jr. The necessity for cellular RNA and protein synthesis

for viral inhibition resulting from interferon. *Biochem. Biophys. Res. Commun.* 15:513-518 (1964).

16. Levine, S. Effect of actinomycin-D and puromycin dihydrochloride on action of interferon. *Virology* 24:586-588 (1964).

17. Nichol, F. R., and Tershak, D. R. Effects of 5 FU and 6-azauridine on interferon action. *J. Virol.* 1:450-451 (1967).

18. Paucker, K., Cantell, K., and Henle, W. Quantitative studies on viral interference in suspended L-cells. III. Effect of interfering viruses and interferon on the growth rate of cells. *Virology* 17:324-334 (1962).

19. Johnson, H. M., Smith, B. G., and Baron, S. Inhibition of the primary in vitro antibody response of mouse spleen cells by interferon preparations. *IRCS (Med. Sci.)* 2:1616 (1974).

20. Sonnenfeld, G., Mandel, A. D., and Merigan, T. C. The immunosuppressive effect of type II mouse interferon preparations on antibody production. *Cell. Immunol.* 34:193-206 (1977).

21. Blalock, J. E., and Stanton, G. J. Common pathways of interferon and hormonal action. *Nature* 283:406-408 (1980).

22. Cantell, K., Hirvonen, S., Mogensen, K. E., and Pyhala, L. Human leukocyte interferon: Production, purification, stability, and animal experiments. In: *The Production and Use of Interferon for the Treatment and Prevention of Human Virus Infections*, In Vitro Monograph Vol. 3 (C. Waymouth, ed.). Tissue Culture Association, Rockville, Maryland, pp. 35-38 (1974).

23. Strander, H., Cantell, K., Ingimarsson, S., Jakobsson, P. A., Wilsonne, U., and Soderberg, G. Interferon treatment of osteogenic sarcoma—a clinical trial. In: *Modulation of Host Immune Resistance in the Prevention or Treatment of Induced Neoplasias*, Fogarty International Center Proceedings (M. A. Chirigos, ed.). U.S. Government Printing Office, Washington, D. C., No. 28, 377-381 (1974).

24. Reynolds, F. H., Jr., Premkumar, E., and Pitha, P. M. Interferon activity produced by translation of human interferon messenger RNA in cell-free ribosomal systems and in *Xenopus* oocytes. *Proc. Natl. Acad. Sci. USA* 72:4881-4885 (1975).

25. Lockart, R. Z. Biological properties of interferons; criteria for acceptance of a viral inhibitor as an interferon. In: *Interferon and Interferon Inducers* (N. B. Finter ed.). Elsevier, New York, pp. 1-20 (1973).

26. Stewart, W. E., II, Blalock, J. E., Burke, D. C., et al. Interferon nomenclature. *Nature* 286:110 (1980).
27. Allen, G., and Fantes, K. H. A family of structural genes for human lymphoblastoid (leukocyte-type) interferon. *Nature* 287:408-411 (1980).
28. Nagata, S., Mantei, N., and Weissmann, C. The structure of one of the eight or more distinct chromosomal genes for human interferon-alpha. *Nature* 287:401-408 (1980).
29. Goeddel, D. V., Leung, D. W., Dull, J. J., et al. The structure of eight distinct cloned human leukocyte interferon cDNAs. *Nature* 290:20-26 (1981).
30. Tavernier, J., Derynck, R., and Fiers, W. Evidence for a unique human fibroblast interferon (IFN-beta$_1$) chromosomal gene, devoid of intervening sequences. *Nucleic Acids Res.* 9:461-471 (1981).
31. Sehgal, P. B. The interferon genes. *Biochim. Biophys. Acta* 695:17-33 (1982).
32. Dianzani, F., Monahan, T. M., Schupham, A., and Zucca, M. Enzymatic induction of interferon production by galactose oxidase treatment of human lymphoid cells. *Infect. Immun.* 26:879-882 (1979).
33. Devos, R., Cheroutre, H., Taya, Y., et al. Molecular cloning of human immune interferon cDNA and its expression in eukaryotic cells. *Nucleic Acids Res.* 10:2487-2501 (1982).
34. Gray, P. W., Leung, D. W., Pennica, D., et al. Expression of human immune interferon cDNA in *E. coli* and monkey cells. *Nature* 295:503-508 (1982).
35. Naylor, S. L., Sakaguchi, A. Y., Shows, T. B., et al. Human immune interferon gene is located on chromosome 12. *J. Exp. Med.* 157:1020-1027 (1983).
36. Degrave, S., Derynck, R., Tavernier, J., et al. Nucleotide sequence of the chromosomal gene for human fibroblast (beta$_1$) interferon and the flanking regions. *Gene* 14:137-143 (1982).
37. Taniguchi, T., Mantei, N., Schwarzstein, M., et al. Human leukocyte and fibroblast interferons are structurally related. *Nature* 285:547-549 (1980).
38. Aguet, M., and Mogensen, K. E. Interferon receptors. In: *Interferons*, Vol. 5 (I. Gresser, ed.). Academic Press, New York, pp. 1-22 (1983).

39. Miyata, T., and Hayashida, H., Recent divergence from a common ancestor of human IFN-alpha genes. *Nature* 295:165-168 (1982).

40. Dianzani, F., Salter, L., Fleischmann, W. R., Jr., and Zucca, M. Immune interferon activates cells more slowly than does virus-induced interferon. *Proc. Soc. Exp. Biol. Med.* 159:94-97 (1978).

41. Degrado, W. F., Wasserman, Z. R., and Chowdhry, V. Sequence and structural homologies among type I and type II interferons. *Nature* 300:379-381 (1982).

42. De Maeyer-Guignard, J., and De Maeyer, E. Immunomodulation by interferons. In: *Interferons*, Vol. 6 (I. Gresser, ed.). Academic Press, New York, pp. 69-91 (1985).

43. Pestka, S. The purification and manufacture of human interferons. *Sci. Am.* 249(2): 36-43 (1983).

44. Pestka, S. (ed.). *Interferons, Part A*. Methods in Enzymology, Vol. 78. Academic Press, New York (1981).

45. Langford, M. P., Weigent, D. A., Stanton, G. J., and Baron, S. Virus plaque-reduction assay for interferon: Microplaque and regular macroplaque reduction assays. In: *Interferons Part A*. Methods in Enzymology, Vol. 78 (S. Pestka, ed.). Academic Press, New York, pp. 339-346 (1985).

46. Armstrong, J. Cytopathic effect inhibition assay for interferon: Microculture plate assay. In: *Interferons, Part A*, Methods in Enzymology, Vol. 78 (S. Pestka, ed.). Academic Press, New York, pp. 381-387 (1985).

47. Familletti, P. C., Rubinstein, S., and Pestka, S. A convenient and rapid cytopathic effect inhibition assay for interferon. In: *Interferons, Part A*, Methods in Enzymology, Vol. 78 (S. Pestka, ed.). Academic Press, New York, pp. 387-394 (1985).

48. Johnston, M. D., Finter, N. B., and Young, P. A. Dye uptake method for assay of interferon activity. In: *Interferons, Part A*, Methods in Enzymology, Vol. 78 (S. Pestka, ed.). Academic Press, New York, pp. 394-399 (1985).

49. Torok-Storb, B., Johnson, G. G., Bowden, R., and Storb, R. Gammainterferon in aplastic anemia: Inability to detect significant levels in sera or demonstrate hematopoietic suppressing activity. *Blood* 69:629-633. (1987).

50. Ichimori, Y., Kurokawa, T., Honda, S., Suzuki, N., Wakimasu, M., and Tsukamoto, K. Monoclonal antibodies to human interferon-gamma. I.

Antibodies to a synthetic carboxyl-terminal peptide. *J. Immunol. Methods 80*:55-66. (1985).

51. Weil, J., Epstein, L. B., and Epstein, C. J. Synthesis of interferon induced polypeptides in normal and chromosome 21-aneuploid human fibroblasts: Relationship to relative sensitivities in antiviral assays. *J. Interferon Res. 1*:11-124 (1980).

52. Weil, J., Epstein, C. J., Epstein, L. B., et al. A unique set of polypeptides is induced by gamma interferon in addition to those induced in common with alpha and beta interferons. *Nature 301*:437-439 (1983).

53. Pitha, P. M., Vengris, V. E., and Reynolds, F. H. The role of cell membrane in the antiviral effect of interferon. *J. Supramol. Struct. 4*:467-473 (1976).

54. Higoshi, Y., and Sokawa, Y. Microinjection of interferon and 2'-5'oligoadenylate into mouse L-cells and their effect on virus growth. *J. Biochem. 91*:2021-2028 (1982).

55. Tan, Y. H., Schneider, E. L., Tischfield, J., et al. Human chromosome 21 dosage: Effect on the expression of the interferon induced antiviral state. *Science 186*:61-63 (1974).

56. Tovey, M. G. Interferon and cyclic nucleotides. In: *Interferons*, Vol. 4 (I. Gresser, ed.). Academic Press, New York, pp. 23-46 (1982).

57. Kushnaryov, V. M., MacDonald, H. S., Sedmak, J. J., and Grossberg, S. E. Murine interferon-beta receptor-mediated endocytosis and nuclear membrane binding. *Proc. Natl. Acad. Sci. USA 82*:3281-3285 (1985).

58. Hovanessian, A. G., Brown, R. E., and Kerr, I. M. Synthesis of low molecular weight inhibitor of protein synthesis with enzyme from interferon treated cells. *Nature 268*:537-540 (1977).

59. Kerr, I. M., and Brown, R. E. pppA'p5'A2'p5'A: An inhibitor of protein synthesis synthesized with an enzyme fraction from interferon-treated cells. *Proc. Natl. Acad. Sci. USA 75*:256-260 (1978).

60. Ratner, L., Weigand, R., Farrell, P., et al. Interferon, double-stranded RNA and RNA degradation. Fractionation of the endonuclease INT system into two macromolecular components; role of a small molecule in nucelase activation. *Biochem. Biophys. Res. Commun. 81*:947-957 (1978).

61. Farrell, P. J., Sen, G. C., Dubois, M. F., et al. Interferon action: Two distinct pathways for inhibition of protein synthesis by double-stranded RNA. *Proc. Natl. Acad. Sci. USA 75*:5893-5897 (1978).

62. Williams, B. R. C., Kerr, I. M., Gilbert, C. S., et al. Synthesis and breakdown of pppA'p5'A2'p5'A and transient inhibition of protein synthesis in extracts from interferon-treated and control cells. *Eur. J. Biochem* 92:455–462 (1978).

63. Schmidt, A., Chernajovsky, Y., Shulman, L., et al. An interferon-induced phosphodiestrerase degrading (2'-5') oliogoisoadenylate and the C-C-A terminus of tRNA. *Proc. Natl. Acad. Sci. USA* 76:4788–4792 (1979).

64. Nilsen, T. W., and Baglioni, C. Mechanisms for discrimination between viral and host mRNA in interferon-treated cells. *Proc. Natl. Acad. Sci. USA* 76:2600–2604 (1979).

65. Krishnan, I., and Baglioni, C. Increased levels of (2'-5')oligo(A) polymerase activity in human lymphoblastoid cells treated with glucocorticoids. *Proc. Natl. Acad. Sci. USA* 77:6506–6510 (1980).

66. Stark, G. R., Dower, W. J., Schimke, R. T., et al. 2-5A synthetase: Assay, distribution and variation with growth or hormone status. *Nature 278*: 471–473 (1979).

67. Lebleu, B., Sen, G. C., Shaila, S., et al. Interferon, double-stranded RNA and protein phosphorylation. *Proc. Natl. Acad. Sci. USA* 73:3107–3111 (1976).

68. Ohtsuki, K., Dianzani, F., and Baron, S. Decreased initiation factor activity in mouse L-cells treated with interferon. *Nature 269*:536–538 (1977).

69. Roberts, W. K., Clemens, M. J., and Kerr, I. M. Interferon-induced inhibition of protein synthesis in L-cell extracts: An ATP dependent step in the activation of an inhibitor by double-stranded RNA. *Proc. Natl. Acad. Sci. USA* 73:3136–3140 (1976).

70. Farrell, P. J., Balkow, K., Hunt, T., et al. Phosphorylation of initiation factor eiF-2 and the control of reticulocyte protein synthesis. *Cell 11*: 87–200 (1977).

71. Lenz, J. R., and Baglioni, C. Inhibition of protein synthesis by double-stranded RNA and phosphorylation of initiation factor eiF-2. *J. Biol. Chem. 253*:4219–4223 (1978).

72. Samuel, C. E. Mechanism of interferon action: Phosphorylation of protein synthesis initiation factor eiF-2 in interferon-treated human cells by a ribosome associated kinase processing site specificity similar to hemin-regulated rabbit reticulocyte kinase. *Proc. Natl. Acad. Sci. USA* 76:600–604 (1979).

73. Kimchi, A., Shulman, L., Schmidt, A., Chernajovsky, Y., Fradin, A., and Revel, M. Kinetics of the induction of three translation-regulatory enzymes by interferon. *Proc. Natl Acad. Sci. USA* 76:3208-3212 (1979).
74. Kimchi, A., Zilberstein, A., Schmidt, A., Shulman, L., and Revel, M. The interferon-induced protein kinase PK-i from mouse L-cells. *J. Biol. Chem.* 254:9846-9853 (1979).
75. Gross, M., Knish, W. M., and Kwan, A. Rabbit reticulocyte double-stranded RNA-activated protein kinase and the hemin-controlled translational repressor phosphorylate the same Mr 1500 peptide of eukaryotic initiation factor 2a. *FEBS Lett.* 125:223-226 (1981).
76. Lindenmann, J. Inheritance of resistance to influenza in mice. *Proc. Soc. Exp. Biol. Med.* 116:506-509 (1964).
77. Krug, R. M., Shaw, M., Broni, B., et al. Inhibition of influenza viral mRNA synthesis in cells expressing the interferon-induced Mx gene product. *J. Virol* 56:201-206 (1985).
78. Friedman, R. M., and Sonnabend, J. A. Inhibition of interferon action by p-fluorophenylalanine. *Nature* 203:366-367 (1964).
79. Weigent, D. A., Langford, M. D., Stanton, G. J., and Blalock, J. E. Interferon-induced transfer of viral resistance by human B and T lymphocytes. *Cell. Immunol.* 87:678-683 (1984).
80. Stewart, W. E., II, Scott, W. D., and Sulkin, S. E. Relative sensitivities of viruses to different species of interferons. *J. Virol.* 4:147-153 (1969).
81. Friedman, R. M. Antiviral activity of interferons. *Bacteriol. Rev.* 41:543-567 (1977).
82. Maheshwari, R. K., Banerjee, D. K., Wechter, C. J., et al. Interferon treatment inhibits glycosylation of a viral protein. *Nature* 287:454-456 (1980).
83. Takemoto, K., and Baron, S. Non-heritable interferon resistance in a fraction of virus populations. *Proc. Soc. Exp. Biol. Med.* 121:670-675. (1973).
84. Fleischmann, W. R., Jr., and Simon, E. H. Effect of interferon on virus production from isolated single cells. *J. Gen. Virol.* 20:127-137 (1973).
85. Gresser, I. In: *Cancer—A Comprehensive Treatise* (F. Becker, ed). Plenum Press, New York pp. 521-571 (1977).
86. Gresser, I., and Tovey, M. G. Antitumor effects of interferon. *Biochim. Biophys. Acta* 516:231-247 (1978).

87. Stewart, W. E., II, Gresser, I., Tovey, M. G., et al. Identification of the cell multiplication inhibitory factors in interferon preparations as interferons. *Nature 262*:300-302 (1976).

88. Baron, S., Merigan, T. C., and McMcKerlie, M. L. Effect of crude and purified interferon on the growth of uninfected cells in culture. *Proc. Soc. Exp. Biol. Med. 121*:50-52 (1966).

89. Gresser, I., Coppey, J., and Bourali, C. Interferon and murine leukemia. VI. Effect of interferon on preparations on the lymphoid leukemia of AKR mice. *JNCI 43*:1083-1089 (1969).

90. Gresser, I., Maury, C., and Tovey, M. G. Interferon and murine leukemia. VII. Therapeutic effect of interferon preparations after diagnosis of lymphoma in AKR mice. *Int. J. Cancer 17*:647-651 (1976).

91. Came, P. E., and Moore, D. H. Inhibition of spontaneous mammary carcinoma of mice by treatment with interferon and poly I:C. *Proc. Soc. Exp. Biol. Med 137*:304-305 (1971).

92. Atanasiu, P., and Chany, C. Action d'un interferon provenant de cellules malignes sur l'infection experimentale du hamster nouveau—ne par le virus du polyme. *C.R. Acad. Sci. Paris 251*:1687-1689 (1960).

93. Lampson, G. P., Tytell, A. A., Nemes, M. M., and Hilleman, M. R. Purification and characterization of chick embryo interferon. *Proc. Soc. Exp. Biol. Med. 112*:468-478 (1963).

94. Kishida, T., Kato, S., and Nagano, Y. Effet due facteur inhibiteur du virus sur le fibroma de Shope. *C. R. Soc. Biol. (Paris) 159*:782-789 (1965).

95. Balkwill, F., and Taylor-Papadimitriou, J. Interferons affect both G_1 and $S + G_2$ in cells stimulated from quiescence to growth. *Nature 274*:798-800 (1978).

96. Collyn-d'Hooghe, M., Broute-Boye, D., Malaise, E. P., and Gresser, I. Interferon and cell division. XII. Prolongation by interferon of the intermitotic time of mouse mammary tumor cells in vitro. Microcinematographic analysis. *Exp. Cell Res. 105*:73-77 (1977).

97. Mataresse, G. P., and Rossi, G. B. Effect of interferon on growth and division cycle of Friend erythroleukemic murine cells in vitro. *J. Cell Biol. 75*:344-354 (1977).

98. Lundbald, D., and Lundgren, E. Block of a glioma cell line in S by interferon. *Int. J. Cancer 27*:749-754 (1981).

99. Leanderson, T., and Lundgren, E. Growth inhibition by IFN achieved by collecting cells in G_0. *J. Interferon Res.* 2:21-29 (1982).

100. Lloyd, R. E., Blalock, J. E., and Stanton, G. J. Cell to cell transfer of interferon-induced antiproliferative activity. *Science* 221:953-955 (1983).

101. Tyring, S., Klimpel, G. R., Fleischmann, W. R., Jr., and Baron, S. Direct cytolysis by partially-purified preparations of immune interferon. *In. J. Cancer* 30:59-64 (1982).

102. Ito, M., and Buffet, R. F. Cytocidal effect of purified human fibroblast interferon on tumor cells in vitro. *JNCI* 66:819-825 (1981).

103. Tyring, S. K., Klimpel, G. R., Brysk, M., et al. Eradication of cultured human melanoma cells by immune interferon and leukocytes. *JNCI* 73: 1067-1073 (1984).

104. Gresser, I., Maruy, C., and Brouty-Boye, D. Mechanism of antitumor effect of interferon in mice. *Nature* 239:167-168 (1972).

105. Braun, W., and Levy, H. B. Interferon preparations as modifiers of immune response. *Proc. Soc. Exp. Biol. Med* 141:769-773 (1972).

106. Johnson, H. M., and Baron, S. The nature of the suppressive effect of interferon and interferon inducers on the in vitro immune response. *Cell. Immunol.* 25:106-115 (1976).

107. Gisler, R. H., Lindahl, P., and Gresser, I. Effects of interferon on antibody synthesis in vitro. *J. Immunol.* 113:438-444 (1974).

108. Schultz, R. M., Chirigos, M. A., and Heine, U. I. Functional and morphologic characteristics of interferon-treated macrophages. *Cell. Immunol.* 35:84-91 (1978).

109. Huang, K. Y., Donahoe, R. M., Gordon, F. B., and Dressler, H. R. Enhancement of phagocytosis by interferon-containing preparations. *Infect. Immun.* 4:581-588 (1971).

110. Degre, M., Sonnenfeld, G., Rollag, H., and Mooland, B. Effect of gamma interferon preparations on in vitro phagocytosis and degradation of *Escherichia coli* by mouse peritoneal macrophages. *J. Interferon Res.* 1:505-512 (1981).

111. Imanishi, J., Yokota, Y., Kishida, T., et al. Phagocytosis-enhancing effect of human leukocyte interferon preparations of human peripheral monocytes in vitro. *Acta Virol. (Praha)* 19:52 (1975).

112. Hamburg, S. I., Cassell, G. H., and Rabinovitch, M. Relationship between enhanced machrophage phagocytic activity and the induction of interferon by Newcastle disease virus in mice. *J. Immunol.* 124:1360-1364 (1980).

113. Schreiber, R. D., Pace, J. L., Russel, S. W., et al. Macrophage-activating factor produced by a T cell hybridoma: Physicochemical and biosynthetic resemblance to gamma-interferon. *J. Immunol.* 131:826-832 (1983).

114. Lindahl. P., Leary, P., and Gresser, I. Enhancement by interferon of the specific cytotoxicity of sensitized lymphocytes. *Proc. Natl. Acad. Sci. USA* 69:721-725 (1972).

115. Kishida, T., Morikawa, K., Ito, H., and Yokota, Y. Influence de l'interferon sur l'inhibition par les macrophages, de la multiplication in vitro de la cellule maligne murine (FM_3A). *C. R. Soc. Biol. (Paris)* 167:1502-1505 (1973).

116. Zarling, J. M., Sosman, J., Eskra, L., et al. Enhancement of T cell cytotoxic response by purified human fibroblast interferon. *J. Immunol.* 121:2002-2004 (1978).

117. Trinchieri, G., Santoli, D., Dee, R. R., and Knowles, B. B. Anti-viral activity induced by culturing lymphocytes with tumor-derived virus-transformed cells. Identification of the antiviral activity as interferon and characterization of the human effector lymphocyte subpopulation. *J. Exp. Med.* 147:1299-1313 (1978).

118. Gidlund, M., Orn, A., Wigzell, H., et al. Enhanced NK activity in mice injected with interferon and interferon inducers. *Nature* 273:759-761 (1978).

119. Svet-Moldavsky, G. J., and Chernyakhovskaya, I. J. Interferon and the interaction of allogeneic normal and immune lymphocytes with L-cells. *Nature* 215:1299-1300 (1967).

120. Chernyakhovskaya, I. Y., Slavina, E. G., and Svet-Moldavsky, G. J. Antitumor effect of lymphoid cells activated by interferon. *Nature* 228:71-72 (1970).

121. Einhorn, S., Blomgren, H., and Strander, H. Interferon and spontaneous cytotoxicity in man. II. Studies in patients receiving exogenous leukocyte interferon. *Acta Med. Scand.* 204:477-483 (1978).

122. Trinchieri, G., and Santoli, D. Antiviral activity induced by culturing lymphocytes with tumor-derived or virus-transformed cells. Enhance-

ment of human natural killer cell activity by interferon and antagonistic inhibition of susceptibility of target cells to lysis. *J. Exp. Med. 147*: 1314–1333 (1978).

123. Rothermel, C. D., Rubin, B. Y., and Murray, H. W. Gamma-interferon is the factor in lymphokine that activates human macrophages to inhibit intracellular *Chlamydia psittaci* replication. *J. Immunol. 131*: 2542–2544 (1983).

124. Pfeffercorn, E. R. Interferon gamma blocks the growth of *Toxoplasma gondii* in human fibroblasts by inducing the host cells to degrade tryptophan. *Proc. Natl Acad. Sci. USA 81*:908–912 (1984).

125. Kierszenbaum, F., and Sonnenfeld, G. Beta interferon inhibits cell infection by *Trypansoma cruzi. J. Immunol. 132*:905–912 (1984).

126. Buckholm, G., and Degre, M. Effect of human leukocyte interferon on invasiveness of *Salmonella* species in Hep-2 cell cultures. *Infect. Immun. 42*:1198–1202 (1983).

127. Niesel, D. W., Hess, C. B., Chou, Y. C., et al. Natural and recombinant IFN inhibit epithelial cell invasion by *Shigella* sp. *Infect. Immun. 52*: 828–833 (1986).

128. Levin, S., and Hahn, T. Interferon deficiency syndrome. *Clin. Exp. Immunol. 60*:267–273 (1985).

129. Benczur, M., Petranyl, G. G., Palffy, G., et al. Dysfunction of natural killer cells in multiple sclerosis: A possible pathogenic factor. *Clin. Exp. Immunol. 39*:657–662 (1980).

130. Minato, N., Reid, L., Neighbor, A., et al. Interferon, NK cells and persistent virus infections. *Ann. N.Y. Acad. Sci. 350*:42–52 (1980).

131. Epstein, L. B., Lee, S. H. S., and Epstein, C. J. Enhanced sensitivity of trisomy 21 monocytes to the maturation-inhibiting effect of interferon. *Cell. Immunol. 50*:191–194 (1980).

132. Skurkovich, S., and Eremkina, E. I. The probable role of interferon in allergy. *Ann. Allergy 35*:356–360 (1975).

133. DeStefano, E., Friedman, R. M., Friedman-Kien, A. E., et al. Acid-labile leukocyte interferon in homosexual men with Kaposi's sarcoma and lymphoadenopathy. *J. Infect. Dis. 146*:451–455 (1982).

134. Preble, O. T., Black, R. J., Friedman, R. M., et al. Systemic lupus erythematosus: Presence in human serum of an unusual acid-labile leukocyte interferon. *Science 216*:429–431 (1982).

135. Todd, I., Pufol-Borell, R., Hammond, L. J., et al. Interferon-gamma induces HLA-DR expression in thyroid epithelium. *Clin. Exp. Immunol.* 61:265-278 (1985).

136. Lonei, M., Lamb, J. R., Bottazzo, G. F., and Feldman, M. Epithelial cells expressing aberrant MHC class II determinants can present antigen to cloned human T cells. *Nature* 312:639-641 (1984).

137. Londei, M., Bottazzo, G. F., and Feldman, M. Human T cell clones from autoimmune thyroid glands: Specific recognition of autologous thyroid cells. *Science* 228:85-89 (1985).

138. Imanishi, J., Karaki, T., Sasaki, O., et al. The preventive effect of human interferon-alpha preparations on upper respiratory disease. *J. Interferon Res.* 1:169-178 (1980).

139. Greenberg, S. B., Harmon, M. W., Couch, R. B., et al. Prophylactic effect of low doses of human leukocyte interferon-alpha against infections with rhinovirus. *J. Infect. Dis.* 145:542-546 (1982).

140. Dekonig. E. W. G., van Bijsterveld, O. P., and Cantell, K. Combination therapy for dendritic keratitis with human leukocyte interferon and trifluorothymidine. *Br. J. Opthalmol.* 66:509-512 (1982).

141. Sundmacher, R., Cantell, K., Skoda, R., et al. Human leukocyte and fibroblast interferon in a combination therapy of dentritic keratitis. *Albrecht Von Graefes Arch. Klin. Exp. Opthalmol.* 208:229-233 (1978).

142. Romano, A., Revel, M., Guarari-Rotman, D., et al. Use of human fibroblast-derived (beta) interferon in the treatment of epidermic adenovirus keratoconjunctivitis. *J. Interferon Res.* 1:169-178 (1980).

143. Armstrong, J. A. Clinical use of interferons: Systemic administration in viral diseases. *Handb. Exp. Pharmacol.* 71:455-469 (1984).

144. Pazin, G. J., Armstrong, J. A., Lem, M. T., et al. Prevention of reactivated herpes simplex infection by human leukocyte interferon after operation on the trigeminal root. *N. Engl. J. Med* 301:225-230 (1979).

145. Greenberg, H. B., Pollard, R. B., Lutwick, L. I., et al. Effect of human leukocyte interferon on hepatitis B virus infection in patients with chronic active hepatitis. *N. Engl. J. Med.* 295:517-522 (1976).

146. Quesada, J. R., Gutterman, J. U., and Hesh, E. M. Treatment of hairy cell leukemia with alpha interferons. *Cancer* 57:1678-1680 (1986).

147. Geffen, J. R., Klein, R. J., and Friedman-Kien, A. E. Intralesional

manifestations of human leukocyte interferon therapy in patients with cancer. *JAMA 252*:938-941 (1984).

173. Honigsberger, L., Fielding, J. W., and Priestman, T. J. Neurological effects of recombinant human interferon (letter). *Br. Med. J. 286*:719 (1983).

174. Mattson, K., Niiranen, A., Iivanianen, M., et al. Neurotoxicity of interferon. *Cancer Treat. Rep. 67*:958-961 (1983).

175. Mattson, K., Niiranen, A., Laaksonen, R., et al Psychometric monitoring of interferon neurotoxicity (letter). *Lancet 1*:275-276 (1984).

176. Rohatnier, A. Z. S., Prior, P. F., Burton, A. C., et al. Central nervous system toxicity of interferon. *Br. J. Cancer 47*:419-422 (1983).

177. Rohatnier, A. Z. S., Balkwill, F. R., Griffin, D. B., et al. A phase I study of human lymphoblastoid interferon administered by continuous intravenous infusion. *Cancer Chemother. Pharmacol. 9*:97-102 (1982).

178. Smedley, H., Katrak, M., Sikora, K., et al. Neurological effects of recombinant human interferon. *Br. Med. J. 286*:262-264 (1983).

179. Fleischmann, W. R., Jr., Georgiades, J. A., Osborne, L. C., and Johnson, H. M. Potentiation of interferon activity by mixed preparations of fibroblast and immune interferon. *Infect. Immun. 26*:248-253 (1979).

180. Fleischmann, W. R., Jr., Kleyn, K. M., and Baron, S. Potentiation of antitumor effect of virus-induced interferon by mouse immune interferon preparations. *JNCI 65*:963-966 (1980).

181. Fleischmann, W. R., Jr. Potentiation of the direct anticellular activity of mouse interferons: Mutual synergism and interferon concentration dependence. *Cancer Res. 42*:869-875 (1982).

182. Koren, S., and Fleischmann, W. R., Jr. Quantitation of in vivo potentiation resulting from combined interferon therapy: Antitumor effect against B-16 melanoma in mice. *J. Interferon Res 6*:473-482 (1986).

183. Chirigos, M. A., and Pearson, J. W. Cure of murine leukemia with drug and interferon treatment. *JNCI 51*:1367-1368 (1973).

184. Gresser, I., Maury, C., and Tovey, M. G. Efficacy of combined interferon cyclophosphamide therapy after diagnosis of lymphoma in AKR mice. *Eur. J. Cancer 14*:97-99 (1978).

185. Slater, L. M., Wetzel, M. W., and Cesario, T. Combined interferon-antimetabolite therapy of murine L1210 leukemia. *Cancer 48*:5-9 (1981).

186. Kuwata, T., Fuse, A., and Morinaga, N. Combined effects of interferon and antitumor drugs on the growth of human transformed cells in vitro. *Int. Soc. Chemother., Proc. 10th Int. Congress of Chemother.* pp. 1103-1106 (1978).

187. Namba, M., Miyoshi, T., Kenemori, T., et al. Combined effects of 5-fluoroacil and interferon on proliferation of human neoplastic cells in culture. *Gann* 73:819-824. (1982).

188. Namba, M., Yamamoto, S., Tanaka, H., et al. In vitro and in vivo studies on potentiation of cytotoxic effects of anticancer drugs or cobalt 60 gamma ray by interferon on human neoplastic cells. *Cancer* 15:2262-2267 (1984).

189. Williamson, B. D., Carswell, E. A., Rubin, B. Y., et al. Human tumor necrosis factor produced by human B-cell lines: Synergistic cytotoxic interaction with human interferon. *Proc. Natl. Acad. Sci. USA* 80: 5397-5401 (1983).

190. Koren, S., Klimpel, G. R., and Fleischmann, W. R., Jr. Macrophage colony stimulating factor (CSF-1) blocks the myeloid suppressive but not the antiviral or antiproliferative activities of murine alpha, beta, and gamma interferons in vitro. *J. Biol. Respir. Modif.* 5:571-580 (1986).

191. Koren, S., Klimpel, G. R., and Fleischmann, W. R., Jr. Treatment of mice with macrophage colony stimulating factor (CSF-1) prevents the in vivo myelosuppression induced by murine alpha, beta, and gamma interferons. *J. Biol. Respir. Modif.* 5:481-489 (1986).

2
Molecular Mechanisms of Interferon Action

BRYAN R. G. WILLIAMS

Hospital for Sick Children, Toronto, Ontario, Canada

There is an increasing amount of evidence to suggest that interferons (IFN), in addition to eliciting antiviral and anticellular activities, may also be involved in the regulation of normal cellular metabolism, growth, and differentiation. These processes are probably regulated at the levels of IFN gene expression, interaction of IFN with specific cell surface receptors, or induction and action of specific mRNAs and proteins by IFN. Although the molecular mechanisms underlying these events are not fully understood, there have been several recent advances in determining IFN-receptor interactions, in the characterization of IFN-regulated genes, and also in the discovery of IFN regulation of growth factor activity and proto-oncogene expression. These are the main emphasis of this review.

IFN were originally characterized because of their ability to protect cells from virus infection. This protection results from a series of biochemical changes that are initiated following exposure to IFN (see Ref 1 for a recent review). It has now become apparent from the detailed analysis of two biochemical pathways (2′,5′-oligoadenylate synthetase and protein kinase) implicated in mediating antiviral activity that there are differences in the responses of different cells at a given biochemical level to the same or different IFN (e.g., IFN-α/β compared with IFN-γ. This is likely to be the case for all activities ascribed to IFN that are controlled initially at the level of IFN-receptor binding.

I. INTERFERON-RECEPTOR INTERACTIONS

The initiation of cellular responses to IFN is mediated through specific high-affinity receptors in the plasma membrane. There are at least two functional types of receptors on most cells. IFN-α or IFN-β (type I IFN) bind to one type of receptor, whereas IFN-γ (type II IFN) binds to a distinct receptor (reviewed in Ref. 2). Affinity labeling experiments that identify IFN-α binding complexes of 140-160 kD (3-5) and IFN-γ binding complexes of about 110 kD (6, 7) in a variety of human cell types further illustrate this difference. However, in at least one human cell line there is evidence for an indirect interaction between type I and type II receptors since prior exposure to IFN-γ reduces the affinity of subsequent IFN-α receptor binding (8). This existence of two functionally distinct IFN receptors makes it possible for different molecular events to be initiated as early as the interaction of IFN with its specific cell surface receptor.

Synergistic responses observed with combinations of type I and type II (reviewed in Ref. 1) IFN are consistent with the activation of distinct pathways in some cells by these IFN. Within the type I IFN, different subtypes of IFN-α display variable affinity for their receptor. These affinities in some cases correlate with the relative biologic efficacies of these subtypes (9, 10).

Heterogeneity in the binding of IFN-a_2, characterized by biphasic Scatchard plots, has been observed in some cells and has been shown to be closely linked to cell proliferation (11-14). A study of the kinetics of IFN-receptor dissociation has indicated that this binding heterogeneity is consistent with the presence of negative cooperative site-site interactions between receptors. Thus high concentrations of IFN induce a lowered affinity of receptors for IFN (11). However, in cells demonstrating the two different forms of binding, there does not appear to be any difference in the receptors that can be chemically cross-linked to IFN. Interestingly, a Daudi lymphoblastoid cell variant that is resistant to the antiproliferative effects of IFN does not show heterogenity and cannot undergo receptor interactions (11). This suggests that these interactions at the cell surface may be necessary to initiate the anticellular activities of IFN through the activation of alternative pathways.

Events subsequent to the binding of IFN by cell surface receptors are not well understood. Both IFN-α and IFN-γ are internalized and degraded intracellularly (15, 16), although the existence of alternative pathways that result in the release of undegraded IFN has also been suggested for some cell types (17, 18). Clearance of IFN-receptor complexes from the cell surface results in receptor down-regulation and desensitization of the cells to further exposure to IFN. No requirement for internalization has been established in the expression of the biologic effects of IFN, and in the case of the 2-5A synthetase and 1-8 genes internalization is not required (see below) (15). Ultrastructural study (2) has shown that a proportion of IFN is internalized and subsequently localized in clathrin-coated pits. This evidence is consistent with IFN entering cells by receptor-mediated endocytosis, a mechanism shared by numerous polypeptide hormones.

The antiviral and growth-inhibitory effects of IFN are detectable (largely because of the nature of the assays involved) only after several hours of incubation. However, increases in the transcription rate of some IFN-induced genes can be detected as early as 5 min after the addition of IFN (18). Therefore, interaction of IFN with receptors must result in the rapid transmission of signals to the nucleus. Recently, we have demonstrated that the transcription of the IFN-induced 2-5A synthetase and 1-8 genes is closely linked to surface receptor occupancy and is most likely mediated by transmembrane signals alone (14). There is a striking coincidence of IFN-receptor binding and transcriptional induction kinetics, which strongly suggests a stoichiometric relationship between the number of surface receptors occupied and the amount of signal that is generated or released. The nature of the signal(s) mediating the transcriptional response to IFN remains to be determined. By using a variety of direct methodologies we have been unable to detect changes in cytoplasmic alkalinization, Ca^{2+} flux, and phosphoinositide turnover during early times of exposure of human cells to IFN (19). These mechanisms have been implicated in the generation of second messengers mediating the mitogenic activation of cells by growth factors and mitogens (20). However, IFN treatment does effect an immediate but transient decrease in the levels of the c-*fos* proto-oncogene (21) mRNA in cells where c-*fos* is constitutively expressed. This decrease and recovery closely parallel IFN receptor binding and down-regulation and suggest that IFN and c-*fos* share part of a common signaling pathway.

II. GENES REGULATED BY INTERFERONS

The effects of IFN on cellular functions are extensive and pleiotropic. These effects are mediated by both inhibition of expression of some genes and induction of expression of other genes. These two phenomena may also be interdependent, with inhibition of gene expression by IFN in some instances requiring the synthesis of new proteins (e.g., inhibition of c-*myc*) (22). Both IFN-α and IFN-γ induce a common set of polypeptides, but in addition there are proteins that are induced only by IFN-α/β (e.g., the Mx protein) (23) and others that are induced to a greater extent by IFN-γ (e.g., class II HLA) (see also Refs. 24 and 25). A number of cDNAs corresponding to IFN-α/β or IFN-γ inducible mRNAs have recently been isolated (18,26-29). The transcription of these RNAs increases rapidly in response to IFN, but they are also subject to varying degrees of posttranscriptional control (18,27-32). Although the proteins encoded by a number of these mRNAs number have no known function, several encode proteins with well-characterized activities. These include both class I and class II histocompatibility antigens, β_2-microglobulin, metallothionein-II (MT II), thymosin b_4, 2-5A synthetase, and the Mx protein (18, 28, 33). Although increased HLA and β_2-microglobulin expression probably contributes to the immunoregulatory and antitumor activities of IFN, the role that metallothionein or thymosin plays in the mechanism of action of IFN remains obscure. In the genes encoding some of these interferon-regulated proteins, a consensus sequence has been demonstrated that may be important for induction by IFN-α. Genes in which this sequence has been found are listed in Table 1.

Table 1 Interferon-Regulated Genes Containing the Consensus IFN-α Response Sequence TTCNC/GNACCTCNGCAGTTTCTCC/TTCT-CT[a]

Gene	Distance 5' of CAP Site
Class II HLA-DR	(567)
Class I HLA-A3	(142)
Class I (mouse)	
H-2Kb	(165)
H-2Kk	
H-2Ld	
Q10 (Qa)	
27.1 (Qa)	
β_2-microglobulin	(3' noncoding)
MT II	(600)
Mouse 202	(first exon)
Thymosin B4	
6-16	

[a] In the class I and II HLA genes and MT II the consensus sequence is found in the 5' flanking regions of the genes. However, in the mouse 202 gene, which encodes a 56 kD protein of unknown function (29), and in β_2-microglobulin, the sequence appears to be transcribed. It has not yet been demonstrated whether this sequence is essential for induction by IFN or whether it can confer IFN inducibility on genes not normally activated by IFN. A sequence with limited similarity has been found in the 2-5A synthetase gene 116 bp upstream of the translation start site (author's unpublished observations). The sequence has not been demonstrated to be present in the 1-8 gene family. Both these genes are under stringent transcriptional regulation by IFN and probably possess alternative IFN-responsive promoter and/or enhancer sequences.

III. INTERFERON-INDUCED CHANGES IN INTRACELLULAR FUNCTIONS

A number of biochemical changes occur in cells following IFN-receptor interactions. An incomplete list is detailed in Table 2, and references can be found in Reference 34. Many of these changes have not been associated with the functional activity of IFN as an antiviral or anticellular agent and are probably secondary effects. However, some result from direct induction by IFN and may have important clinical implications.

It has been known for some time that IFN stimulates prostaglandin production in human fibroblasts (35). More recently it has been demonstrated that IFN appears to act as an endogenous pyrogen by directly stimulating prostaglandin E_2 production by the hypothalamus (36). This appears to account for the febrile response seen in patients on IFN therapy. The IFN-mediated depression of hepatic cytochrome P_{450}-linked mono-oxygenases also appears to be a direct effect and can alter drug biotransformation (37). However, perhaps the most marked direct effect of IFN that has been demonstrated to dramatically alter tumorigenicity is the modulation of class I antigen expression. Human adenovirus 12-transformed cells express only low levels of class I antigens and are highly tumorigenic in syngeneic hosts. However, if the cells are exposed to IFN before inoculation in immunocomponent hosts, they have a much reduced tumorigenic capacity (38). Furthermore, the administration of IFN to animals following the introduction of a tumorigenic dose of adenovirus 12-transformed cells resulted in the effective rejection of the tumor. Although these experiments do not exclude the involvement of a number of host responses (cytotoxic T cells, natural killer cells, and activated macrophages), there is little doubt that the IFN induction of the major histocompatibility complex (MHC) locus is essential to its antitumor effect in this case. An equally striking case of direct induced expression of a protein by IFN resulting in a virus-resistant phenotype occurs with the Mx protein (reviewed in Ref. 39). This is a 75 kD protein that appears only in mouse cells bearing the Mx^+ allele following treatment with IFN-α or IFN-β but not IFN-γ (40,41). Similar proteins have been detected in human cells.

Table 2 Changes in Cellular Functions Induced by Interferons

<table>
<tr><td colspan="2" align="center">Enhanced gene expression</td></tr>
<tr><td>2-5A synthetase</td><td>2'-Phosphodiesterase</td></tr>
<tr><td>2-5A-dependent RNase</td><td>Class I and II HLA</td></tr>
<tr><td>dsRNA-dependent protein kinase</td><td>β_2-Microglobulin</td></tr>
<tr><td>b-Tubulin</td><td>Thymosin b_4</td></tr>
<tr><td>Platelet factor 4/b-thromboglobulin</td><td>Mx protein</td></tr>
<tr><td>Guanylate binding protein</td><td>Metallothionein</td></tr>
<tr><td colspan="2" align="center">Enhancement of activity or synthesis</td></tr>
<tr><td>Arylhydrocarbon hydroxylase</td><td>Type IV collagenase</td></tr>
<tr><td>Prostaglandin E_2, F_2</td><td>Histamine</td></tr>
<tr><td>Fc receptors</td><td>tRNA methylase</td></tr>
<tr><td>Cyclic AMP</td><td>Cyclic GMP</td></tr>
<tr><td>Carcinoembryonic antigen</td><td>Indoleamine dioxygenase</td></tr>
<tr><td colspan="2" align="center">Decreased activity or synthesis</td></tr>
<tr><td>Glycosyltransferase</td><td>Hexose monophosphate shunt</td></tr>
<tr><td>Glucocorticoid inducible enzymes</td><td>Unsaturated fatty acids</td></tr>
<tr><td>Ornithine decarboxylase</td><td>Thymidine transport</td></tr>
<tr><td>s-Adenosylmethionine decarboxylase</td><td>Protein phosphatases</td></tr>
<tr><td>Cytochrome P_{450} mono-oxygenases</td><td>Cell surface IgM</td></tr>
<tr><td>Transferrin receptors</td><td>EGF receptors</td></tr>
<tr><td>IL-2 receptors</td><td></td></tr>
</table>

The resistance conferred by Mx is specific for influenza virus, and experiments using the constitutive expression of Mx cDNA in mouse cells have shown that the Mx protein is solely responsible for this resistance (41). The mechanism of resistance conferred by Mx is unknown. The Mx protein accumulates in the nucleus, and it is speculated that it interferes with an obligatory nuclear event in influenza virus replication (42).

Investigation of the biochemical basis of the antiviral activity of IFN has led to the elucidation of two pathways that are activated by double-stranded RNA (dsRNA). These are the protein kinase and $2',5'$-oligoadenylate synthetase (2-5A synthetase) pathways that when activated in vitro or in IFN-treated virus-infected cells result in the inhibition of protein synthesis. This is acieved in the case of the protein kinase through the phosphorylation of the a subunit of protein synthesis initiation factor eIF2. The 2-5A synthetase, once activated by dsRNA, utilizes ATP to synthesize a novel series of $2',5'$-linked oligonucleotides that in turn activate an RNase (2-5A-dependent RNase, RNase F, and RNase L). This RNase, which is ubiquitous in higher vertebrates, degrades both mRNA and rRNA, cleaving 3' of UA or UU sequences and effectively halting protein synthesis. The 2-5A is rapidly degraded by a $2'$-phophodiesterase (which itself may in some cases be regulated by IFN) such that activation of the nuclease and inhibition of protein synthesis are transient. Oligomers of 2-5A have been found to occur naturally in a variety of IFN-treated cells infected with a wide variety of both RNA and DNA viruses, although this does not always correlate with the development of an antiviral state (43). Nevertheless, both the protein kinase and 2-5A synthetase (reviewed extensively in Ref. 30) pathways are active in mediating the antiviral effects of IFN in some virus-cell systems. In other virus infections, particularly where dsRNA is not formed, alternative biochemical mechanisms probably operate but are little understood.

IV. THE 2-5A SYSTEM

Although the principal regulators of the 2-5A system are IFN and dsRNA, the occurrence of 2-5A synthetase in a wide variety of mammalian and avian cells and tissues and its regulation in response to hormone treatment (44) have led to the suggestion that the 2-5A system may be involved in more general aspects of cell growth and metabolism. Moreover, it has been demonstrated recently that PDGF can directly activate the 2-5A synthetase gene (45), leading to the suggestion that the 2-5A system may be involved in the control of cellular proliferation induced by PDGF. Interestingly, 2-5A synthetase can, in vitro, $2'$-adenylate a number of important metabolites, including NAD, ADP ribose, $A5'pppp5'A$, and tRNA, although none of these products have been detected in vivo. However, a number of 2-5A-related compounds are found in normal cells and tissues in addition to IFN-treated simian virus 40- (SV40), vaccinia-, and herpesvirus-infected cells. The function of these compounds and whether they are in fact products of 2-5A synthetase has yet to be elucidated.

The 2-5A system is important in mediating the effects of IFN in some virus-cell interactions. Oligonucleotides of 2-5A introduced into intact cells also inhibit protein and DNA synthesis, enhance RNA breakdown, and inhibit virus replication. As in cell-free protein-synthesizing systems (46), this effect of 2-5A is transient as 2-5A is rapidly degraded. The most definitive evidence for the importance of the 2-5A system in vivo comes from an analysis of the effect of an analog inhibitor of 2-5A in preventing the antiviral activity of IFN against encephalomyocarditis (EMC) virus. A partial reversion of the antiviral state and inhibition of the characteristic 2-5A-mediated cleavage of ribosomal RNA is seen when this analog is introduced into IFN-treated EMC virus-infected cells (47). Since the 2-5A system is composed of at least three enzymes, the synthetase, the 2-5A-dependent RNase, and the $2'$-phosphodiesterase, the potential for regulation at different levels of the pathway is possible. Little is known about the role of the $2'$-phosphodiesterase in controlling 2-5A levels; however, both IFN treatment and mitogenic stimulation can result in increased enzyme levels (48). The 2-5A-dependent RNase is not regulated by IFN in most cell lines, but in certain cells it can be induced as much as 20-fold (49) and its levels can also vary with the differentiation state of the cells. Affinity labeling experiments indicate the 2-5A-dependent RNase is a 2-5A binding protein between 77,000 and 85,000 daltons (50,51) that may be regulated independently of the 2-5A-synthetase or 2'-phosphodiesterase during cell growth or differentiation (52,53). The activity of the 2-5A-dependent RNase can also be regulated by virus infection. This virus-mediated inhibition of the nuclease activity can be prevented by treatment of the cells with IFN (54). Thus one of the actions of IFN is to maintain an active (2-5A-dependent RNase through an as yet undefined mechanism.

Purification of the 2-5A synthetase to apparent homogeneity by two groups (55,56) suggested that there was a single 2-5A synthetase. However, experiments measuring synthetase mRNA levels indicate that at least two forms of the enzyme exist in mouse and human cells. Mouse Ehrlich ascites cells express mRNAs encoding both a large (85,000–100,000 daltons) and a smaller enzyme (20,000–30,000 daltons) (57). Gel filtration and oocyte injection experiments have also identified enzymes of 60,000–80,000 daltons and 30,000 daltons in human SV80 and HeLa cells. It is still unclear whether the two different sizes of 2-5A synthetase are derived from different genes or are different forms of the same polypeptide and are thus derived from the same gene. The molecular cloning, characterization, and chromosomal localization of the 2-5A synthetase gene suggests the latter is more likely. The isolation of cDNAs encoding the 2-5A synthetase, analysis of both phage and cosmid genomic clones, and comparison with genomic DNA indicate that there is a single gene for the 2-5A synthetase. This comprises eight exons and seven introns that can undergo a novel form of alternative RNA processing depending on cell type (58–60). The unique form of RNA processing of the 3' end of this gene results in transcripts differing in size and sequence at the 3' end. Either one or both mRNAs may be present in different cell types. The deduced C terminus of the smaller (1.6 kilobase, kb) mRNA appears to be hydrophobic whereas that of the larger mRNA (1.8 kb) is acidic (60). This may lead to differences in the interaction with other cellular proteins or in the localization of the two enzymes (the larger, approximately 46,000 daltons; the smaller, 40,000 daltons) encoded by the two mRNAs.

Several cDNA clones encoding the the mouse 2-5A synthetase have been isolated (61). These hybridize to two mRNAs in IFN-treated mouse cells, one of 1.8 kb and a larger mRNA of about

4 kb present following 15 hr of IFN treatment. The structure of the mouse gene and relationship of these two mRNAs remain to be determined. The presence of large RNAs that correlate with a peak of synthetase activity in the S phase of synchronized mouse embryo fibroblasts has been described and the suggestion made that the product of these transcripts may be involved in cell cycle-related functions (62).

Using rodent-human somatic cell hybrids and filter hybridization analysis of cell hybrid DNA, the hyman 2-5A synthetase gene has been mapped to chromosome 12 (63). This contrasts with a previous assignment of this gene to chromosome 11 using an enzyme activity assay. The reason for this discrepancy remains unclear, although the presence of different enzyme activities with different hydrophobic properties would make any analysis based on chromotography difficult to interpret.

Analyses of proteins from IFN-treated cells using Western blots and antibodies raised against synthetic peptides derived from the 2-5A synthetase sequence (62,64) reveal in addition to the 40,000 and 46,000 dalton proteins additional larger polypeptides that may represent the larger forms of the enzyme described above. Thus the possibility exists of further alternative processing of transcripts from the synthetase gene that share the 3' terminus but differ toward the 5' end.

The 5' flanking region of the 2-5A synthetase gene has been sequenced but not yet analyzed in functional assays. The sequence data reveal significant homology to the human IFN-β_1 promoter (58), but interestingly, this lies outside the inducer-responsive element essential for virus induction of the IFN-β_1 gene (65). Transcription of the IFN-β_1 gene is also regulated by IFN itself, a phenomenon termed priming (66,67). Recent evidence suggests this activation requires an IFN-induced trans-acting factor (68). It remains to be determined whether the same or a similar factor interacts with the region of shared homology in the IFN-β_1 and 2-5A synthetase genes.

Measurement of 2-5A synthetase activity in peripheral blood lymphocytes (PBL) has provided a useful means of monitoring individual responses to both viral infection and IFN therapy

(69-72). A quick cell blot assay of 2-5A synthetase RNA has also been described in which treatment of PBL with as little as 10 U/ml of IFN resulted in a signal detectable by hybridization (73). The development of antibodies against the synthetase should enable other forms of rapid assay to be evaluated. This may prove to be particularly useful in the development of a prognostic assay for patients with AIDS-related complex, a pre-AIDS syndrome in individuals infected with the virus HIV. Measurement of 2-5A synthetase activity in PBL from these patients appears to be particularly useful in predicting the outcome of asymptomatic contacts with antibodies to HIV (74).

V. THE PROTEIN KINASE

An enhanced protein kinase activity dependent on dsRNA has been identified in extracts from many different human and mouse cell lines treated with interferon. This kinase activity phosphorylates an endogenous 65,000-67,000 dalton protein (p65) in mouse cells and a 68,000-72,000 dalton protein (p68) in human cells. The kinase also phosphorylates either the endogenous or exogenous 34,000 dalton a subunit of the protein synthesis initiation factor eIF2 and added histones. Phosphorylation of the a subunit of eIF2 prevents the repeated formation of methionyl-tRNA-40S ribosome subunit initiation complexes, thus inhibiting protein synthesis initiation. The kinase appears to be active in a number of IFN-treated virus-infected cell systems, but the significance of the protein kinase system to the antiviral activity of IFN remains unclear (see Ref. 1 for a recent review). Vaccinia virus-infected cells appear to contain a factor that inhibits dsRNA-activated protein kinase (75-78). There is also evidence that the virus-associated (VA) RNAs of adenovirus can inhibit the activity of the kinase (79-82). An understanding of the mechanisms of inhibition involved in these systems should aid in determining the role of the kinase in IFN action.

There was some uncertainty as to whether p65 and p68 were substrates of the dsRNA-dependent protein kinase or the enzymes themselves (83,84). However recent descriptions of polyclonal and monoclonal antibodies against p68 (85,86) have allowed this protein to be measured directly and show there is a tight correlation between p68 protein and kinase activity. The p68 protein purified on monoclonal antibody (MOAb)-Sepharose can be activated with dsRNA and ATP and is capable of phosphorylating exogenous eIF2 and histones. Heparin is also a very efficient activator of the kinase, which suggests that activators other than dsRNA may also exist in intact cells. The kinase activity on exogenous substrates can be correlated with the degree of phosphate saturation of p68 and removal of this phosphate leads to the loss of kinase activity. An ATP binding site also exists on p68. Despite these data, there remain unanswered questions about the p68 protein. The p68 isolated from the MOAb column shows no protein kinase activity on itself or on added substrates and on the MOAb column appears to be dependent on another protein of 48,000 daltons (p48) for activity. However, reconstitution experiments using these two isolated proteins have not been successful and there remains the possibility that an as yet unidentified protein is required for the activation of p68 in the presence of dsRNA or heparin.

A MOAb (10A5, IgM) that specifically binds a protein of approximately 68,000 daltons has been used to characterize this antigen as IFN induced, dsRNA binding, localized to the cytoplasm, and encoded on chromosome 12 (87,88). This antigen is also a phosphoprotein, but no evidence for kinase activity has been obtained because of the difficulty of utilizing IgM molecules for affinity chromotography. The 10A5 MOAb has been used to isolate a cDNA clone from a λ-gtll expression library, and this clone has been used to identify the 10A5 transcript as 3.2 kb in length and to comprise approximately 0.05% of cellular mRNA (88). Somatic cell hybrid analysis has confirmed the gene transcribing the 10A5 epitope is on chromosome 12 although there are also homologous sequences on chromosome 7 and on other chromosomes. Activity assays of human-rodent somatic cell hybrids have shown the 10A5 antigen is not the p68 kinase. The possbility remains, however, that more than one kinase may be regulated by IFN.

VI. REGULATION OF ONCOGENE EXPRESSION BY INTERFERON

Activation of proto-oncogene expression is important in initiating and maintaining the transformed cell phenotype (89). Although the molecular mechanisms responsible for the antiproliferative activity of IFN are unknown, an increasing amount of evidence suggests that at least part of this activity may result from selective inhibition or regulation of expression of specific proto-oncogenes.

The human lymphoblastoid cell line Daudi, which expresses high levels of c-*myc*, is unusually sensitive to growth inhibition by IFN. This inhibition of growth is accompanied by a selective reduction in c-*myc* RNA (90). There is some controversy about the mechanism by which IFN mediates this effect. IFN either has a direct inhibitory effect on the transcription of the c-*myc* gene (91) or reduces the level of c-*myc* RNA by a posttranscriptional mechanism 992,93). Interferon also inhibits the PDGF-mediated increase in c-*myc* in quiescent BALB/c3T3 cells by a mechanism that is partly dependent on protein synthesis. It is therefore possible that IFN may act to inhibit c-*myc* expression through independent pathways that act at either a transcriptional or a posttranscriptional level. A number of IFN-resistant Daudi cell lines have been independently isolated, and in all cases the resistance to the antiproliferative effect of IFN appears to correlate with a loss in the sensitivity of c-*myc* to regulation by IFN. In lymphoblastoid cell lines (Namalva and Raji) naturally resistant to the antigrowth activity of IFN, the steady-state levels of c-*myc* RNA are unaltered following IFN treatment. Therefore there is a strong correlation between the antigrowth activity of IFN and the negative regulation of the c-*myc* proto-oncogene. Although less work has been reported, it appears that N-*ras* RNA may also be changed quantitatively and qualitatively in Daudi cells exposed to IFN (94).

Regulation of human *ras* oncogene expression has also been observed in cells transformed with the Ha-MuSV LTR-activated c-HA-*ras*1 protogene. This resulted in a phenotypic reversion of transformed cells accompanied by a reduction in the *ras*-encoded p21 protein (95,96). When IFN was omitted from the reverted cell cultures, retransformed foci appeared. However, a monolayer of persistent revertants surrounding the foci could be maintained and isolated to yield stable cell lines. These persistent revertants resisted transformation by a variety of oncogenes but could be retransformed by treatment with azacytidine. These results suggest an alternative mechanism of action of IFN causing alterations in the methylation state of DNA.

Recent advances in determining the nature of the molecular and biochemical events that occur when IFN with cells suggest these are as diverse as the biologic activities of IFN. An understanding of the mechanisms of regulation of IFN-responsive genes and further characterization of the products of these genes should not only elucidate the multiple mechanisms of IFN action but may also provide insight into the control of normal cell growth and differentiation.

REFERENCES

1. Williams, B. R. G., and Fish, E. N. In: *Interferons. Their Impact in Biology and Medicine* (J. Taylor-Papadimitriou, ed.) Oxford University Press, Oxford, p. 40 (1985).
2. Zoon, K. C., and Arnheiter, H. *Pharmacol. Ther.* 24:259 (1984).
3. Joshi, A. R., Sarkar, F. H., and Gupta, S. L. *J. Biol. Chem.* 257:13884 (1982).
4. Faltynek, C. R., Branca, A. A., McCandless, S., and Baglioni, C. *Proc. Natl. Acad. Sci. USA* 80:3269 (1983).
5. Sarkar, F. H., and Gupta, S. L. *Eur. J. Biochem.* 140:461 (1984).
6. Littman, S. J., Faltynek, C. R., and Baglioni, C. *J. Biol. Chem.* 260:1191 (1985).
7. Anderson, P., and Nagler, C. *Biochem. Biophys. Res. Commun.* 120:828 (1984).
8. Hannigan, G. E., Fish, E. N., and Williams, B. R. G. *J. Biol. Chem.* 259:8084 (1984).
9. Hannigan, G. E., Gewert, D. R., Fish, E. N., Read, S. E., and Williams, B. R. G. *Biochem. Biophys. Res. Commun.* 110:537 (1983).

10. Aguet, M., Grobke, M., and Dreiding, P. *Virology, 132*:211 (1984).

11. Hannigan, G. E., Gewert, D. R., and Williams, B. R. G. *J. Biol. Chem. 259*:9456 (1984).

12. Williams, B. R. G., Hannigan, G. E., Gelfand, E. W., and Freedman, M. H. In: *The Biology of the Interferon System* (H. Kirchner and H. Schellekens, eds.). Elsevier, Amsterdam (1984), p. 99.

13. Hannigan, G. E., Lau, A. S., and WIlliams, B. R. G. *Eur. J. Biochem. 157*: 187 (1986).

14. Hannigan, G. E., and Williams, B. R. G. *EMBO J. 5*:1607 (1986).

15. Branca, A. A., Faltynek, C. R., D'Allesandro, S. B., and Baglioni, C. *J. Biol. Chem. 257*:13291 (1982).

16. Anderson, P., Yip, Y. K., and Vilcek, J. *J. Biol. Chem. 258*:6497 (1983).

17. Aguet, M., and Blanchard, B. *Virology, 115*:249 (1981).

18. Friedman, R. L., McMahon, M., Kerr, I. M., and Stark, G. R. *Cell 38*:745 (1984).

19. Mills, G. B., Hannigan, G., Stewart, D., Mellors, A., Williams, B., and Gelfand, E. W. In: *The 2-5A System: Molecular and Clinical Aspects of the Interferon-Regulated Pathway* (B. R. G. Williams and R. H. Silverman, eds.). Alan R. Liss, New York, p. 357 (1985).

20. Macara, I. G. *Am. J. Physiol. (Cell Physiol. 17)*: C3-C11 (1985).

21. Williams, B. R. G., and Hannigan, G. E. In: *Interferons as Cell Growth Inhibitors and Antitumor Factors*, UCLA Symposia on Molecular and Cellular Biology, Vol. 50 (R. Friedman, T. Merigan, and T. Sreevalsan, eds.). Alan R. Liss, New York (1986), p. 279.

22. Einat, M., Resnitzky, D., and Kimichi, A. *Proc. Natl. Acad. Sci. USA 82*: 7608 (1985).

23. Staeheli, P., Horisberger, M. A., and Haller, O. *Virology 132*:456 (1984).

24. Weil, J., Epstein, C. J., Epstein, L. B., Sedmak, J. J., Sabran, J. L., and Grossberg, S. E. *Nature 301*:437 (1983).

25. Weil, J., Epstein, C. J., and Epstein, L. B. *Nat. Immun. Cell Growth Regulation 3*(1):51 (1984).

26. Chebath, J., Merlin, G., Metz, R., Benech, P., and Revel, M. *Nucleic Acids Res. 11*:1213 (1983).

27. Larner, A. C., Jonak, G., Cheng, Y.-S. E., Korant, B., and Knight, E., Jr. *Proc. Natl. Acad. Sci. USA 81*:6733 (1984).

28. Merlin, G., Chebath, J., Benech, P., Metz, R., and Revel, M. *Proc. Natl. Acad. Sci. USA 80*:4904 (1983).

29. Samanta, H., Dougherty, J. P., Brawner, M. E. B., Smidtlz, H., and Lengyel, P. In: *Chemistry and Biology of Interferons* (T. C. Merigan and R. M. Friedman, eds.). Academic Press, New York (1982).

30. Williams, B. R. G., Hannigan, G. E., and Saunders, M. E., et al. In: *The 2-2-5A System: Molecular and Clinical Aspects of the Interferon-Regulated Pathway* (B. R. G. Williams and R. H. Silverman, eds.). Alan R. Liss, New York, p. 227 (1985).

31. Friedman, R. L., and Stark, G. R. *Nature 314*:637 (1985).

32. Larner, A. C., Chaudhuri, A., and Darnell, J. E. *J. Biol. Chem. 261*:453 (1986).

33. Staehli, P., Dreiding, P., Haller, O., and Lindermann, J. *J. Biol. Chem. 260*:1821 (1985).

34. Williams, B. R. G. In: *Interferon and Cancer* (K. Sikora, ed.). Plenum Press, New York, p. 33 (1983).

35. Fitzpatrick, F. A., and Stringfellow, D. A. *J. Immunol. 125*:431 (1980).

36. Dinerello, C. A., Bernheim, H. A., Duff, G. W., Le, H. V., Nagabhushan, T. L., Hamilton, N. C., and Coceani, F. *J. Clin. Invest. 74*:906 (1984).

37. Singh, G., Renton, K. W., and Stebbing, N. *Biochem. Biophysics. Res. Commun. 106*:1256 (1982).

38. Hayashi, H., Tanaka, K., Jay, F., Khoury, G., and Jay, G. *Cell 43*:263 (1985).

39. Haller, O. *Curr. Topics Microbiol. Immunol. 92*:25 (1981).

40. Horisberger, M. A., and Hochkeppel, H. K. *J. Biol. Chem. 260*:1730 (1985).

41. Staehli, P., Haller, O., Boll, W., Lindenmann, J., and Weissman, C. *Cell 44*:147 (1986).

42. Krug, R. M., Shaw, M., Broni, B., Shapiro, G., and Haller, O. *J. Virol. 56*:201 (1985).

43. Rice, A. P., Roberts, W. K., and Kerr, I. M. *J. Virol. 50*:220 (1984).

44. Stark, G. R., Dower, W. J., Shimke, R. T., Brown, R. E., and Kerr, I. M. *Nature 278*:471 (1980).

45. Zullo, J. N., Cochran, B. H., Huang, A. S., and Styles, C. D. *Cell 43*:793 (1985).

46. Williams, B. R. G., Kerr, I. M., Gilbert, C. S., White, C. N., and Ball, L. A. *Eur. J. Biochem.* 92:455 (1978).

47. Watling, D., Serafinowska, H. T., Reese, C. B., and Kerr, I. M. *EMBO J.* 4:431 (1985).

48. Kimichi, A., Shure, H., and Revel, M. *Eur. J. Biochem.* 114:5 (1981).

49. Jacobsen, H., Czarniecki, C. W., Krause, D., Friedman, R. M., and Silverman, R. H. *Virology* 125:496 (1983).

50. Wreschner, D. H., Silverman, R. H., James, T. C., Gilbert, C. S., and Ker, I. M. *Eur. J. Biochem.* 124:261 (1982).

51. Floyd-Smith, G., Yoshie, O., and Lengyel, P. *J. Biol. Chem.* 257:8584 (1982).

52. Krause, D., Silverman, R. H., Jacobsen, H., Leisy, S. A., Dieffenbach, C. W., and Friedman, R. M. *Eur. J. Biochem.* 146:611 (1985).

53. Krause, D., Panet, A., Arad, G., Dieffenbach, C. W., and Silverman, R. H. *J. Biol. Chem.* 260:9501 (1985).

54. Cayley, P. J., Silverman, R. H., Balkwell, F. R., McMahon, M., Knight, M., and Kerr, I. M. In: *Interferons*, UCLA Symposia on Molecular and Cellular Biology (T. C. Merigan and R. M. Friedman, eds.). Academic Press, New York, p. 143 (1982).

55. Yang, K., Samanta, H., Dougherty, J., Jayaram, B., Broeze, R., and Lengyel, P. *J. Biol. Chem.* 256:9324 (1981).

56. Wells, J. A., Swyryd, E. A., and Stark, G. R. *J. Biol. Chem.* 259:1363 (1984).

57. St. Laurent, G., Yoshie, O., Floyd-Smith, G., Samantha, H., Sehgal, P., and Lengyel, P. *Cell* 33:95 (1983).

58. Benech, P., Merlin, G., and Revel, M. *Nucleic Acids Res.* 13:1267 (1985).

59. Saunders, M. E., Gewert, D. R., Tugwell, M. E., McMahon, M., and Williams, B. R. G. *EMBO J.* 4:1761 (1985).

60. Benech, P., Mory, Y., Revel, M., and Chebath, J. *EMBO J.* 4:2249 (1985).

61. Saunders, M., Gewert, D., Castellino, M., Rutherford, M., Flenniken, A., Willard, H., and Williams, B. R. G. In: *The 2-5A System: Molecular and Clinical Aspects of the Interferon-Regulated Pathway* (B. R. G. Williams and R. H. Silverman, eds.). Allan R. Liss, New York, p. 163 (1985).

62. Revel, M., Chebath, J., Benech, P., Wells, V., and Malluci, L. *J. Cell. Biochem. (Suppl.) 10C*:219 (1986).

63. Williams, B. R. G., Saunders, M. E., and Willard, H. F. *Somatic Cell Mol. Genet.* in press (1986).

64. Chebath, J., Benech, P., Mory, Y., Federman, P., Berlissi, H., Gesang, C., Forman, J., Danovitch, S., Lehrer, R., Aloni, N., and Revel, M. In: *The 2-5A System: Molecular and Clinical Aspects of the Interferon-Regulated Pathway* (B. R. G. Williams and R. H. Silverman, eds.). Alan R. Liss, New York, p. 149 (1985).

65. Goodbourn, S., Zinn, K., and Maniatis, T. *Cell 41*:509 (1985).

66. Stewart, W. E., II, Gosser, L. B., and Lockart, R. Z. *J. Virol.* 7:792 (1971).

67. Nir, U., Cohen, B., Chen, L., and Revel, M. *Nucleic Acids Res 12*:6979 (1984).

68. Enoch, T., Zinn, K., and Maniatis, T. *Mol. Cell. Biol.* 6:801 (1986).

69. Williams, B. R. G., and Read, S. E. In: *The Biology of the Interferon System* E. De Maeyer, G. Galasso, and H. Schellekens, eds.). Elsevier, Amsterdam, p. 111 (1981).

70. Williams, B. R. G., Read, S. E., Freedman, M. H., Carver, D. H., and Gelfand, E. W. In: *Chemistry and Biology of Interferons*, UCLA Symposia on Molecular and Cellular Biology, Vol. XXV (T. C. Merigan and R. M. Friedman, eds.). Academic Press, New York, p. 253 (1982).

71. Schattner, A., Merlin, G., Wallach, D., Rosenberg, Bino, T., Hahn, T., Levin, S., and Revel, M. *J. Interferon Res. 1*:587 (1981).

72. Merritt, J. A., Meltzer, D. M., Ball, L. A., and Borden, E. C. In: *The 2-5A System: Molecular and Clinical Aspects of the Interferon-Regulated Pathway* B. R. G. Williams and R. H. Silverman, eds.). Alan R. Liss, New York, p. 423 (1985).

73. Chebath, J., Benech, P., Mory, Y., Federman, P., Berissi, H., Gesang, C., Forman, J., Danavitch, S., Lehrer, R., Aloni, N., and Revel, M. In: *The 2-5A System: Molecular and Clinical Aspect of the Interferon Regulated Pathway* B. R. G. Williams and R. H. Silverman, eds.). Alan R. Liss, New York, p. 149 (1985).

74. Read, S. E., Williams, B. R. G., Coates, R. A., Evans, W. K., Fanning, M. M., Garvey, M. B., and Shepherd, F. A. *J. Infect. Dis. 152*:466 (1985).

75. Whitaker-Dowling, P. A., and Younger, J. S. *Virology 131*:128 (1983).
76. Whitaker-Dowling, P. A., and Younger, J. S. *Virology 137*:171 (1984).
77. Rice, A. P., and Kerr, I. M. *J. Virol. 50*:229 (1984).
78. Paez, E., and Esteban, M. *Virology 134*:12 (1984).
79. Siekierka, J., Mariano, T. M., Reichel, P. A., and Mathews, M. B. *Proc. Natl. Acad. Sci, USA 82*:1959-1963 (1985).
80. Reichel, P. A., Merrick, W. C., Siekierka, J., and Mathews, M. B. *Nature 313*:196 (1985).
81. Schneider, R. J., Safer, B., Munemitsu, S. M., Samuel, C. E., and Shenk, T. *Proc. Natl. Acad. Sci. USA 82*:4321 (1985).
82. O'Malley, R. P., Mariano, T. M., Siekierka, J., and Mathews, M. B. *Cell 44*:391 (1986).
83. Revel, M. In: *Interferon* 1979 (I. Gresser, ed.). Academic Press, London, p. 102 (1979).
84. Krust, B., Galabru, J., and Hovanessian, A. G. *J. Biol. Chem. 259*:8494 (1984).
85. Laurent, A. G., Krust, B., Svab, J., and Hovanessian, A. G. *Biochem. Biophys. Res. Commun. 125*:1 (1984).
86. Laurent, A. G., Krust, B., Svab, J., and Hovanessian, A. G. *Proc. Natl. Acad. Sci. USA 82*:4341 (1985).
87. Penn, L. J. Z., and Williams, B. R. G. *Proc. Natl. Acad. Sci. USA 82*:4959 (1985).
88. Penn, L. J. Z., Willard, H. F., and Williams, B. R. G. In: *Interferons as Cell Growth Inhibitors and Antitumor Factors*, UCLA Symposia on Molecular and Cellular Biology, Vol. 50 (R. Friedman, T. Merigan, and T. Sreevalsan, eds.). Alan R. Liss, New York (1986).
89. Land, H., Parada, L. F., and Weinberg, R. A. *Science 304*:596 (1983).
90. Jonak, G., and Knight, E., Jr. *Proc. Natl. Acad. Sci. USA 81*:1747 (1984)
91. Einat, M., Resnitzky, D., and Kimchi, A. *Nature 313*:597 (1985).
92. Knight, E., Jr., Anton, E. D., Fahey, D., Friedland, B. K., and Jonak, G. *Proc. Natl. Acad. Sci. USA 82*:1151 (1985).
93. Dani, C., Mechti, N., Piechaczyk, M., Lebleu, B., Jeanteur, P., and Blanchard, J. M. *Proc.Natl. Acad. Sci. USA 82*:4896 (1985).

94. Jonak, G., Friedland, B. K., Anton, E. D., and Knight, E., Jr. *J. Cell. Biochem. (Suppl.) 10C*:237 (1986).
95. Samid, D., Chang, E. H., and Friedman, R. M. *Biochem. Biophys. Res. Commun. 119*:21 (1984).
96. Samid, D., Chang, E. H., and Friedman, R. M. *Biochem. Biophys. Res. Commun. 126*:509 (1985).

3
The Immunologic Basis for the Use of Interferons

JEAN E. MERRILL and STEPHAN R. TARGAN

University of California–Los Angeles School of Medicine, Los Angeles, California

I. CLASSES OF INTERFERONS AND LEUKOCYTES THAT PRODUCE THEM

Interferon (IFN) was discovered in 1957 by Isaacs and Lindenmann, with the earliest report demonstrating interferon produced in chick chorioallantoic membrane. One of the first inducers of IFN identified was heat-inactivated influenza virus. Around the same time, Trinchieri et al. described viral inhibitors in supernatants of lymphocytes cocultured with tumor- or virus-transformed cells (1). We now know that most cell types [fibroblasts, epithelial cells, macrophages (Mϕ), and other differentiated cells], in addition to lymphocytes, can make IFN. IFN-a is produced by leukocytes, IFN-β by fibroblasts. These two IFN are induced by a variety of agents, including double-stranded RNAs, intracellular microorganisms, lipopolysaccharides (LPS), low-molecular-weight substances, and organic polymers. Viruses induce IFN-a by B, non-B/non-T, and Mϕ and IFN-β in fibroblasts and epithelial cells (2,3). In the presence of tumor cells, Mϕ and natural killer (NK) cells make IFN-a (2,4). Lymphoblastoid cell lines produce a mixture of a and β with a predominating. These IFN are stable at pH 2 and are coded for on chromosome 9. The genes for 14 distinct subtypes of IFN-α have been cloned, and these bear 85% homology with each other but only 15% homology with IFN-β. IFN-β also distinguishes itself from IFN-α by being a glycoprotein.

The different IFN-α species (labeled IFN-α A–M) can be distinguished in part by their molecular weight (MW), immunoregulatory properties, and antiviral properties. The molecular weight spectrum of these species is from 16.6 to 23.5 kilodaltons (5), the two lower species, 16.6 and 16.9 kD, being less efficient than the higher MW species at stimulating NK cells (5). Ortaldo et al. have found IFN-α J will not boost NK activity even at 10,000 U/ml after 2 hr (6). This species has normal antiviral and antiproliferative activity. It may act by competitively inhibiting other IFN-α species from binding shared receptors, thus reducing their efficacy. In terms of antiviral activity, all species are augmented by a slight temperature increase (to 38 ro 39°C) (7); IFN-α A is preferentially induced over IFN-α B by Sendai virus (8). IFN-α A and D have similar effects on NK cells but IFN-α D may have less antiviral activity than IFN-α A (9).

IFN-γ is a glycoprotein produced by T cells in a Mφ-dependent manner after stimulation with mitogens, specific antigens, antibodies to the T3 antigen, or phorbol myristate acetate (PMA). In distinct contrast to IFN-α or IFN-β, IFN-γ is pH 2 labile, coded for by a separate single gene, and antigenically distinct from α or β. It potentiates α or β in a synergistic manner but is more potent than α or β in its antitumor, anticellular, antiviral, and immunomodulatory actions (2). It has been determined by limiting dilution analysis that after phytohemmaglutinin (PHA) stimulation only 1 in 1000 T cells respond by making IFN-γ (3). By cytofluorographic analysis using a panel of monoclonal antibodies, the phenotype of the IFN-producing cell induced by PHA is Fc γ R+, Fc μ R−, OKM1+, OKT4−, OKT8−, OK11a+ (E rosette marker), suggesting an immature T cell or NK cell (10) Interleukin-2 (IL2) with or without Concanavalin A (ConA) enhancement stimulated OKT4+ and OKT8+ cells to produce IFN-γ (11). Thus IFN-γ does not seem to be produced by a distinct T-cell subset.

II. GENERAL BIOLOGIC EFFECTS OF IFN

IFN induced by viral infections, such as pox, herpes, myxo, or paramyxo-viruses, can be detected within hours in serum and target organs although its local concentration is more important than elevated, transient circulating levels. Typically, IFN-a is produced by Mϕ and NK cells within the first day of infection followed by IFN-γ production by activated T cells 1-2 days later (12). It binds to membrane-bound receptors (either shared or separate for the different IFN classes), and these receptors are internalized and degraded. These events trigger the synthesis of cellular mRNA and antiviral proteins through which a variety of mechanisms limit the spread of virus and reduce disease severity. The interferons' immunoregulatory effects occur through mechanisms altering plasma membrane and cytoskeletal elements, growth and proliferation, and differentiation (2). Anticellular effects are separable from antiviral effects (13-15). Cell growth and proliferation are probably controlled by the effects of IFN on both the plasma membrane and the cell cycle. For example, IFN-β is associated with decreased cellular locomotion, cell enlargement, and an increased rigidity of the plasma membrane (2,16). Abortive proliferation could then result from the reorganization of actin-containing microfilaments into a dense, submembraneous meshwork (2). IFN-a and IFN-γ interfere with the passage of cells into S phase, lengthening the duration of the G_1 and $S + G_2$ phases. However, IFN-γ blocks cells at the G_0/G_1 transition 20 times more efficiently than IFN-a. Growth inhibition is independent of induction of DNA, RNA, or protein and is reversible by washing IFN away from the cells. This is in contrast to the antiviral effect and the antivirally associated growth inhibition of IFN, which is not reversible by washing the cells exposed to IFN. Antivirally associated growth inhibition may be blocked by actinomycin D and ouabain (15).

Induction of cytoplasmic enzymes characteristic of activated, differentiated cells such as 2',5'-oligoadenylate synthetase (2,17, 18) or membrane receptors or antigens required for differentiated functions are examples of the effect of IFN on cellular differentiation.

III. INDUCTION AND SUPPRESSION OF IFN BY IMMUNOREGULATORY MECHANISMS

The participation and regulation of the different IFN in the immune response are schematically depicted in Figure 1. Although there is not much information on the immunologic mechanisms of IFN-α induction, it appears not to require the accessory Mϕ. In recent studies, fibroblast IFN-β has been shown to be induced by a factor like interleukin-1 (19). Whether this is an absolute requirement for IFN-β production is not known. The macrophage seems to be required for maximal production of IFN-γ (20). Mϕ-derived interleukin-1 stimulates IL-2, which in turn induces de novo IFN-γ or augments that already being produced. Farrar and Humes have shown lipoxygenase dependency of IL-2 regulation of IFN-γ secretion. By using the specific lipoxygenase inhibitor nor-dihydroguaiaretic acid (NDGA), it was shown that leukotriene B4 (LTB4) could replace IL-2 in the induction of IFN (21). Inducers of IL-1 and LTB4 production by Mϕ, such as calcium ionophore A-23187 (22,23) and galactose oxidase or sodium peroxidate (23, 24), augmented Mϕ-dependent IFN-γ production.

Interferon-γ can be induced in T cells by antigens or mitogens. Presentation of antigen in the context of the Mϕ HLA–DR antigen provides signal 1, and IL-1 induction of IL-2 provides signal 2. Monoclonal antibody to HLA–DR suppresses IFN-γ production in response to such stimuli as *Mycoplasma arthritidis* or virus but not to PHA-induced IFN production(25). IL-2 induction of proliferation and induction-augmentation of IFN-γ seem to be independent events. Inhibition of blastogenesis (26) or the use of 50 times less than the minimum concentration required of IL-2 to stimulate proliferation (27) still resulted in IFN-γ production. The capacity of IL-2 to actually induce the de novo synthesis of IFN-γ in immature T cells is illustrated by its effect on unstimulated T cells in vitro (11), in vivo in young adult nude mice (28), and on NK cell clones (29). In more mature T cells the requirements for IL-2 in IFN-γ augmentation have been demonstrated by its ability to replace the requirement for Mϕ-derived IL-1 (30,31) and inhibition of IFN-γ production by antibody to the IL-2 receptor (27). IL-2 alone produces no or low levels of IFN-γ (22,23) and thus must act in concert with antigen or mitogen (27,32,33). At

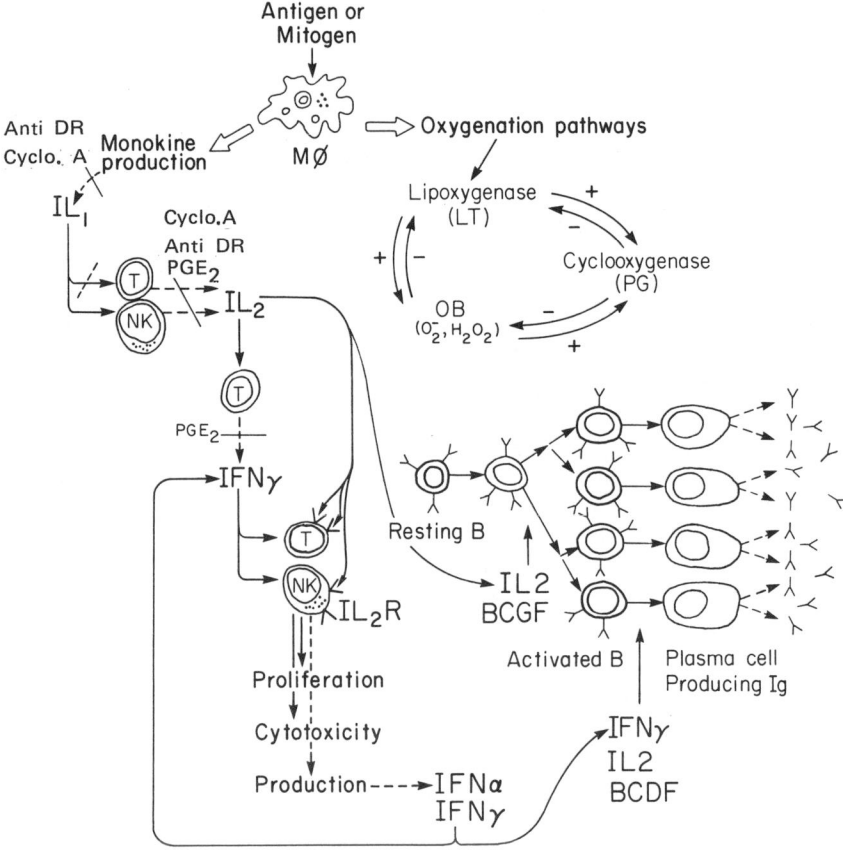

Figure 1 Participants and regulation of the different IFN in the immune response.

optimal concentrations of IL-2 (100 U/ml) in the presence of PHA, a 3- to 40-fold increase in IFN-γ will occur in 48–72 hr. One mechanism of IL-2 augmentation of IFN-γ has been suggested to be its ability to abrogate suppressor cell (Ts) inhibition of IFN production. Sequestration of IL-2 by Ts (34) could be overcome by the addition of more exogenous IL-2 (35).

Other stimuli that induce IFN-γ production by T cells are monoclonal antibodies recognizing T-cell surface protein complexes. Several investigators have shown induction of IFN-γ by xOKT3, an antibody recognizing the T-cell receptor complex. There is still some controversy as to whether the concentration of antibody need be mitogenic (36,37). Antibodies directed at OKT4 or OKT8 antigens had marginal or no effect on IFN-γ production (36). Bhayani and Falcof have shown that pan-T monoclonal antibodies recognizing another T-cell protein complex stimulated both IL-2 and IFN-γ and were mitogenic (38). Requirement of both Mϕ accessory cells (37,38) and an intact Fc portion of the monoclonal antibody suggests that these antibodies work by binding to the FcR on Mϕ. The Mϕ then presents a palisade of repeating specific antigen binding sites to the T cell. These bind and cross-link T-cell antigens, activating the T cell to IFN-γ production (37, 38).

IFN-γ production is regulated by feedback suppression by T cells at days 6–8 of culture (34). Prostaglandin $E_{1,2}$ ($PGE_{1,2}$) probably also controls IFN-γ production by interfering with IL-2 production (see Fig. 1) (39–42) or indirectly through induction of Ts cells. In contrast, although IFN-α and IFN-β are not suppressed by PGE (43), they are negatively regulated by retinoic acid (vitamin A acid) (44).

IV. IFN EFFECTS ON CELL GROWTH AND PROLIFERATION

The presence of IFN in normal bone marrow and its abnormal production in aplasmic anemia suggests IFN has a normal regulatory role in hematopoiesis and implicates it in the pathophysiology of bone marrow failure (45–47). Zoumbas et al. found a positive correlation between the concentration of IFN used and suppression of myeloid colony-forming units (CFU-C) and erythroid burst-forming units (BFU-E). Both IFN-α and IFN-γ were inhibitory, although IFN-α was less inhibitory (45). Raefsky and colleagues showed that as little as 5 U/ml of recombinant IFN-γ could synergize with IFN-α to inhibit CFU-C three times more than IFN-α alone (46). In contrast, rIFN-α did not synergize with rIFN-γ. Auxiliary cells may be required for synergy to occur. The mediation of inhibition by IFN-γ requires the DR antigen and activated Mϕ or NK cells (46). Others have shown that IFN-γ can synergize with IFN-β to suppress proliferation of granulocyte and erythroid progenitors, but IFN-α did not synergize with IFN-β (47).

At concentrations from 10 to 1000 U/ml, IFN-α or IFN-β in vitro suppressed proliferation induced by PHA stimulation or mixed lymphocyte reaction (MLR). In contrast, IFN-γ suppressed MLR only at 1 U/ml and suppressed PHA-induced proliferation at 1000 U/ml (48). Einhorn et al. claim that although the inhibitory effect of IFN-α can be seen in vitro, it is only inhibitory in vivo during the first 24 hr of treatment, suggesting that there is no long-term effect in vivo (49).

B-lymphocyte transformation, cell outgrowth, and the ability to produce immunoglobulin (Ig) in response to Epstein-Barr virus (EBV) is limited to different degrees by IFN. Recombinant IFN-α, IFN-β, IFN-γ when added before EBV infection act directly on B cells to limit virus replication. IFN-γ exerted a 7–10 times more potent antiviral effect than IFN-α or IFN-β (50). When added early after EBV infection, all three IFN reduced B-cell outgrowth and Ig secretion (50,51). Although IFN-α and IFN-β were effective only within the first 24 hr, the inhibitory effect of IFN-γ lasted 3–4 days postinfection (50). B-lymphoblastoid lines already transformed by EBV were insensitive to the antiproliferative effects of all three types of IFN. In addition, rIFN-γ inhibits B-cell proliferation induced by soluble anti-Ig (xIgM and xIgD) activation but not by Sepharose-bound anti-Ig (52). The different mechanisms of actions of IFN depend on the stimulus and stage of differentiation of the B cell. Cerebrospinal fluid (CSF) induced Mφ proliferation initiates an antiproliferative production of IFN-α or IFN-β (53). Down-regulation of clonal expansion of Mφ during functional activation is controlled by IFN-γ, which reduces the number of surface transferrin receptors (54).

V. EFFECTS OF IFN ON DIFFERENTIATION

A. Alterations in Membrane and Cytoplasmic Markers of Differentiation

Changes in T-cell subsets in vivo after treatment with IFN-α seem to be related to the dose. At low doses, cytotoxic suppressor

OKT8+ cells rise proportionately with no change in helper-inducer OKT4+ cells. At high doses, the OKT8+ cells are depressed, resulting in an increase in the OKT4/OKT8 ratio (55-57). The OKT4 cells are less sensitive to the inhibitory effects of IFN than are OKT8+ cells (58). This effect may relate to the inhibition of expansion of OKT8+ cells. Clonal expansion is required prior to differentiation of CD8+ cells to functional suppressor cells. In vitro, and perhaps at very high local concentrations in vivo, OKT4+ cells involved in MLR are decreased in the presence of IFN-a. There is a decreased expression of the surface antigen, as determined by fluorescence intensity, as well as a decrease in the actual percentage of OKT4+ cells (59). The effects of IFN-a, in vivo and in vitro, are to induce an increase in the numbers of immature T cells bearing the surface marker OKT10. IFN-a also increases the density of this antigen per cell (59-61).

Although IFN prevents the proliferation of cells, it induces differentiation. For cells of myelomonocytic lineage, this includes the increased expression of Fc receptors for IgG (FcγR) and DR antigens. Increases in these markers lead to more differentiated functions by these cells, as will be discussed.

IFN-γ induces FcγR for IgG$_{2a}$ and IgG$_3$ (but not IgG$_1$ and IgG$_{2b}$) on the monocytelike cell line U937 (62-64). As the result of 10 U/ml of rIFN-γ for 18 hr, U937 acquires a sevenfold increase in FcγR (63) as well as enhanced ADCC (62,63). Recombinant IFN-a $_D$ and IFN-γ $_A$ augment FcγR on blood monocytes (65). The effect of IFN-γ on the promyelocytic line HL60 is to inhibit growth and increase the expression of monocyte-related surface antigens, including FcR (66-68). Immature myeloid cells of the bone marrow and leukemia cells of peripheral blood of patients with chronic myelogenous leukemia can be induced with IFN to differentiate to macrophages (66). Even myeloid cells as immature as metamyelocytes or band cells will be driven to monocyte differentiation (66). These changes are not induced by IFN-a or IFN-β (66,67,69).

Certain cytoplasmic enzymes and oxygen intermediates that correlate with cellular differentiation are altered by IFN. IFN-γ induces N-acetylglucouronidase and alkaline phosphatase in U937 cells (64) and an increase in lysosomal enzymes (68) and naphthyl acetate esterase (66,69) in myeloid cells. IFN-γ induces the release of hydrogen peroxide in U937 and HL60 (64,68). IFN-β and IFN-γ increase cell volume (67,69). In contrast, IFN-α at 50-300 U/ml inhibits cell volume, phagocytosis, acid phosphatase, and leucine aminopeptidase in developing macrophages (70). The enzyme 2',5'-oligoadenylate synthetase, which correlates with cytotoxicity in T cells and PMN, is increased in the presence of IFN (17,18).

IFN-γ is critical in the induction of class II (DR) antigens on a wide variety of lymphoid and nonlymphoid cells. Induction of DR on nonlymphoid tissue-bound cells occurs in many organs, including the kidney, brain, liver, and skin (71). This is usually associated with inflammation in situ and the presumed need to facilitate presentation of antigen at that local site. The induction of DR on thymic epithelium (72) illustrates the importance of IFN-γ in T-cell education for self-recognition. IFN-γ induces or increases DR on fetal monocytes, myeloid cell lines (73,74), neonatal cord blood monocytes (75), B lymphomas and lymphoblastoid cell lines (74,86), and peripheral blood monocytes (74,77, 78). IFN-γ increases the number of cells with DR, the density per cell, and the shedding of this antigen by monocytes and B cells. Shed DR may exhibit antigen-presenting functions in conjunction with exogenous antigens (76). Natural and rIFN-α also induce DR antigens on monocytes in vivo (79) and in vitro (75,78). In contrast, IFN-β shows an antagonistic effect to IFN-γ induction of class II antigens on murine macrophages. Although by itself rIFN-α induces class II antigens, it inhibits IFN-γ induction of these markers (80). IFN-γ also results in an increase in HLA and β_2-microglobulin on leukocytes (2).

B. Regulation of Secreted Immunoregulatory Molecules

Upon activation, leukocytes secrete soluble immunoregulatory products that in turn actively induce or suppress subsequent steps of the immune response (Fig. 1). Interferons can enhance, suppress, or mimic these immunoregulatory molecules. IFN-γ has the capacity to mimic certain lymphokines such as macrophage inhibitory factor (MIF) (81), macrophage activating factor (MAF), class II antigen induction factor, and B-cell helper factor (82). As such, it has been difficult to distinguish IFN from these proteins even at the biochemical level. These monokines may alternatively be one species or produced under the control of one gene. Human peripheral blood leukocytes, activated by PHA in culture, produce lymphotoxin (LT), which both induces IFN and is induced by it (83,84). In synergy with RIL2 or mitogens, tumor necrosis factor (TNF-α or β) is induced by IFN (85) and it in turn synergizes with IFN-γ or IFN-α in its cytotoxic effect on target cells (86). After stimulation with IFN-γ, Mφ release neopterin. This factor is a precursor of biopterin, derived from GTP, and is an essential cofactor of neurotransmitter synthesis (87). Both IFN-γ and IFN-α induce suppressor factors in humans (88).

The effects of IFN in vivo and in vitro on antibody production are both time and dose dependent relative to administration of antigen (89). The effects of IFN-α in vivo, if administered to animals before antigen, are to decrease the primary T-independent and secondary T-dependent antibody responses (2). IFN-γ given under similar condition is 20–250 times as suppressive. The suppression is due to the antiproliferative effects on B cells and the activation of T-suppressor cells, which interfere with Mφ processing of antigen (2,69). If IFN-α or IFN-β is added 24–48 hr after antigen stimulation in vivo, antibody production goes up owing to the inhibitory effect of IFN on Ts cells (2).

In vitro, IFN-α added in high doses (2) or before antigen (90) results in inhibition of induction of antibody synthesis. Nevertheless, at low doses IFN-α increases Ig production: in the presence or absence of pokeweed mitogen (PWM) or EBV, B cells can be induced to secrete both IgG and IgM (90–93). Purified B cells can respond to IFN-α in the absence of PWM by secreting IgM (91). Maximal responses, however, require PWM and T cells and result in both IgM and IgG (91,92). B cells must be preincubated or cultured from time 0 with IFN-α for it to be effective (91,93). As with IFN-α or IFN-β, if IFN-γ is added to B cells that have already undergone clonal expansion, it acts as a B-cell differentiation factor inducing a 10-fold increase in IgG- and IgM-secreting plasma cells (94,95).

At very low concentrations of IFN (α, β, or γ), adherent leukocytes showed an enhanced potential of IL-1 synthesis. This secretion was only revealed by a second signal provided by poly I:C, K562 tumor cells or endotoxin (96-98). IFN-γ has a greater effect on IL-1 secretion than IFN-α or IFN-β. It has the capacity, if added at day 4 in vitro, to reverse the loss of IL-1 production that normally occurs by day 12 in culture (98).

C. Modulation of Cytotoxic Functions of Leukocytes

Interferon enhances cytotoxicity by a wide variety of effector cells (T cells, Mϕ, PMN, NK, and K cells), including activated killer (AK) cells (99), toward a broad spectrum of target cells (2). Activation of such cytolytic effectors can be by a variety of means, including MLR (100), exposure to yeast, parasites, or tumor- or virus-transformed cell lines, or conjugation to targets by a specific antibody or nonspecific lectin. Both IFN-α (101, 102) and IFN-γ (103, 104) activate monocytes to tumoricidal activity. Mϕ can kill adherent and nonadherent tumor targets while leaving nonmalignant cells unharmed (102,103). Activiation in vitro takes 24 hr and 1000 U/ml IFN-α (101,102). As in most systems, IFN-γ is more efficient than IFN-α or IFN-β in the activation of Mϕ to antimicrobial killing (105,106). This may be related to the proportion of Mϕ-bearing receptors for IFN-γ and/or the density of IFN-γR per cell (107,108), the ability of IFN-γ to affect both recruitment and recycling of Mϕ effectors (109), and its ability to decrease the sensitivity of activated Mϕ to the negative regulatory effects of PGE$_2$ (110).

All three IFN affect natural and antibody-mediated cytotoxicity of granulocytes (PMN) and promyelocytic cell lines (111-114). Clearly, IFN increases FcγR and thus augments ADCC (67-69, 113). The IFN effect was maximal if antibody concentration was suboptimal (113,114). The increase in oxidative burst products induced in Mϕ and PWM by IFN (64,68,69) is the likely explanation for the increase in natural as well as antibody-mediated lysis.

Interferons have a defined effect on the lytic capacity of natural killer cells (115-117). In general, most interferons enhance the ability of these cells to lyse and to kill sensitive target cells. All three classes of interferon (α, β, and γ) have been used to study the effects in vitro (118,119). Several recent studies have examined the relative effectiveness of these classes of interferons in enhancing cytotoxic activity (118,120,121). Interferon-α and IFN-β are less efficient than IFN-γ in activating NK lysis (118, 120). This activation is produced through direct action with interferon on the natural killer cell. Enriched, purified populations of NK cells are able to respond directly to interferon induction (122). The use of recombinant DNA-produced interferons to activate NK lysis confirms that the interferon molecules within the "purified" preparations are responsible for enhanced NK lysis (6,118,120). It appears that the mechanism of activation of these interferons is interactive. That is, simultaneous addition of IFN-α and IFN-β in vitro results in additive activation of NK cells (118, 120). On the other hand, if one takes either IFN-α or IFN-β and mixes it with IFN-γ, rather than an additive effect, there is a synergistic enhancement of NK lytic activity (118). The potential mechanisms of these interactions is considered following the discussion of the actual NK lytic mechanism enhancement by a single type of interferon (123,124).

An understanding of the mechanism of NK cytotoxicity is required in order to comprehend the mechanism by which interferon can enhance NK lysis. The killing of one cell by another occurs in a very orderly sequence of events. Initially the NK cell must recognize the target cell and be capable of binding to its membrane (125). Once the target cell binds, a series of complicated interactions results in the triggering of the NK cell (126). A series of events follows within the NK cell, termed programing for lysis, and probably culminates with the transfer of a proteinaceous lytic material from the NK cell onto the target cell (127,128). Following this transfer is the final stage of the lytic process, which is termed killer cell-independent lysis. It is during this stage that a series of events occurs within the target cell that are independent of the killer cell. These events lead to the disintegration and death of the target (125). Each individual effector cell is then capable of detaching from the target cell and seeking out and finding a second target cell and repeating the lytic cycle as described (129–131). There is a refractory period before the effector cell is capable of going on to kill a second, third, or fourth target. This latter event is termed the rate of recycling of the lytic process (129,130).

One could propose that the enhancement of NK lysis by interferon may occur at one of several of these stages in the lytic cycles. IFN could induce a greater number of cells capable of performing lysis, that is, produce new killer cells. It may enhance the rate of the lytic sequence of events and therefore allow cells to recycle such that the same number of cells would now kill more targets in a given period of time. The mechanism of interferon enhancement of NK lysis has been demonstrated at the cellular and molecular levels. The enhancement of the lytic process at the cellular level has been determined using whole peripheral blood as well as enriched NK populations. It was established, using a single-cell cytotoxic assay and chromium-release assay, that two events resulted in cytotoxic activation (123,124). Among those cells capable of recognizing targets, there was an increase in the lytically active cells: with no increase in the cells capable of binding the target cells, there was an increase in the number of those binding that were now lytically active. There was a recruitment of new effector cells capable of binding targets (132). In addition, there was an acceleration of the lytic process such that all the measurable lytic events occurred much more rapidly (123).

In further studies using a calcium pulse technique, it was established that, after interferon activation, the kinetics of the programming phase of the lytic process was enhanced but the killer cell-independent phase was not. This suggested that the NK cell was activating and processing the release of factors and transferring them to the target cell more rapidly (125). It was demonstrated that pretreatment of natural killer cells with interferon enabled more cytotoxic factors to be released (133,134). These factors released from natural killer cells are capable of killing NK targets in the absence of effector cells (135). Thus, interferon enhanced the programming process and made available more lytic moieties for potential transfer onto the target cells. It was also shown that there was an enhanced ability to recycle and to kill again in a given period of time (129,130).

The molecules within the NK cell that are induced by interferon, affecting this enhancement of the programming process, have not specifically been determined. However, it has been shown that protein synthesis is required for this enhancement to occur (136). There is induction of NK-associated phospholipase A_2 activity (137). This molecule has recently been suggested as playing a role in triggering NK lysis (138) and correlates with the enhanced rate of programming for lysis associated with interferon activation (125).

In addition to enhancement of the NK lytic process, treatment of the target cells alone with all classes of IFN can decrease the ability of those cells to be killed by NK cells (1,139–141). IFN-γ, however, is much more efficient in this cytoprotection (141). It is capable of protecting certain target cells at concentrations less than those required to protect cells from viral infection (141). The mechanism of this inhibition at the cellular level appear to be inhibition of the postbinding events. NK cells bind interferon-treated or untreated targets equally well (141,142). It appears as if treated targets do not induce the subsequent lytic programming in the NK cell (142). This has been further documented by demonstrating that interferon-pretreated target cells do not induce the release of natural killer cytotoxic factors from effector cells (143). The mechanism of this protection may well be related to certain proteins that are induced by interferon in the target cells. Nevertheless, the actual mechanism and proteins involved in this protection remain to be elucidated.

Among the large granular lymphocytes there are cells that can mediate ADCC. Since ADCC is probably mediated by the same effector cell as NK lysis (144), interferon should enhance ADCC as well as NK cytotoxicity. However, the results are not as clear as those with NK-mediated lysis. Whether one is able to see augmentation with interferon in the system is very much dependent upon the concentration of the antibody used during the in vitro assay (113,145). Only with a suboptimal concentration of antibody that produces a lower level of antibody-dependent cytotoxicity is enhancement of this lytic activity demonstrable (113,145). Since the mechanism of ADCC-mediated cytotoxicity is not as clearly defined as NK-mediated cytotoxicity, it is difficult to determine the mechanism for the enhancement.

In summary, the family of biologic response modifiers, the interferons, have several potential roles in the modification of NK or K cell-mediated cytotoxicity. Interferon-γ appears to be the most potent of the classes of interferon in their ability to enhance cytotoxicity. Combinations of these modulators as well as other potential modulators, such as interleukins, may indeed potentiate these effects.

VI. PRODUCTION AND RESPONSE TO IFN IN PATIENTS WITH MULTIPLE SCLEROSIS

Because of the debate over the nature of the exogenous infectious agent(s) triggering the disease onset and/or perpetuating the pathologic condition, much attention has been paid to IFN production and response in multiple sclerosis (MS) patients. Special attention has been paid to natural killer cells since their presence would benefit the host by eliminating virus-infected cells whereas their absence would lead to viral persistence. Virally modified tissue could then be the target of both specific and nonspecific cellular and humoral autoreactivity (146,147). NK cells could be reduced by two distinct mechanisms. Exogenous antigen may stimulate antibody production, and the resulting immune complexes may bind to and inhibit NK cells (148-150). Alternatively, immune complexes could inhibit NK through the induction of PGE (145, 151-153). In addition, PGE could feedback-suppress IL-2 and IFN-γ (39-42,153). Thus in MS, for which viral etiology has been suggested although no virus specific to MS has been isolated, NK cells and IFN produced by NK and other cells (154,155) are of relevance and perhaps importance in the primary etiology and secondary immune imbalances in these patients.

In vitro production of the IFN-a response to a variety of viral stimuli has been shown by some investigators (156-158) to be normal in MS patients. Other investigators have shown depressed IFN-a in vitro in response to tumor target cells, poly I:C, and such viruses as measles, Newcastle disease, mumps, rubella, herpes simplex, and influenza (159-168). IFN-a production has been shown to be depressed in both peripheral blood and cerebrospinal fluid cells (161). Vervliet et al. have published a series of articles investigating IFN-γ production in vitro (157,169–174) in which they identified a segment of the MS patient population who were nonresponders to induction by ConA or PHA. Only 40-50% of all MS patients produced IFN-γ compared with 85–90% of normal controls (157,169). Those MS patients who did respond made normal levels of IFN-γ (157); those that did not respond could not be induced to do so even with increasing doses of ConA (170). A low IFN-γ response and lack of induction by higher mitogen concentrations were also seen in cerebrovascular accident and meningoencephalitis patients (170).

The controversy over HLA-related defects in NK cell activity and IFN production in MS patients continues. Abb and colleagues have documented that low responsiveness by peripheral blood lymphocytes of any individual to inducers of IFN-α (flu virus, Molt 4 cells) is associated with DR_2, though they found no association of IFN-γ production and DR_2 (172). Vervliet and colleagues showed that the lower IFN-γ response rate was more pronounced in DR_{2+} carriers, as were lower spontaneous and IFN-stimulated NK activities (157). It has been shown that MS patients show a higher than normal frequency of DR_2 antigen (159,165, 173,174), and thus studies have been conducted to link DR_2 antigen as the sole source for defective NK and IFN production in MS patients. An association of DR_2 and low NK and IFN production in the general populace would make trivial the findings in MS. Such an association has not been upheld, however; nor has a firm association between DR and defective NK and IFN circuits been established. Initial work correlating low NK cell activity and DR_2 in MS patients (159,173) apparently is not statistically significant (165,174). The finding that low NK cell activity occurs in DR_2 MS patients but not in normal DR_2 controls (173) or in normal DR_{2+} monozygotic MS twins with normal NK activity (167,175, 176) makes this HLA association an unlikely explanation for defects in MS patients. That low IFN production is the cause of low NK cell activity in MS (160,162, 168,174) also seems unlikely since IFN-α is not always low (167, 175,176). When it is low it does not correlate with NK cell activity

(162,165). It would appear that NK and IFN activities are independent phenomena.

In the realm of autoimmune disorders of unknown but probably infectious etiologies, MS has been the topic of many papers and reviews on NK cell activity because of the disease association with a possible virus, such as measles. Two reports found no defect in ADCC, NK, or IFN-inducible NK (157,158). However, there seem to be overwhelming data that MS patients are defective in NK cell activity to a variety of tumor and virus-infected targets (159,162-165,167,173-175,177-184). In one study, the defect was target cell related, with lower NK cell killing to virus-infected targets (173). There also seems to be general agreement that activity is lowest during active disease (159,162-164,177-179). NK activity is lower in an acute relapse than in chronic progressive or remission stages (163,164,178,179). Nor can NK cell activity be detected in the cerebrospinal fluid of MS patients by a sensitive single-cell assay (163,164,177-179), but it is detectable in the CSF of patients with acute infections of the central nervous system (177,178).

Decreased NK cell activity in MS has been demonstrated using the 51Cr release assay (159,163,164,173,177-180), but the underlying defect responsible for this result may reside in the defect at the level of target cell binding or killing or effector recycling. At the single-cell level, acute relapse patients have fewer peripheral blood NK cells during an exacerbation; the defect is at both the level of binding to and lysis of the target (177). There is an apparent defect in recycling as well (177,178). By a similar assay, there are no binders or killers in CSF, that is, no detectable functional NK cells (177,178). Both the defect in IFN production and NK activity in MS may be due to elevated PGE in vivo (163,164,171, 179).

Even though 0.5 IU/ml of IFN could have been detected in CSF or serum of MS patients, none was ever seen in two separate studies (173,183); in yet another article it was elevated compared with controls (184). Jacobs et al. treated MS patients with intrathecal injections of purified IFN-β and documented that the rate of relapse of IFN recipients was less than before treatment and less than control (185,186). Huddlestone et al. showed similar results with IFN-a treatment of MS patients (187). Rice et al. reported that 9 of 12 MS patients receiving 9×10^6 IU IFN-a showed an increase in NK activity in vitro within the first 48 hr. By the first week this had dropped back to baseline. Despite continuous IFN over the next 6 months there were no further changes in NK (188). Kamin-Lewis examined in vitro IFN responsiveness of IFN-a-treated MS patients to Newcastle disease virus (NDV) or measles virus and poly I:C, as well as proliferation in response to ConA. IFN-treated patients exhibited normal proliferative responses but a decreased IFN production to all in vitro inducers (189).

VII. CONCLUSIONS

There is in response to exogenous viral infections an immediate production of IFN-a by Mϕ, NK cells, and B cells and IFN-β by fibroblasts. The response is swift because there is no need for an accessory cell in the production of IFN-a or IFN-β. However, antiviral and anticellular effects are short-lived. IFN-γ production takes longer to reach a maximum, but its effects are 20-200 times stronger than those of IFN-a or IFN-β and last much longer IFN-β, if anything, prolongs the waning effects of IFN-a and IFN-β by synergizing with low concentrations. The concentration and kinetic complexities of IFN-γ production by T cells is dependent on the Mϕ accessory cell, for both induction (through the IL-1-IL-2 circuit) and inhibition (through PGE and Ts induction). This is not true of IFN-a or IFN-β, which are not suppressed by prostaglandins. IFN-γ inhibits precursor cells from clonal expansion and thus causes a buildup of immature cells, such as OKT10+ cells in the blood and granulocyte and erythroid progenitors in bone marrow. In contrast, IFN-γ promotes differentiation of resting cells of intermediate maturity or of committed but immature cells. It does so by decreasing proliferation: while cells are slowed down in G_0 there is increased induction of membrane and cytoplasmic changes. Induction of membrane DR antigens enhances antibody production and cytotoxicity because of effective antigen presentation. Induction of IL-1 and IL-2 secretion leads to expansion and maturation of B and T cells. IFN-γ, in addition to inducing growth factors of differentiated cells (such as LT, TNF, IL-1, MIF, and IL-2), synergizes with these factors to enhance their effects. IFN-γ may mimic such factors as MAF and BCDF to promote differentiation of Mφ and B cells, respectively. IFN-γ prevents the senescence of Mφ in vivo and in vitro. IFN-γ ultimately enhances Ts cell differentiation and thus suppresses itself by a feedback inhibition. IFN-α and IFN-β do not induce differentiation; in fact, they inhibit cytoplasmic enzymes and surface antigens and receptors required for differentiated interactions.

Care must be taken in extrapolating the in vivo effects of IFN from in vitro data. To date relatively few assays are able to demonstrate changes in vitro that may have been induced in vivo after prolonged interferon therapy. Many in vivo changes are seen in vitro for only a short while after initiation of therapy. The body may thus adjust to IFN therapy by returning to a homeostatic level. Alternatively, current assays may not be sensitive enough. Thus, the effects of IFN in long-term intervention in immune abnormalities in diseases like MS may be impossible to measure in vitro or even maintain in vivo.

REFERENCES

1. Trinchieri, G., Santoli, D., Dee, R. R., and Knowles, B. B. Antiviral activity induced by culturing lymphocytes with tumor-derived or virus-transformed cells: Identification of the anti-viral activity as interferon and characterization of the human effector lymphocyte subpopulations. *J. Exp. Med.* 147:1299-1313 (1978).

2. Preble, O. T., and Friedman, R. M. Biology of disease: Interferon-induced alterations in cells: Relevance to viral and nonviral disease. *Lab. Invest.* 49:4-48 (1983).

3. Wiranowska-Stewart, M., and Stewart, W. E. II. Determination of human leukocyte populations involved in production of interferons alpha and gamma. *J. Interferon Res.* 1:233-243 (1981).

4. Ronnblom, L., Ramstedt, U., and Alm, G. V. Properties of human natural interferon-producing cells stimulated by tumor cell lines. *Eur. J. Immunol.* 13:471-476 (1983).

5. Heron, I., Hokland, M., and Berg, K. 13 Native human interferon alpha species assessed for immunoregulatory properties. *J. Interferon Res.* 3: 231-239 (1983).

6. Ortaldo, J. R., Herberman, R. B., Harvey, C., Osheroff, P., Pan, Y.-C., Kelder, B., and Pestka, S. A species of human alpha interferon that lacks the ability to boost human natural killer activity. *Proc. Natl. Acad. Sci. USA 81*:4926-4929 (1984).

7. Hirai, N., Hill, N. O., and Osther, K. Temperature influences on different human alpha interferon activities. *J. Interferon Res.* 4:507-516 (1984).

8. Imai, M., Sano, T., Yanase, Y., Miyamoto, K., Yonehara, S., Mori, H., Honda, T., Fukuda, S., Nakamura, T., Miyakawa, Y., and Maymi, M. Demonstration of two subtypes of human leukocyte interferon (IFN) by monoclonal antibodies. *J. Immunol.* 128:1824-2825 (1982).

9. Hawkins, M. J., Borden, E. C., Merritt, J. A., Edwards, B. S., Ball, L. A., Grossbard, E., and Simon, K. J. Comparison of the biologic effects of two recombinant human interferons alpha (rA and rD) in humans. *J. Clin. Oncol.* 2:221-226 (1984).

10. O'Malley, J. A., Nussbaum-Blumenson, A., Sheedy, D., Grossmayer, B. J., and Ozer, H. Identification of the T cell subset that produces interferon. *J. Immunol.* 128:2522-2526 (1982).

11. Kasahara, T., Hooks, J. J., Dougherty, S. F., and Oppenheim, J. T. Interleukin 2 mediated immune interferon (IFN) production by human T cells and T cell subsets. *J. Immunol.* 130:1784-1789 (1983).

12. Ronnblom, L., Forsgren, A., and Alm, G. V. Characterization of interferons induced by bacteria and interferon producing leukocytes in human peripheral blood. *Infect. Immun.* 40:126-132 (1983).

13. Dahl, H. Human interferon and cell growth inhibition. IV. The effect of isolated interferon components on the growth of different human cell lines. *J. Interferon Res.* 3:327-332 (1983).

14. Dahl, H. Human interferon and cell growth inhibition. IV. Effect of different inhibitors of cellular functions on interferon activities. *J. Interferon Res.* 3:333-339 (1983).

15. Dahl, H. Human interferon and cell growth inhibition. VII. Reversibility of interferon activities. *J. Interferon Res.* 3:387-393 (1983).

16. Chatterjee, S., Cheung, H. C., and Hunter, E. Interferon inhibits Sendai-virus induced cell fusion: An effect on cell membrane fluidity. *Proc. Natl. Acad. Sci. USA* 79:835-839 (1981).

17. Schattner, A., Merlin, G., Bregman, V., Hahn, T., Levin. S., Revel, R., and Wallach, D. (2'-5')-oligo A synthetase in human polymorphonuclear cells increased activity in interferon treatment and in viral infections. *Clin. Exp. Immunol.* 57:265-270 (1984).

18. Gazitt, Y., Ben-Bassat, H., Wallach, D., Revel, M., and Schattner, A. Interferon induced cytotoxity (2'-5') oligo (A) synthetase activity in T cells. *Clin. Immunol. Immunopathol.* 30:71-79 (1984).

19. Billiau, A., Opdenakker, G., Van Damme, J., Deley, M., Volckaert, G., Van Beeuman, J. Interkeukin 1: Amino acid sequencing reveals microheterogeneity and relationship with an interferon inducing monokine. *Immunol. Today* 6:235-236 (1985).

20. Ratliff, T. L., MacDermott, R. P., Poepping. N. J., Oakley, D. M., Shapiro, A., and Catalona, W. J. Production of gamma interferon by human T and null cells and its regulation by macrophages. *Cell. Immunol.* 74:111-119 (1982).

21. Farrar, W. L., and Humes, J. L. The role of arachidonic acid metabolism in the activities of interleukin 1 and 2. *J. Immunol.* 135:1153-1159 (1985).

22. Braude, J. A. A simple and efficient method for the production of human gamma interferon. *J. Immunol. Methods* 63:237-246 (1983).

23. Langford, M. P., Weigent, D. A., Georgiades, J. A., Johnson, H. M., and Stanton, G. J. Antibody to staphylococcal enterotoxin A induced human immune interferon (IFN γ). *J. Immunol.* 126:1620-1623 (1981).

24. Antonelli, G., Blalock, J. E., and Dianzani, F. Generation of a soluble IFN γ inducer by oxidation of galactose residues on macrophages. *Cell. Immunol.* 94:440-440 (1985).

25. Cole, B. C., and Thorpe, R. N. Induction of human gamma interferons by a mitogen derived from *Mycoplasma arthritides* and by phytohemagglutinin: Differential inhibition with monoclonal anti-HLA DR antibodies. *J. Immunol.* 131:2392-2396 (1983).

26. Ng, W. S., Ng, M. H., Inoue, M., and Tan, Y. H. Kinetics of human immune interferon production and blastogenesis. *Clin. Exp. Immunol.* 44:594-602 (1981).

27. Vilcek, J., Henriksen-Destefano, D., Siegel, D., Klion, A., Robb, R. J., and Le, J. Regulation of IFN induction in human peripheral blood cells by exogenous and endogenously produced interleukin 2. *J. Immunol.* 135:1851-1856 (1985).

28. Klein, J. R., and Bevan, M. J. Secretion of immune interferon and generation of cytotoxic T cell activity in nude mice are dependent on interleukin 2: Age-associated endogenous production of interleukin 2 in nude mice. *J. Immunol. 130*:1780-1783 (1983).

29. Handa, K., Suzuki, R., Matsui, H., Shimizu, Y., and Kumagai, K. Natural killer (NK) cells as a responder to-interleukin 2 (IL2). II. IL2 induced interferon production. *J. Immunol. 130*:988-992 (1983).

30. Farrar, W. L., Johnson, H. M., and Farrar, J. L. Regulation of the production of immune interferon and cytotoxic T lymphocytes by interleukin 2. *J. Immunol. 126*:1120-1125 (1981).

31. Kawase, I., Brooks, C. G., Kuribayashi, K., Olabuenaga, S., Newman, W., Gillis, S., and Henney, C. S. Interleukin 2 induces interferon production: Participation of macrophages and NK-like cells. *J. Immunol. 131*:288-292 (1983).

32. Pearlstein, K. T., Palladino, M. A., Welte, K., and Vilcek, J. Purified human interleukin 2 enhances induction of immune interferon. *Cell. Immunol. 80*:1-9 (1983).

33. Hecht, T. T., Longo, D. L., and Matis, L. A. The relationship between immune interferon production and proliferation in antigen-specific, MHC restricted T cell lines and clones. *J. Immunol. 131*:1049-1055 (1983).

34. Papermaster, V., Torres, B. A., and Johnson, H. M. Evidence for suppressor T cell regulation of human gamma interferon production. *Cell. Immunol. 79*:279-287 (1983).

35. Torres, B., Farrar, W. L., and Johnson, H. M. Interleukin 2 regulates immune interferon (IFN γ) production by normal and suppressor cell cultures. *J. Immunol. 128*:2217-2219 (1982).

36. von Wussow, P., Platsoucas, C. D., Wiranowska-Stewart, M., and Stewart, W. E., II. Human γ interferon production by leukocytes induced with monoclonal antibodies recognizing T cells. *J. Immunol. 127*:1197-1200 (1981).

37. Chang, T.-W., Testa, D., Kung, P. C., Perry, L., Dreskia, H. J., and Goldstein, G. Cellular origin and interactions involved in γ-interferon production induced by OKT3 monoclonal antibody. *J. Immunol. 128*: 585-589 (1985).

38. Bhayani, H., and Falcof, R. T cell surface antigens defined by monoclonal antibodies involved in the induction of human interferon-γ and interleukin 2. *Cell. Immunol. 94*:536-546 (1985).

39. Zlotnik, A., Shimon-Kevitz, R., Kappler, J., and Marr, P. Effect of prostaglandin E_2 on the interferon induction of antigen presenting ability in P388D1 cells and on IL2 production by T cell hybridomas. *Cell. Immunol.* 90:154-166 (1985).

40. Aoki, N., Maruyama, Y., Ohno, Y., and Azuma, Y. Indomethacin augmented inhibitory effects of interferons on lymphoproliferative response. *Immunol. Lett.* 7:321-324 (1984).

41. Rappaport, R. S., Dodge, G. R. Prostaglandin E inhibits the production of human interleukin 2. *J. Exp. Med.* 155:943-948 (1982).

42. Walker, C., Kristensen, F., Bettens, F., and de Weck, A. L. Lymphokine regulation of activated (G_1) lymphocyte to prostaglandin E_2-induced inhibition of interleukin 2 production. *J. Immunol.* 130:1770-1773 (1983).

43. Forti, R. L., Mitchell, W. M., Workman, R. J., Forbes, J. T., Hubbard, W. R., A functional cyclooxygenase enzyme is not required for mediation of the pleiotropic effects of human alpha or beta interferon. *Prostaglandins* 26:409-420 (1983).

44. Rhodes, J. Human interferon action: Reciprocal regulation by retinoic acid and beta carotene. *JNCI* 70:833-837 (1983).

45. Zoubmos, N. C., Djeu, J. Y., and Young, N. W. Interferon is the suppressor of hematopoiesis generated by stimulated lymphocytes in vitro. *J. Immunol.* 133:769-774 (1984).

46. Raefsky, E. L., Platanias, L. C., Zoumbos, N. C., and Young, N. S. Studies of interferon as a regulator of hematopoietic cell proliferation. *J. Immunol.* 135:2507-2512 (1985).

47. Broxmeyer, H. E., Cooper, S., Rubin, B. Y., and Taylor, M. W. The synergistic influences of human interferon γ and interferon α on suppression of hematopoietic progenitor cells is additive with the enhanced sensitivity of these cells to inhibition by interferons at low oxygen in vitro. *J. Immunol.* 135:2502-2506 (1985).

48. Shalaby, M. R., Weck, P. K., Rinderknecht, E., Harkins, R. N., Frane, J. W., and Ross, M. J. Effects of bacteria produced human alpha, beta, and gamma interferons on in vitro immune functions. *Cell. Immunol.* 84:380-392 (1984).

49. Einhorn, S., Blomgren, H., Einhorn, N., and Strander, H. In vitro and in vivo effects of interferon on the response of human lymphocytes to mitogens. *Clin. Exp. Immunol.* 51:369-377 (1983).

50. Lotz, M., Tsoukas, C. D., Fong, S., Carson, D. A., and Vaughn, J. H. Regulation of Epstein-Barr virus infections by recombinant interferons. Selected sensitivity to interferon gamma. *Eur. J. Immunol.* 15:520-525 (1985).

51. Torsteinsdottir, S., Masucci, M. G., Bejarano, M. T., Berthold, W., Klein, E., and Klein, G. Selective inhibitory effect of the IFN gamma on the agarose clonability of tumor derived lymphoid cell lines. *Cell. Immunol.* 9:65-73 (1985).

52. Mond, J. J., Finkelman, F. D., Sarma, C., O'Hara, J., and Serrate, S. Recombinant interferon γ inhibits the B cell proliferative response stimulated by soluble but not by Sepharose bound anti-immunoglobulin antibody. *J. Immunol.* 135:2513-2517 (1985).

53. Moore, R. N., Larsen, H. S., Horohov, D. W., and Rouse, B. T. Endogenous regulation of macrophage proliferative expansion by colon stimulating factor-induced interferon. *Science* 223:178-181 (1984).

54. Hamilton, T. A., Gray, P. W., and Adams, D. O. Expression of the transferrin receptor on murine peritoneal macrophages modulated by in vitro treatment with interferon gamma. *Cell. Immunol.* 89:478-488 (1984).

55. Silver, H. K., Connors, J. M., Karim, K. A., Kong, S., Spinell, J. J., deJong, G., McClean, D. M., and Salinas, F. A. Effect of lymphoblastoid interferon on lymphocyte subsets in cancer patients. *J. Biol. Resp Mod.* 2:428-440 (1983).

56. Ernstoff, M. S., Fusi, S., and Kirkwood, J. M. Parameters of interferon action. II. Immunological effects of recombinant leukocyte interferon (IFN alpha 2) in phase I-II trials. *J. Biol. Respir. Mod.* 2:546-547 (1983).

57. Hersey, P., Hasic, E., MacDonald, M., Edwards, A., Spurling, A., Coates, A. S., Milton, G. W., and McCarthy, W. H. Effects of recombinant leukocyte interferon (rIFN-alpha A) on tumor growth and immune response in patients with metastatic melanoma. *Br. J. Cancer* 51:815-826 (1985).

58. Knop, S., Stremmer, R., Taborski, U., Freitag, W., deMaeyer-Grugnard, J., and Nacher, E. Inhibition of the T suppressor circuit of delayed-type hypersensitivity by interferon. *J. Immunol.* 133:2412-2416 (1984).

59. Hokland, M., Hokland, P., Heron, I., and Schlossman, S. F. Selective effects of alpha interferon on human T lymphocyte subsets during mixed lymphocyte cultures. *Scand. J. Immunol.* 17:559-567 (1983).

60. Hokland, M., Ritz, J., and Hoklund, P. Interferon induced changes in expression of antigens defined by monoclonal antibodies on malignant and nonmalignant mononuclear hematopoietic cells. *J. Interferon Res.* 3: 199-210 (1983).

61. Maluish, A. E., Leavitt, R., Sherwin, S. A., Oldham, R. K. and Herberman, R. B. Effects of recombinant interferon alpha on immune function in cancer patients. *J. Biol. Respir. Mod.* 2:470-481 (1983).

62. Akiyama, Y., Lubeck, M. D., Steplowski, Z., and Koprowski, H. Induction of mouse IgG2 and IgG3 dependent cellular cytotoxicity in human monocytic cells (U937) by immune interferon. *Cancer Res.* 44:5127-5131 (1984).

63. Shen, L., Guyre, P. M., and Fanger, M. W. Direct stimulation of ADCC by cloned gamma interferon is not ablated by glucocorticoids: Studies using a human monocyte-like cell line (U937). *Mol. Immunol.* 21:167-173 (1984).

64. Harris, P. E., Ralph, P., Litcofsky, P., and Moore, M. A. Distinct activities of interferon gamma lymphokine and cytokine differentiation inducing factors acting on the human monoblastic leukemia cell line U937. *Cancer Res.* 45:9-13 (1985).

65. Fertsch, D., and Vogel, S. N. Recombinant interferons increase macrophage Fc receptor capacity. *J. Immunol.* 132:2436-2439 (1984).

66. Perussia, B., Dayton, E. T., Fanning, V., Thiagarajan, P., Hoxie, J., and Trinchieri, G. Immune interferon and leukocyte-conditioned medium induce normal and leukemic myeloid cells to differentiate along the monocytic pathway. *J. Exp. Med.* 158:2058-2080 (1983).

67. Hatton, T., Pack, M., Bougnoux, P., Chang, L. L., and Hoffman, T. Interferon induced differentiation of U937 cells: Comparison with other agents that promote differentiation of human myeloid or monocyte like cell lines. *J. Clin. Invest.* 72:237-244 (1983).

68. Harrison, P. E., Ralph, P., Gabrilove, J., Welte, K., Karmali, R., and Moore, M. A. Distinct differentiation inducing activities of gamma interferon and cytokine factors acting on human promyelactic leukemia cell line HL60. *Cancer Res.* 45:3090-3095 (1985).

69. Ball, E. D., Guyre, P. M., Shen, L., Glynn, J. M., Maliszewski, R., Baker, P. E., and Fanger, M. W. Gamma interferon induces monocytoid differentiation in the HL60 cell line. *J. Clin. Invest.* 73:1072-1077 (1984).

70. Becker, S. Influence of interferon on human monocyte to macrophage development. *Cell. Immunol.* 84:145-153 (1984).

71. Aubock, J., Niedewieser, D., Remani, N., Fritsch, P., and Huber, C. Human interferon gamma induces expression of HLA-DR on kera— tinocytes and melanocytes. *Arch. Dermatol. Res.* 277:270-275 (1985).

72. Berrih, S., Arenzana-Seisdedos, F., Cohen, S., Devos, R., Charron, D., and Virelizier, J. L. Interferon gamma modulates HLA class II antigen expression on cultured human thymic epithelial cells. *J. Immunol.* 135: 1165-1171 (1985).

73. Kelley, V. E., Fliers, W., and Strom, T. B. Cloned human interferon γ but not interferon α or β induces expression of HLA-DR determinants by fetal monocytes and myeloid leukemic cell lines. *J. Immunol.* 132:240-245 (1984).

74. Wong, G. H. W., Clark-Lewis, I., McKimm-Breschkin, J. L., Haris, A. W. and Schrader, J. W. Interferon γ induces enhanced expression of Ia and H2 antigens on B lymphoid, macrophage, and myeloid cell lines. *J. Immunol.* 131:788-793 (1983).

75. Stiehm, E. R., Sztein, M. B., Steeg, P. S., Mann, D., Newland, C., Blaese, M., and Oppenheim, J. J. Deficient DR antigen expression on human cord blood monocytes: Reversal with lymphokines. *Clin. Immunol. Immunopathol.* 30:430-436 (1984).

76. Gershon, H. E., Kuang, Y.-D., Scala, G., and Oppenheim, J. J. Effects of recombinant interferon γ on HLA-DR antigen shedding by human peripheral adherent mononuclear cells. *J. Leuko. Biol.* 38:279-291 (1985).

77. Becker, S. Interferon gamma accelerates immune proliferation via its effects on monocyte HLA-DR expression. *Cell. Immunol.* 91:301-307 (1985).

78. Sztein, M. D., Steeg, P. S., Johnson, H. M., and Oppenheim, J. J. Regulation of human peripheral blood monocyte DR antigen expression in vitro by lymphokines and recombinant interferons. *J. Clin. Invest.* 73:556-565 (1984).

79. Rhodes, J., Jones, D. H., and Bleehen, N. M. Increased expression of human monocyte HLA DR antigens and Fc gamma receptors in response to human interferon in vivo. *Clin. Exp. Immunol.* 53:739-743 (1983).

80. Ling, P. D., Warren, M. K., and Vogel, S. N. Antagonistic effect of interferon on the interferon induced expression of Ia antigen in murine macrophages. *J. Immunol. 135*:1857-1863 (1985).

81. Thurman, G. B., Braude, I. A., Gray, P. W., Oldham, R. K., and Stevenson, H. C. MIF like activity of natural and recombinant interferon gamma and their neutralization by monoclonal antibody. *J. Immunol. 134*:305-309 (1985).

82. Zlotnick, A., Roberts, W. K., Vasil, A., Blumbenthal, E., Larosa, F., Liebson, H. J., Endres, R. O., Graham, S. D., Jr., White, J., Hill, J., Henson, P., Klein, J. R., Bevan, M. J., Marrack, P., and Kappler, J. W. Coordinate production by a T cell hybridoma of gamma interferon and three other lymphokine activities: Multiple activities of a single lymphokine? *J. Immunol. 131*:1-794-800 (1983).

83. Wallach, D., and Hahn, T. Enhanced release of lymphotoxins by interferon treated cells. *Cell. Immunol. 76*:390-396 (1983).

84. Robbins, C. H. Immunoregulation by lymphokines: Immune interferons and lymphotoxin induction of lymphokine activity in human peripheral blood leukocyte cultures. *Adv. Exp. Med. Biol. 166*:37-44 (1983).

85. Nedwin, G. E., Svedersky, L. P., Bringman, T. S., Palladino, M. A., Jr., and Goeddel, D. V. Effect of interleukin 2 interferon γ, and mitogens on the production of tumor necrosis factors α and β. *J. Immunol. 135*: 2492-2497 (1985).

86. Williamson, B. D., Carswell, E. A., Rubin, B. Y., Prendergast, J. S., and Old, L. J. Human tumor necrosis factor produced by human B cell lines: Synergistic cytotoxic interaction with human interferon. *Proc. Natl. Acad. Sci. USA 80*:5397-5401 (1983).

87. Huber, C., Batchelor, J. R., Fuchs, D., Hausen, A., Lang, A., Niederwieser, D., Reibnegger, G., Swetly, P., Troppmair, J., and Wachter, H. Immune response associated production of neopterin release from macrophages primarily under control of interferon gamma. *J. Exp. Med. 160*:310-316 (1984).

88. Schnaper, H. W., Pierce, C. W., and Aune, T. M. Identification and initial characterization of conconavalin A and interferon induced human suppressor factors: Evidence for a human equivalent of murine soluble immune response suppressor (SIRS). *J. Immunol. 132*:2429-2435 (1984).

89. Johnson, H. M., and Torres, B. A. Recombinant mouse interferon gamma regulation of antibody production. *Infect. Immun.* 41:546-548 (1983).

90. Pelton, B. K., and Denman, A. M. Immunoregulatory effects of alpha interferon. Effects on in vitro antibody synthesis by lymphocytes from patients with rheumatoid arthritis. *Ann. Rheum. Dis.* 44:143-147 (1985).

91. Neubauer, R. H., Goldstein, L., Rabin, H., and Stebbing, N. Stimulation of in vitro immunoglobulin production by interferon alpha. *J. Immunol.* 134:299-304 (1985).

92. Rodriquez, M. A., Prinz, W. A., Sibbitt, W. L., Bankhurst, A. D., and Williams, R. C. Jr. Alpha interferon increases immunoglobulin production in cultured human mononuclear leukocytes. *J. Immunol.* 130:1215-1219 (1983).

93. Rodriquez, M. A., Prinz, W. A., Bankhurst, A. D., and Williams, R. C., Jr. Human alpha interferon enhances in vitro IgM rheumatoid factor synthesis by lymphocytes from normal subjects and rheumatoid arthritis patients. *Arthritis Rheum.* 26:1091-1097 (1983).

94. Sidman, C. L., Marshall, J. D., Shultz, L. D., Gray, P. W., and Johnson, H. M. Interferon is one of several direct B cell-maturing lymphokines. *Nature* 309:801-803 (1984).

95. Nakagawa, T., Hirano, T., Nakagawa, N., Yashizaka, K., and Kishimoto, T. Effect of recombinant IL2 and gamma IFN on proliferation and differentiation of human B cells. *J. Immunol.* 134:959-966 (1985).

96. Arenzana-Seisdedos, F., and Virelizier, J.-L. Interferons as macrophage activating factors. II. Enhanced secretion of interleukin 1 by lipopolysaccharide-stimulated human monocytes. *Eur. J. Immunool.* 13:437-440 (1983).

97. Herman, J., Kew, M. C., and Rabson, A. R. Defective interleukin 1 production by monocytes from patients with malignant disease. Interferon increases IL1 production. *Cancer Immunol. Immunother.* 16:182-185 (1984).

98. Arenzana-Seisdedos, F., Virelizier, J. L., and Fiers, W. Interferons as macrophage-activating factors. III. Preferential effects of interferon gamma on the interleukin 1 secretory potential of fresh or aged human monocytes. *J. Immunol.* 134:2444-2448 (1985).

99. Itoh, K., Shiiba, K., Shimizu, Y., Suzuki, R., and Kumagai, K. Generation of activated killer (AK) cells by recombinant interkeukin 2 (IL2) in collaboration with interferon gamma (IFN gamma). *J. Immunol.* 134:2444-2448 (1985).

100. Oshimi, K., Oshimi, Y., Motoji, T., Kobayashi, S., and Mizoguchi, H. Lysis of leukemia and lymphoma cells by autologous and allogeneic interferon activated blood mononuclear cells. *Blood* 61:790-798 (1983).

101. Sone, S., Utsugi, T., Shirahama, T., Ishii, K., Matsuura, S., and Ogawara, M. Induction by interferon alpha of tumorcidal activity of adherent mononuclear cells from human blood: Monocytes as responder and effector cells. *J. Biol. Respir. Mod.* 4:134-140 (1985).

102. Dean, R. T., and Virelizier, J. L. Interferon as a macrophage activating factor. I. Enhancement of cytotoxicity by fresh and matured human monocytes in the absence of other soluble signals. *Clin. Exp. Immunol.* 51:501-510 (1983).

103. Koff, W. C., Fogler, W. E., Gutterman, J., and Fidler, I. J. Efficient activation of human blood monocytes to a tumorcidal state by liposomes containing recombinant gamma interferon. *Cancer Immunol. Immunother.* 19:85-89 (1985).

104. Schreiber, R. D., Hicks, L. J., Celada, A., Buchmeier, N. A., and Gray, P. W. Monoclonal antibodies to murine gamma interferon which differentially modulate macrophage activation and antiviral activity. *J. Immunol.* 134:1609-1618 (1985).

105. Territo, M., Sarna, G., and Figlin, R. Effect of in vivo administration of interferon on human monocyte function. *J. Biol. Respir. Mod.* 2:450-457 (1983).

106. Wilson, C. B., and Westall, J. Activation of neonatal and adult human macrophages by alpha, beta, and gamma interferons. *Infect. Immun.* 49:351-356 (1985).

107. Celada, A., Gray, P. W., Rinderknecht, E., and Schreiber, R. D. Evidence for a gamma interferon receptor that regulates macrophage tumorcidal activity. *J. Exp. Med.* 160:55-74 (1984).

108. Finbloom, D. S., Hoover, D. L., and Wahl, L. M. The characteristics of binding of human recombinant interferon to its receptor on human

monocytes and human monocyte like cell lines. *J. Immunol. 135*: 300-305 (1985).

109. Fischer, D. C., Golightly, M. G., and Koren, H. S. Potentiation of the cytolytic activity of peripheral blood monocytes by lymphokines and interferon. *J. Immunol. 130*:1220-1225 (1983).

110. Russell, S. W., and Pace, J. L. Gamma interferon interferes with the negative regulation of macrophage activation by prostaglandin E_2. *Mol. Immunol. 21*:249-254 (1984).

111. Einhorn, S., Wasserman, J., Lundell, G., Blomgren, H., Cedermark, B., Jarstrand, C., Petrini, B., Strander, H., Theve, T., and Ohman, U. Treatment of patients with disseminated colorectal cancer with recombinant human alpha 2 interferon: Studies on the immune system. *Int. J. Cancer 33*:251-256 (1984).

112. Buessow, S. C., Gillespie, G. Y., and Malaley, M. S. Tumoricidal activity of an acute pro-myelocyteic leukemia cell line (HL-60) is augmented by human interferon alpha 1. *Leuko. Res. 8*:801-811 (1984).

113. Basham, T. Y., Smith, W. K., and Merigan, T. C. Interferon enhances antibody-dependent cellular cytotoxicity when suboptimal concentrations of antibody are used. *Cell. Immunol. 88*:393-400 (1984).

114. Hokland, P., and Berg, K. Interferon enhances the antibody dependent cellular cytotoxicity (ADCC) of human polymorphonuclear leukocytes. *J. Immunol. 127*:1585-1588 (1981).

115. Trinchieri, G., and Santoli, D. Antiviral activity induced by culturing lymphocytes with tumor-derived or virus-transformed cells. Enhancement of natural killer cell activity by interferon and antagonistic inhibition of susceptibility of target cells to lysis. *J. Exp. Med. 147*: 1314-1333 (1978).

116. Gidund, M., Orn, A., Wigzell, H., Senik, A., and Gresser, I. Enhanced NK cell activity in mice injected with interferon and interferon inducers. *Nature 273*:759-761 (1978).

117. Boraschi, D., Soldateschi, D., and Tagliabue, A. *Eur. J. Immunol. 12*: 320-326 (1982).

118. Weigent, D. A., Langford, M. P., Fleischmann, W. R., and John G. Potentiation of lymphcyte natural killer by mixtures of alpha or beta interferon with recombinant gamma interferon. *Infect. Immun. 40*(1): 35-38 (1983).

119. Ortaldo, J. R., Mason, A., Rehberg, E., Moscher, J., Kelder, B., Pestka, S., and Herberman, R. B. Effects of recombinant and hybrid recombinant human leukocyte interferons on cytotoxic activity of natural killer cells. *J. Biol. Chem.* 158(24):15011-15015 (1983).

120. Targan, S., and Stebbing, N. In vitro interactions of purified cloned human interferons on NK cells: Enhanced activation. *J. Immunol.* 129(3):934-935 (1982).

121. Edwards, B. S., Hawkins, M. J., and Borden, E. C. Comparative in vivo and in vitro activation of human natural killer cells by two recombinant α-interferons differing in antiviral activity. *Cancer Res.* 44:3135-3139 (1984).

122. Ortiz de Landazuri, M., Lopez Botet, M., Timonen, T., Ortaldo, J. R., and Herberman, R. B. Human large granular lyphocytes: Spontaneous and interferon-boosted NK activity against adherent and nonadherent tumor cell lines. *J. Immunol.* 127:1380 (1981).

123. Targan, S., and Dorey, F. Interferon activation of pre-spontaneous killer' (pre-SK) cells and alteration in kinetics of lysis of both 'pre-Sk and active sk cells. *J. Immunol.* 124(5):2157-2161 (1980).

124. Silva, A., Bonavida, B., and Targan, S. Mode of action of interferon-mediated modulation of natural killer cytotoxicity activity: Recruitment of pre-NK cells and enhanced kinetics of lysis. *J. Immunol.* 125(2):479-484 (1980).

125. Hiserodt, J. C., Britvan, L. J., and Targan, S. R. Characterization of the cytolytic reaction mechanism of the human natural killer (NK) lymphocyte: Resolution into binding, programing, and natural killer cell-independent steps. *J. Immunol.* 129(4):1782-1787 (1982).

126. Targan, S. R., and Newman, W. Definitions of a 'trigger' stage in the NK cytotolic reaction sequence by a monoclonal antibody to the glycoptrotein T-200. *J. Immunol* 131(3):1149-1153 (1983).

127. Hiserodt, J. C., Britvan, L. J., and Targan, S. R. Studies on the mechanism of the human natural killer cell lethal hit: Evidence for transfer of protease-sensitive structures requisite for target cell lysis. *J. Immunol.* 131: (1983).

128. Hiserodt, J. C., Britvan, L. J., and Targan, S. R. Studies on the mechanism of the human natural killer cell lethal hit: Analysis of the mechanism of protease inhibition of the lethal hit. *J. Immunol.* 131(6): 2705-2709 (1983).

129. Ullberg, M., and Jondal, M. Recycling and target-binding capacity of human natural killer cells. *J. Exp. Med.* 153:615 (1981).

130. Targan, S. R. The dual interaction of prostaglandin E_2 (PGE_2) and interferon (IFN) on NK lytic activation: Enhanced capacity of effector-target lytic interactions (recycling) and blockage of pre-NK cell recruitment. *J. Immunol.* 127(4):1424-1428 (1981).

131. Targan, S. R., Britvan, L., and Dorey, F. Activation of human NKCC by moderate exercise: Increased frequency of NK cells with enhanced capability of effector-target lytic interactions. *Clin. Exp. Immunol.* 45: 352-360 (1981).

132. Timonen, T., Ortaldo, J. R., and Herberman, R. B. Analysis by a single cell cytotoxicity assay of natural killer (NK) cell frequencies among human large granular lymphocytes and the effects of interferon on their activity. *J. Immunol.* 128(6):2514-2521 (1982).

133. Wright, S. C., and Bonavida, B. Studies on the mechanism of natural killer cell-mediated cytotoxicity. III. Activation of NK cells by interferon augments the lytic activity of released natural killer cytotoxic factors (NKCF). *J. Immunol.* 130:2690 (1983).

134. Farram, E., and Targan, S. R. Identification of human natural killer soluble cytotoxic factor(s) (NKCF) derived from NK-enriched lymphocyte populations: Specificity of generation and killing. *J. Immunol.* 130 (3):1252-1256 (1983).

135. Wright, S. C., and Bonavida, S. Selective lysis of NK-sensitive cells by a solumble mediator released from murine spleen cells and human peripheral blood lymphocytes. *J. Immunol.* 126:1516 (1981).

136. Targan, S., and Dorey, F. Dual mechanism of interferon augmentation of natural killer cytotoxicity (NKCC). *Ann. N.Y. Acad. Sci.* 350:121-129 (1980).

137. Hoffman, T., Bougnoux, P., Hattori, T., Chang, Z., and Herberman, R. B. Phospholipid metabolism during NK cell activity: Possible role for transmethylation and phospholipase A_2 activation in recognition and lysis. In: *NK Cells and Other Effector Cells* (R. B. Herberman, ed.). Academic Press, new York, pp. 955-959 (1982).

138. Targan, S., and Deem, R. NK-target cell interactions in binding, triggering, programing, and lethal hit stages of NK cytotoxicity. In. *Natural Cell Mediated Immunity* (R. Herberman, ed.). Academic Press, New York, pp. 155-172 (1985).

139. Welsh, R. M. *Antiviral Res. 1*:5 (1981).

140. Hansson, M., Kiessling, R., Anderson, B., and Welsh, R. M. Effect of interferon and interferon inducers on the NK sensitivity of normal mouse thymocytes. *J. Immunol. 125*:2225 (1980).

141. Wallach, D. Interferon-induced resistance to the killing by NK cells: A preferential effect of IFN-γ. *Cell Immunol. 75*:390–395 (1983).

142. Gronberg, A., Kiessling, R., Masucci, G., Guevara, L. A., Eriksson, E., and Klein, G. Gamma interferon (IFN-γ) produced during effector and target interactions renders target cells less susceptible to NK-cell-mediated lysis. *Int. J. Cancer 32*:609–616 (1983).

143. Wright, S. C., and Bonavida, B. Studies of the mechanism of natural killer cell-mediated cytotoxicity. IV. Interferon-induced inhibition of NK target cell susceptibility to lysis is due to a defect in their ability to stimulate release of natural killer cytotoxic factors (NKCF). *J. Immunol. 130*:2965 (1983).

144. Bradley, P. T., and Bonavia, B. Mechanism of cell-mediated cytotoxicity at the single cell level. IV. Natural killer and antibody dependent cellular cytotoxicities are mediated by the same effector cell. *J. Immunol. 129*:2260 (1982).

145. Merrill, J. E. Natural killer (NK) and antibody dependent cellular cytotoxicity (ADCC) activities can be differentiated by their different sensitivities to interferon and prostaglandin E_1. *J. Clin. Immunol. 3*: 42–50 (1983).

146. Lampert, P. W. Autoimmune and virus-induced demyelinating diseases. *Am. J. Pathol. 91*:176–207 (1978).

147. Dal Canto, M., and Lipton, H. L. Ultrastructural immunohistochemical localization of virus in acute and chronic demyelinating Theiler's virus infection. *Am. J. Pathol. 106*:20–29 (1982).

148. Saksela, E., Timonen, T., Ranki, A., and Hayry, P. Morphological and functional characterization of isolated effector cells responsible for human natural killer activity to fetal fibroblasts and to cultured cell line targets. *Immunol. Rev. 44*:71–95 (1979).

149. Pape, G. R., Moretta, L., Troye, M., and Perlmann, P. Natural cytotoxicity of human Fc γ receptor positive T lymphocytes after surface modulation with immune complexes. *Scand. J. Immunol. 9*:291–299 (1979).

150. Merrill, J. E., Ullberg, M., and Jondal, M. Influence of IgG and IgM receptor triggering on human natural killer cell cytotoxicity measured on the level of the single effector cell. *Eur. J. Immunol.* 11:536-541 (1980).

151. Passwell, J., Rosen, F. S., and Merler, E. The effect of Fc fragments of IgG on human mononuclear cell responses. *Cell. Immunol.* 52:395-403 (1980).

152. Poleshuck, L. C., and Strausser, H. R. Immune complex induced prostaglandin production by monocytes of normal human subjects and cancer patients. *Prostaglandins Med.* 4:363-375 (1980).

153. Baker, P. E., Fahey, J. V., and Munck, A. Prostaglandin inhibition of T cell proliferation is mediated at two levels. *Cell. Immunol.* 61:52-58 (1981).

154. Herberman, R. B., and Ortaldo, J. R. Natural killer cells: Their role in defense against disease. *Science* 214:24-25 (1981).

155. Welsh, R. M. Natural killer cells in virus infections in current topics. In: *Microbiology and Immunology* (O. Haller, ed.). Springer-Verlag, Berlin, pp. 739-765 (1980).

156. Tovell, D. R., McRobbie, I., Warren, K. G., and Tyrrell, D. L. Interferon production by lymphocytes from multiple sclerosis and non MS patients. *Neurology* 33:640-643 (1983).

157. Vervliet, G., Claeys, H., Van Hauer, H., Carton, H., Vermylen, C., Meulepos, E., and Billiau, A. Interferon production and natural killer (NK) activity in leukocyte cultures from multiple sclerosis patients. *J. Neurol. Sci.* 60:137-150 (1983).

158. Santoli, D., Hall, W., Kastrokoff, L., Lisak, R. P., Perussia, B., Trinchieri, G., and Koprowski, H. Cytotoxic activity and interferon production by lymphocytes from patients with multiple sclerosis. *J. Immunol.* 126:1274-1278 (1981).

159. Benczur, M., Petranyi, G. G., Palffy, G., Varga, M., Talas, M., Kotsy, B., Foldes, I., and Hollan, S. R. Dysfunction of natural killer cells in multiple sclerosis: A possible pathogenic mechanism. *Clin. Exp. Immunol.* 39:657-662 (1980).

160. Neighbour, P. A. Studies of interferon production and natural killing by lymphocytes from multiple sclerosis patients. *Ann. N.Y. Acad. Sci.* 436:181-191 (1984).

161. Merrill, J. E., Ellison, G. W., and Myers, L. W. Cytotoxic activity of

peripheral blood and cerebrospinal fluid lymphocytes from patients with multiple sclerosis and other neurological diseases: Analysis at the single cell level of the relationship of cytotoxic effectors and interferon producing cells. *Clin. Immunol. Immunopathol. 31*:390-402 (1984).

162. Neighbour, P. A., Grayzel, A. I., and Miller, A. E. Endogenous and interferon-augmented natural killer cell activity of human peripheral blood mononuclear cells in vitro. Studies of patients with multiple sclerosis, septemic lupus erythematosus, or rheumatoid arthritis. *Clin. Exp. Immunol. 49*:11-21 (1982).

163. Merrill, J. E., Gerner, R. H., Myers, L. W., and Ellison, G. W. Regulation of natural killer cell cytotoxicity by prostaglandin E in the peripheral blood and cerebrospinal fluid of patients with multiple sclerosis and other neurological diseases. Part I. Association between amount of prostaglandin produced, natural killer, and endogenous interferon. *J. Neuroimmunol. 4*:223-237 (1983).

164. Merrill, J. E., Myers, L. W., and Ellison, G. W. Regulation of natural killer cell cytotoxicity by prostaglandin E in the peripheral blood and cerebrospinal fluid of patients with multiple sclerosis and other neurological diseases. Part 2. Effect of exogenous PGE_1 on spontaneous and interferon induced natural killer. *J. Neuroimmunol. 4*:239-251 (1983).

165. Gyodi, E., Benczur, M., Palffy, G. G., Tálas, M., Petrányi, G., Foldes, I., and Hollan, S. R. Association between HLA B7, DR2 and dysfunction of natural and antibody-mediated cytotoxicity without connection with the deficient interferon production in multiple sclerosis. *Hum. Immunol. 4*:209-217 (1982).

166. Salonen, R., Ilonen, J., Reunanen, M., and Salmi, A. Defective production of interferon associated with HLA DW2 antigen in stable multiple sclerosis. *J. Neurol. Sci. 55*:197-206 (1982).

167. Kaudewitz, P., Zander, H., Abb, J., Ziegler-Heitbrock, H. W., and Reithmuller, G. Genetic influence on natural cytotoxicity and interferon production in multiple sclerosis studies in monozygotic discordant twins. *Hum. Immunol. 7*:51-58 (1983).

168. Haahr, S., Møller-Larson, A., and Pederson, E. Immunological parameters in multiple sclerosis patients with special reference to the herpes virus group. *Clin. Exp. Immunol. 51*:197-206 (1983).

169. Vervliet, G., Carton, H., Meulepas, E., and Billiau, A. Interferon production by cultured peripheral leukocytes of MS patients. *Clin. Exp. Immunol. 58*:116-126 (1984).

170. Vervliet, G., Carton, H., and Billiau, A. Interferon gamma production by peripheral blood leukocytes from patients with multiple sclerosis and other neurological diseases. *Clin. Exp. Immunol.* 59:391-399 (1985).

171. Vervliet, G., Deckmyn, H., Carton, H., and Billiau, A. Influence of prostaglandin E_2 and indomethacin on interferon gamma production by cultured peripheral blood leukocytes of multiple sclerosis patients and healthy donors. *J. Clin. Immunol.* 5:102-108 (1985).

172. Abb, J., Zander, H., Abb, H., Albert, E., and Diehnardt, F. Associating human leukocyte low responsiveness to inducers of interferon alpha with HLA-DR2. *Immunology* 49:239-244 (1983).

173. Hauser, S. L., Ault, K. A., Levin, M. J., Garavoy, M. R., and Weiner, H. L. Natural killer cell activity in multiple sclerosis. *J. Immunol.* 127:1114-1118 (1981).

174. Benczur, M., Gyodi, E., Petranyi, G., Hollan, S. R., Palffy, G., Talas, M., Stoger, I., and Foldes, I. Impaired natural killer cell function in multiple sclerosis and association with the HLA system. In: *NK Cells and Other Natural Effector Cells* (R. B. Herberman, ed.). Academic Press, New York, pp. 1227-1232 (1982).

175. Abb, J., Kaudewitz, P., Zander, H., Ziegler, H.-N. L., Dienhardt, F., and Riethmuller, R. Interferon (IFN) production and natural killer (NK) cell activity in patients with multiple sclerosis: Influence of genetic factors assessed by studies of monozygotic twins. In: *NK Cells and Other Natural Effector Cells* (R. B. Herberman, ed.). Academic Press, New York, pp. 1233-1240 (1982).

176. Zander, H., Abb, J., Kaudewitz, P., and Riethmuller, G. Natural killing activity and interferon production in multiple sclerosis. *Lancet* 1:280-283 (1982).

177. Merrill, J. E., Jondal, M., Seeley, J., Ullberg, M., and Siden, A. Decreased NK killing in patients with multiple sclerosis: An analysis on the level of the single effector cell in peripheral blood and cerebrospinal fluid in relation to disease activity. *Clin. Exp. Immunol.* 47:419-430 (1981).

178. Merrill, J. E., Scott, A., Myers, L., and Ellison, G. Cytotoxic activity of peripheral blood and cerebrospinal fluid lymphocytes from patients with multiple sclerosis and other neurological diseases. *J. Neuroimmunol.* 3:123-138 (1982).

179. Merrill, J. E., Gerner, R. H., Myers, L. W., and Eillison, G. W. Regula-

tion of NK activity and IFN production by PGE in the peripheral blood and cerebrospinal fluid of patients with multiple sclerosis and other neurological diseases. In: *Intercellular Communication in Leukocyte Function* (J. W. Parker and R. L. O'Brien, eds.). John Wiley & Sons, Chichester, England, pp. 79-83 (1983).

180. McGarry, R. C., Rodier, J. C., and Brunet, D. Mechanisms of natural killer cell depression in multiple sclerosis. In: *NK Cells and Other Natural Effector Cells* (R. B. Herberman, ed.). Academic Press, New York, pp. 1219-1225 (1982).

181. Uchida, A., Maida, E. M., Lenzhofer, R., and Micksche, M. Natural killer cell activity in patients with multiple sclerosis: Interferon and plamapheresis. *Immunobiology* 160:392-402 (1982).

182. Hirsch, R. L., and Johnson, K. P. The effect of recombinant alpha 2 interferon on defective natural killer cell activity in multiple sclerosis. *Neurology (N.Y.)* 35:597-600 (1985).

183. Salonen, R. CSF and serum interferon in multiple sclerosis: A longitudinal study. *Neurology (N.Y.)* 33:1604-1606 (1983).

184. Degre, M., Dahl, H., and Vandvik, B. Interferon in the serum and cerebrospinal fluid of patients with multiple sclerosis and other neurological disorders. *Acta Neurol. Scand.* 53:152-156 (1976).

185. Jacobs, L., O'Malley, J., Freeman, A., and Ekes, R. Intrathecal interferon reduces exacerbations in multiple sclerosis. *Science* 214:1026-1028 (1981).

186. Jacobs, L., O'Malley, Freeman, A., Murawski, J., and Ekes, R. Intrathecal interferon in multiple sclerosis. *Arch. Neurol.* 39:609-615 (1982).

187. Huddlestone, J. R., Francis, G. S., Hooper, C. K., Kramin-Lewis, R. M., Johnson, K. P., *et al.* Systemic alpha interferon therapy of multiple sclerosis. *Neurology (N.Y.)* 34:1273-1279 (1984).

188. Rice, G. P., Casali, P., Merigan, T. C., and Oldstone, M. B. Natural killer cell activity in patients with MS given alpha interferon. *Ann. Neurol.* 14:333-338 (1983).

189. Kamin-Lewis, R. M., Danitch, H. S., Merigan, T. C., and Johnson, K. P. Decreased interferon synthesis and responsiveness to interferon by leukocytes from multiple sclerosis patients given natural alpha interferon. *J. Interferon Res.* 4:423-432 (1984).

4
Pharmacokinetics of Interferons

ROBERT J. WILLS

Hoffmann-La Roche Inc., Nutley, New Jersey

RICHARD ALAN SMITH

Center for Neurologic Study, San Diego, California

I. INTRODUCTION

Successful drug therapy is the optimal balance of unwanted side effects and desired pharmacologic effect(s). Both the side effect response and the therapeutic response are a function of the drug concentration at the respective site(s) of action. Since concentrations at these sites are difficult if not impossible to measure, the plasma has been used as an alternate site for measurement. This assumes that plasma concentrations reflect concentrations at the site(s) of action. Drug concentrations in plasma rise and fall with time as the drug absorbs, distributes, metabolizes, and eliminates. Knowledge of the mechanisms and the time-related processes involved in absorption, distribution, metabolism, and elimination is called pharmacokinetics.

In the case of neurologic disorders, the blood-brain barrier represents a significant factor that must be considered along with other treatment variables. Under normal circumstances the blood-brain barrier prevents proteins from reaching the nervous system from the general circulation, but in some conditions, for example neoplasia, this obstacle may be breached. In each clinical instance it is hoped that pharmacokinetic studies may shed light on the optimum therapeutic strategy. It is the intent of this preview to facilitate the task of those who choose to undertake such studies—first by reviewing general pharmacokinetic concepts and then by review of what is known about the pharmacokinetic behavior of interferons in animals and humans.

II. PHARMACOKINETIC CONCEPTS

Many parameters and concepts are related to pharmacokinetics. The major parameters and concepts are discussed here as they relate to the clinical setting. More complete and detailed reviews of all the pharmacokinetic parameters and concepts are available (1-4).

A. Bioavailability

The U.S. Food and Drug Administration defines bioavailability as "the rate and extent to which the active drug ingredient or therapeutic moiety is absorbed from a drug product and becomes available at the site of drug action" (5). For most drugs, which are dosed chronically in the clinical setting, the rate of absorption is not as important as the extent. The bioavailability of drugs given intravenously is 100% since the total dose is delivered directly to the general circulation. Drug administered by any other route must pass through membranes prior to reaching the general circulation, thus being burdened with the additional process of absorption. Absorption or the ability to absorb is a function of the physical and chemical properties of the drug, the release properties of the dosage form, the solubilization of released drug, and the surrounding environment, such as the presence of food, antacids, or other medications in the case of oral administration.

The extent of drug that reaches the general circulation is estimated by the pharmacokinetic parameter AUC, or simply the mathematical area under the plasma concentration-time curve. The most common way of calculating this parameter is by trapezoidal summation (3). The absolute bioavailability F_{abs} can be determined from any route of delivery if the extent of absorption can be compared with that following intravenous administration [Eq. (1)]:

$$F_{abs} = \frac{AUC_{nonintravenous}}{AUC_{intravenous}} \times \frac{dose_{intravenous}}{dose_{nonintravenous}} \quad (1)$$

For most drugs, intravenous dosage forms are not developed. Therefore, the bioavailability F_{rel} must be assessed relative to an alternate standard, such as a solution, suspension, or other manufactured product [Eq. (2)]:

$$F_{rel} = \frac{AUC_{test}}{AUC_{standard}} \times \frac{dose_{standard}}{dose_{test}} \quad (2)$$

In the clinical setting, it may not be practical to obtain enough data to generate AUC. In these situations, comparisons of the observed maximum concentration and the time to reach that concentration may be used an estimate.

B. Elimination Half-Life

The elimination half-life $t_{1/2}$ is the time it takes plasma concentrations to decrease by one-half during the elimination phase of a drug. Estimates of half-life can be obtained from concentration-time profiles. If logarithmic concentrations are plotted against time, the terminal linear slope can be used to estimate half-life by approximating the time it takes the concentration to decrease by one-half anywhere on the terminal linear line. A more objective approach is to determine the slope β of the best-fit terminal line using a statistical nonlinear method of least-squares regression. Half-life is then calculated using Equation (3):

$$t_{1/2} = \frac{\ln 2}{\beta} \quad (3)$$

Half-life can be used to estimate the time to reach steady-state conditions. Dosing over a time span of approximately five half-lives produces plasma concentrations that are 97% of steady-state concentrations. Similarly, once therapy has been discontinued, a time span equivalent to five half-lives results in a 97% reduction of the body burden.

C. Clearance

Clearance can be defined as the volume of plasma or urine that is cleared of drug over a given period of time and is expressed as volume per unit of time. Clearance can also be viewed as loss of drug across an organ of elimination, such as the liver, kidney, or lung. The latter view has a physiologic meaning that can be used to evaluate the effects of changes in blood flow, plasma protein binding, enzyme activity, or secretory processes on the clearance of a drug. The total clearance Cl of a drug from the body is a function of organ clearance, such as renal or liver, saturated enzyme processes, and protein binding.

Under the simplest conditions in which there is no saturable elimination, Cl is directly proportional to concentration. That is, the amount of drug cleared is equal to the amount of drug delivered to the body:

$$Cl = F_{abs} \frac{dose}{AUC} \tag{4}$$

Hepatic clearance Cl_H can be defined in terms of blood flow Q through the liver and the drug concentration in blood:

$$Cl_H = QE \tag{5}$$

As drug in blood flows through the liver, a certain amount of drug is extracted or cleared such that the amount of drug in blood flowing out of the liver is less than that flowing in. The hepatic extraction ratio E is defined as the concentrations of drug flowing into the liver minus the concentration of drug flowing out of the liver divided by that flowing in.

The hepatic extraction ratio can be further modified to include protein binding and the inherent or intrinsic ability Cl_I of the liver to clear drug:

$$Cl_H = Q \frac{f_u Cl_I}{Q + f_u Cl_I} \qquad (6)$$

In Equation (6), f_u is the unbound fraction of drug in the blood. The limits of Cl_H are dependent upon the Cl_I for a particular drug. If the intrinsic ability of the liver to clear a drug is large, the Cl_H approximates liver blood flow. On the other hand, if the intrinsic ability of the liver to clear drug in small, the Cl_H relates to f_u and Cl_I.

Renal clearance Cl_R of a drug depends upon the physical and chemical properties of the drug, upon plasma protein binding, and upon the physiology of the kidney. There are three factors of renal physiology that control the renal handling of drugs: glomerular filtration, tubular secretion, and tubular reabsorption.

Renal clearance of a drug can be determined by dividing the rate of urinary excretion by the plasma concentration:

$$Cl_R = \frac{UC_u}{tC_p} \qquad (7)$$

In practice, the total volume of urine voided U over the entire time interval t for the elimination of the drug is multiplied by the concentration of drug in that volume C_u and divided by the entire time interval and the plasma concentration determined at the midpoint of that time interval.

D. Apparent Volume of Distribution

Apparent volume of distribution has been misunderstood and misrepresented. The apparent volume of distribution does not represent a true physiologic volume but is in fact a proportionality constant relating drug concentrations in plasma to the amount of drug in the body. True distribution volumes, such as plasma volume, 3 liters, and total body water, 42 liters, as well as other physiologic volumes, can be used as reference points. The apparent volume of distribution can be determined by several means that are dependent on the complexity of the concentration-time profile. For the simple case of a single exponential decline, the apparent volume of distribution V_{app} is described by Equation (8):

$$V_{app} = \frac{Cl}{\beta} \qquad (8)$$

More complex profiles are commonly described by Equation (9) or by other approaches (3).

$$V_{area} = \frac{F \times dose}{\beta \times AUC} \qquad (9)$$

The apparent volume of distribution is influenced by binding. Protein-bound drugs have apparent volumes of distribution that are smaller than the true distribution volume. Tissue-bound drugs have apparent volumes of distribution that are larger than the true distribution volume.

III. INTERFERON PHARMACOKINETICS

There are three famlies of interferons: (α), (β), and (γ). The α interferons can be further divided into subtypes of which 15 have been cloned thus far (6). In addition, the interferons exist as natural or as recombinantly derived moieties. For further delineation of these moieties, the reader is referred to several texts that cover the chemistry in proper detail (7-9).

The development of an assay for determining drug concentrations in biologic fluids and tissues is essential before embarking on any pharmacokinetic program. Without accurate and reliable concentrations, pharmacokinetics is a meaningless discipline. For biologically active moieties, such as interferons, a biologic assay would be the assay of choice. However, bioassays are not practical for routine pharmacokinetic use because precise quantification of serial dilutions becomes labor intensive. Under these circumstances a secondary assay, such as a monoclonal antibody sandwich assay, is more conducive to quantitative assay validation. It is necessary to compare concentrations generated by both assays to ensure that the secondary assay is measuring biologically active material.

A. Animals

The majority of work involving interferons has been with natural or cloned human interferon preparations. Biologic research in animals has been complicated by the species-specific biologic activity shared to some degree by all interferons (7). This is in contrast to most conventional drugs, for which activity in animals is used as an in vivo predictor for similar activity in humans. On the other hand, the pharmacokinetics of conventional drugs commonly demonstrates species-specificity. What is interesting with the interferons is that the overall handling, primarily catabolism and excretion, are similar across most species. This is not surprising if one considers that the handling of proteins is natural to all living creatures. This suggests that animals may serve as suitable models for pharmacokinetics of interferons in humans.

1. Absorption

Absorption in the classic sense refers to oral absorption. Oral absorption of intact proteins, such as the interferons, is unlikely because of the natural proteolytic digestive capabilities of the gastrointestinal tract. As expected, studies in dogs (10) and monkeys (11) showed no measurable serum interferon concentration after administration of an oral solution of recombinant interferon-α. However, Yoshikawa et al. (12,13) presented preliminary evidence of mixed micelle absorption enhancement of interferon-α and β from the large intestine of a rat through the lymphatic system, and Bocci et al. (14) reported enteric absorption of both α and β interferons in rats using an absorption enhancer. Although research is still ongoing in the area of oral delivery of peptides and proteins, success is not anticipated in the near future for large proteins, such as interferons.

Alternate sites for absorption have been explored with the interferons. The systemic absorption of interferons from sites other than the gastrointestinal tract has been remarkably good considering the size of these molecules. The α and β interferons have shown the greatest success for absorption. Absorption of α interferons from intramuscular (10,11,15-19), subcutaneous (10,15), intraperitoneal (15,20), intradermal (21), duodenal (16), and rectal (16) sites has been reported. In general, interferon-α absorption from these sites is prolonged. Maximum plasma or serum concentrations occur 1-6 hr postinjection, followed by measurable concentrations through 8-24 hr postinjection. The concentration-time profile appears to be independent of the purity of source of interferon-α, that is, partially purified (17,19,20), natural (15,16), or recombinant (11,18,22). In addition, the disposition profiles (Fig. 1) are similar across the tested species of mice (15,20), rabbits (16,19,22), dogs (10), and monkeys (11,17, 18). Several of these studies have determined the absolute bioavailability from the intramuscular site in dogs, 42% (10), and monkeys, 93% (11) and 56% (18).

The absorption of interferon-β from intramuscular (14,23-28), subcutaneous (16), and intraperitoneal (25) sites is similar to that of α interferons. The concentration profiles (Fig. 1) are also similar to that seen with interferon-α, namely, prolonged absorption with concentrations persisting from 9 to 24 hr after injection. Again, absorption appears to be independent of species and interferon source. Estimates of absolute bioavailability from the intramuscular site can be obtained from published data: 60% in rats (20), 33% (24) and 60% (23) in rabbits, and 43% in monkeys (24). Recently, a bioavailability of 2.2% was reported for interferon-β following intranasal administration to rabbits (29).

The absorption of interferon-γ has not been studied as extensively as that of the α and β interferons. In relevant papers by Cantell et al. (19,30), absorption from an intramuscular site and from subcutaneous sites was observed in rabbits and monkeys after injection of natural human interferon-γ. The resultant profiles (Fig. 1) were similar to that observed with interferon-α with concentrations measurable through 7-9 hr (30) and at least 24 hr (19) postinjection. In contrast, serum concentrations were very low or nondetectable following intramuscular injection of nonglycosylated interferon-γ in monkeys (31).

PHARMACOKINETICS OF INTERFERONS

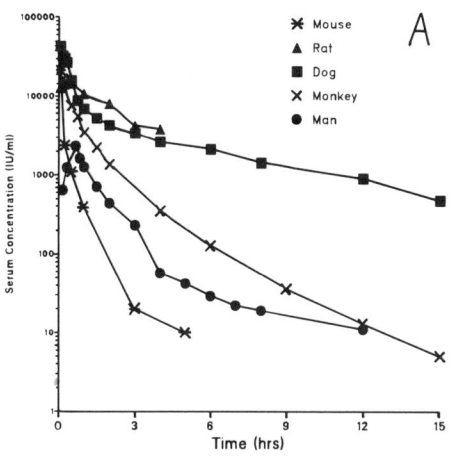

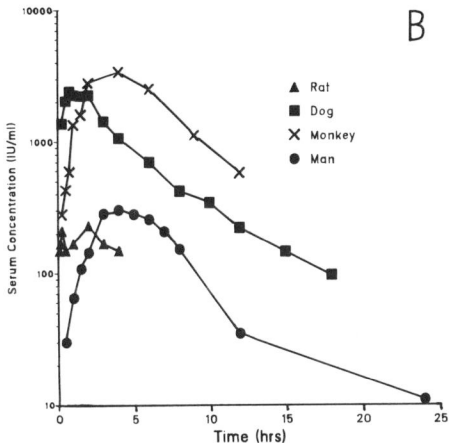

Figure 1 Serum concentrations of recombinant human interferon-α following intravenous (A) and intramuscular (B) doses of 7.65×10^5 IU to mice (32), 5×10^6 IU/kg to rats (35), 3×10^6 IU/kg to dogs (10), 3×10^6 IU/kg to monkeys (11), and 36×10^6 IU to humans (65). Serum concentrations of recombinant human interferon-β following intravenous (C) and intramuscular (D) doses of 5×10^6 IU/kg to rats (35) and 10^7 IU/kg to rabbits (24) and monkeys (24). Serum concentrations of recombinant human interferon-γ following intravenous (E) and intramuscular (F) doses of 3×10^5 IU to rabbits (30), 3×10^5 IU to monkeys (30), and 50×10^6 IU/m² to humans (75).

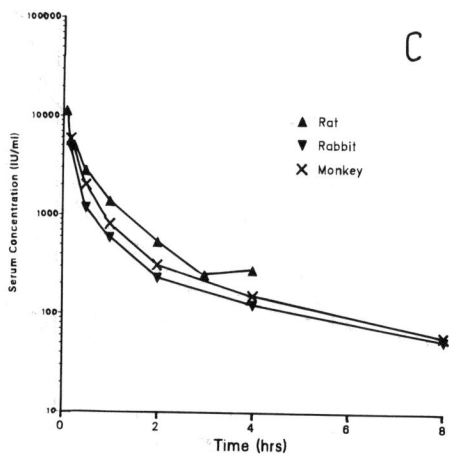

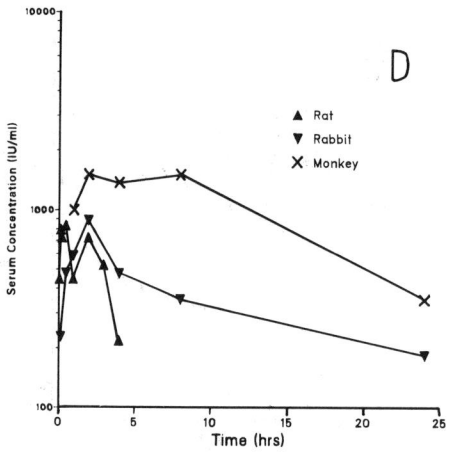

Figure 1 (continued).

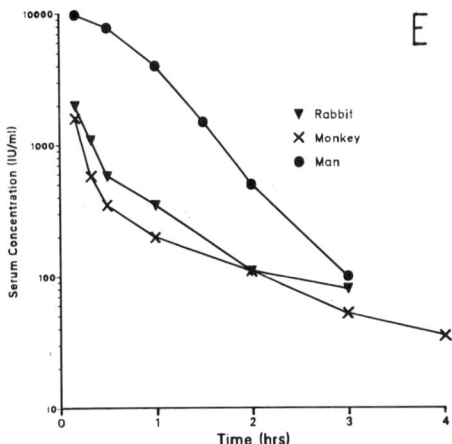

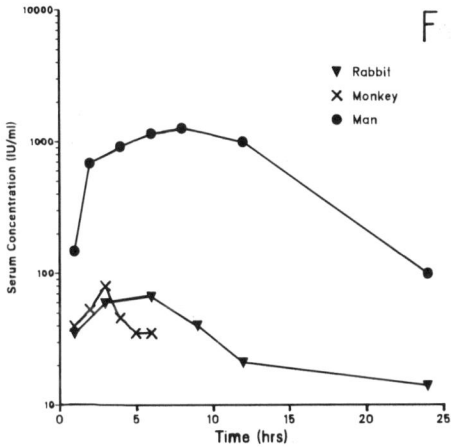

Figure 1 (continued).

2. Distribution

The initial decline in serum concentrations following intravenous administration, independent of the species used, is rapid for α, β, and γ interferons (10,11,18,23–26,30,32–34). The half-lives of this initial distribution are of the order of minutes. Serum concentrations (Fig. 1) then decline more slowly with terminal elimination half-lives ranging from minutes—30–40 min for interferon-α in mice (32)—to hours—7–12 hr for interferon-β in rabbits (23,24)—depending on the species selected and the type of interferon given (10,11,18,23,24,30,32,33,35).

The distribution of α and β interferons is similar. Both α and β interferon have a volume of distribution following intravenous administration that ranges from 20 to 100% of body weight in mice (32), rats (25), rabbits (23,24,33), dogs (10), and monkeys (11,18), suggesting distribution into a volume that approximates total body water. There is no reason to think interferon-γ would behave any differently, but there are no data at this time.

The tissue content of the interferons generally parallels that found in serum or plasma. Measurable concentrations or titers of the interferons have been demonstrated in brain (20,32), spleen (20,25,27,32), lung (20,25,27,32), liver (20,22,32,34), and kidney (25,32,34). For β and γ interferon, the amount of interferon determined in specific organs or tissue reflected the amount found in the serum or plasma, suggesting no uptake of these interferons into the sample organs or tissues (25,34). The tissue distribution of interferon-α has been mixed. Heremans et al. (20) reported liver, lung, and spleen uptake of intraperitoneally administered homologous mouse interferon-α in mice that had implications for the uptake of a species-active interferon-α. In contrast, Bohoslawec et al (32) showed no appreciable uptake into brain, liver, lung, or spleen following intravenous administration of mouse murine interferon-α to mice. However, the kidney showed an appreciable uptake of mouse murine interferon-α. In that same paper (32), two human α subtypes, A and D, and one human hybrid, A/D (Bgl), displayed a tissue distribution profile (Fig. 2) similar to that of biologically active mouse murine interferon-α, supporting the species-independent pharmacokinetic behavior of α interferons.

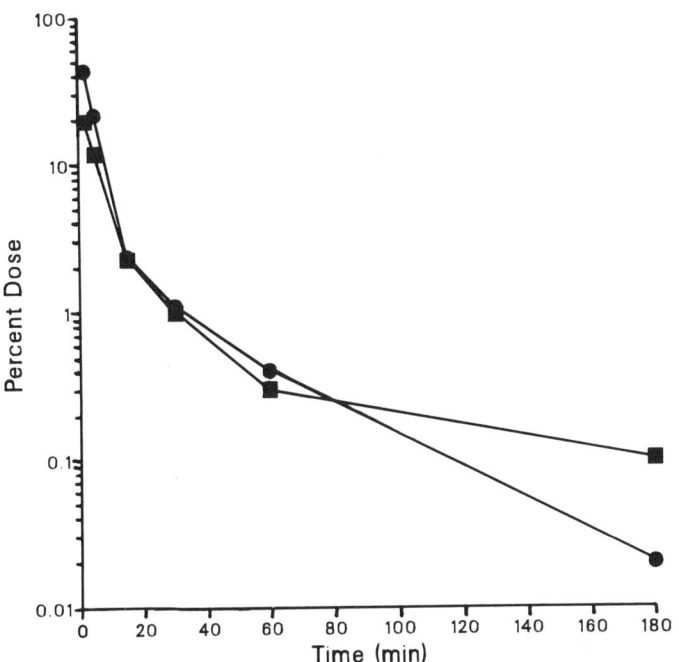

Figure 2 Total interferon-α serum content as a percentage of the administered intravenous dose of recombinant human interferon-α (●, 7.6×10^5 IU) and mouse murine interferon-α (■, 8.7×10^5 IU) (32).

Owing to the potential clinical benefit of a central nervous system (CNS)-active molecule and to the understanding of the CNS adverse drug reactions common to interferons, cerebrospinal fluid (CSF) penetration has been an area of special interest. Penetration of CSF could be achieved with high intravenous doses of both α and β interferons (17,18,25,26,36). However, the data are clear in that α and β interferons do not readily penetrate the CSF. Given the failure of interferon to readily cross the blood-brain barrier, some workers have elected to explore intrathecal or intraventricular administration (18,26). High concentrations of α and β interferon in the CSF were obtained, with measurable concentrations persisting through 24-48 hr (Fig. 3). Billiau (37)

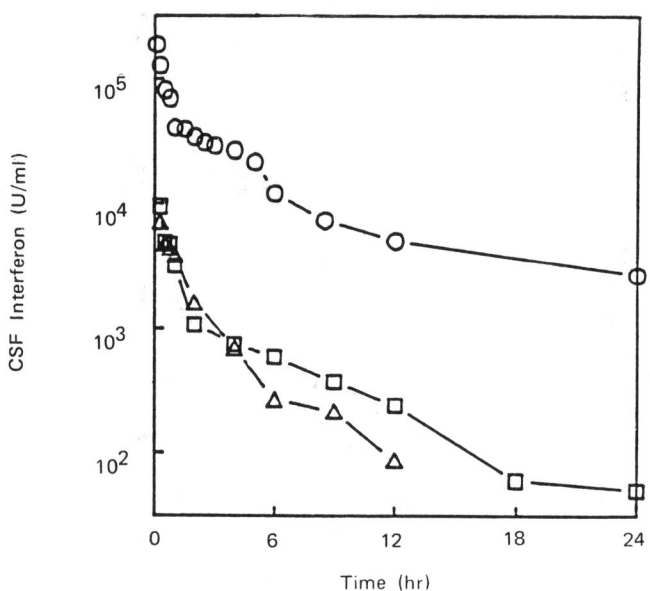

Figure 3 Cerebrospinal concentrations of rIFN-αA following intraventricular doses of 5000 IU/kg to two monkeys (□, △) and 120,000 IU/kg to one monkey (○) (18).

found that interferon-β equilibrated throughout the CSF pathway after intrathecal injection to monkeys, but upon sacrifice at 3 hr postadministration, interferon was not detected in the substance of the brain. Re-examining this question, Smith and Landel sought to map the action of interferon in the brain using molecular biologic techniques (38). Partially purified interferon-α was administered to juvenile Rhesus monkeys as a 7.5×10^6 IU intravenously or 1×10^6 IU intracisternally. Analysis of brain tissue suggested that interferon could reach the parenchyma of the brain from both the vascular and CSF compartments. Thus, the intrathecal or intraventricular route of administration may provide an alternate route to systemic delivery insofar as attaining high interferon concentrations in the CSF. There are no data regarding interferon-γ.

3. Catabolism

The catabolism, or breakdown to by-products that are then biochemically reused, of interferons has been the most widely researched area of interferon pharmacokinetics. Not suprisingly, the interferons are handled in a manner similar to that used for other proteins of the same size. Most of the work detailing the physiologic handling of plasma proteins was done beginning in the late 1960s and continuing through today. A good review is provided by Maack et al. (39). Another important aspect of protein catabolism is that it is similar across all species.

Undoubtedly, the most effective and efficient system for catabolizing proteins is the gastrointestinal tract. However, restricting this discussion to internal systems, the kidney becomes the major catabolizing organ for low-molecular-weight ($<$60,000 daltons) proteins (40). The liver has been shown to play a role in the catabolism of glycosylated proteins (41). Other organs and tissue, such as the lungs and muscle, are thought to play minor roles in protein catabolism (42).

The catabolism of the three types of interferon, whether natural or cloned, falls within the natural handling of proteins. The catabolism of interferon-a including subtypes, has been the most extensively studied of the three types. In general, a interferons are filtered through the glomeruli of the kidney via luminal endocytosis followed by proximal tubular reabsorption (43–47). During reabsorption, the a interferons undergo proteolytic degradation by lysosomal enzymes (46–49), rendering negligible amounts of intact interferon-a excreted in the urine. Several studies assessed the effect of nephrectomy on the pharmacokinetics of interferon-a. As expected, the clearance of interferon-a was significantly decreased (Fig. 4) in nephrectomized rabbits (45) and rats (35). Consistent with these findings, the liver has been shown to play a small role in the catabolism of a interferons (50,51).

Both β and γ interferons undergo renal catabolism (34,51,52) but to a much smaller extent than the a interferons. The work generated thus far suggests that liver catabolism is the predominant pathway of elimination (34,51) for β and γ interferons.

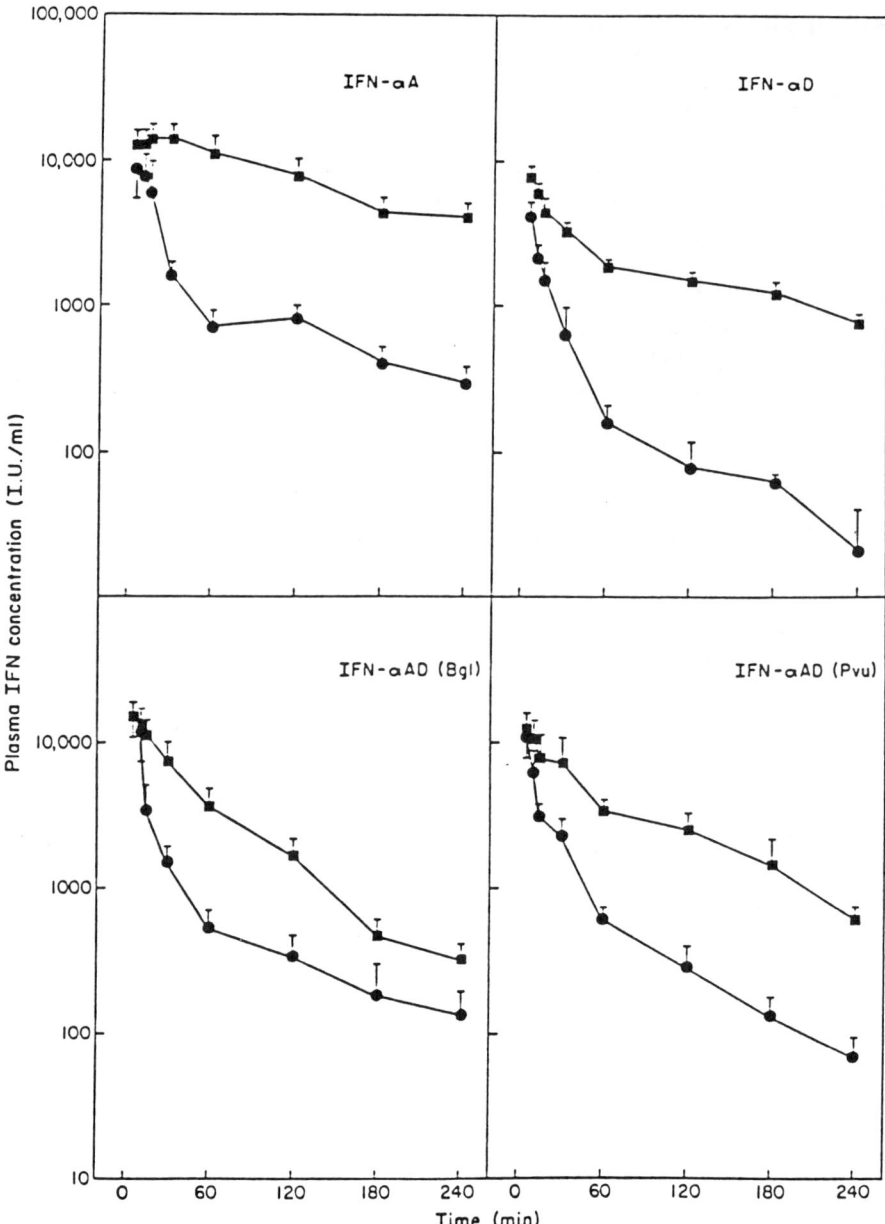

Figure 4 Plasma concentrations of recombinant human a interferons following a 5×10^6 IU/kg injection to sham-operated (●) and bilaterally nephrectomized rats (■) (35).

Natural β and γ interferon contain sialic acids groups, classifying them as glycosylated proteins. The literature supports liver catabolism of glycosylated proteins (40). In one study (35), the clearance of interferon-β, both natural (glycosylated) and cloned, was unaltered in nephrectomized rats, supporting a nonrenal pathway for catabolism. Other organs, such as lung and muscle, have been suggested as potential catabolic sites for interferons. A more detailed review of interferon catabolism is provided by Bocci (53). In contrast to the catabolic profile of interferons, there has been evidence that recombinant subtypes of α interferons reduce hepatic drug metabolism activity in mice (54-56). Further, it has been demonstrated that the greater the antiviral activity of a given clone in murine cells, the greater is the ability to depress hepatic microsomal cytochrome P_{450} content in the mouse (54).

B. Human

In the 1970s, human testing of interferons was restricted by the limited availability, purity (generally less than 1%), and specific activity (of the order of 10^6 U/mg of protein) of interferon material. The advent of genetic engineering in 1980, permitting the production of interferon using recombinant DNA technology, made available highly pure (99+%) and highly specific (2×10^8 U/mg of protein) preparations for large-scale human testing (6). Human leukocyte interferon was the first preparation available. Early phase I studies targeted a host of viral and oncologic diseases with the intent of establishing the safety, tolerance, pharmacokinetics, and efficacy of interferon (57-64). Although the clinical results were often disappointing, it was learned that the route and the rate of administration were important treatment variables.

The pharmacokinetic profiles of interferons vary considerably with the route of administration, as was observed in animals. The route-dependent differences in the concentration-time profiles, which actually reflect the rate of delivery, govern the safety and efficacy profiels (Fig. 5). During the early investigations of recombinant interferon-α, it was quickly realized that intravenous administration, despite the large serum concentrations, was better

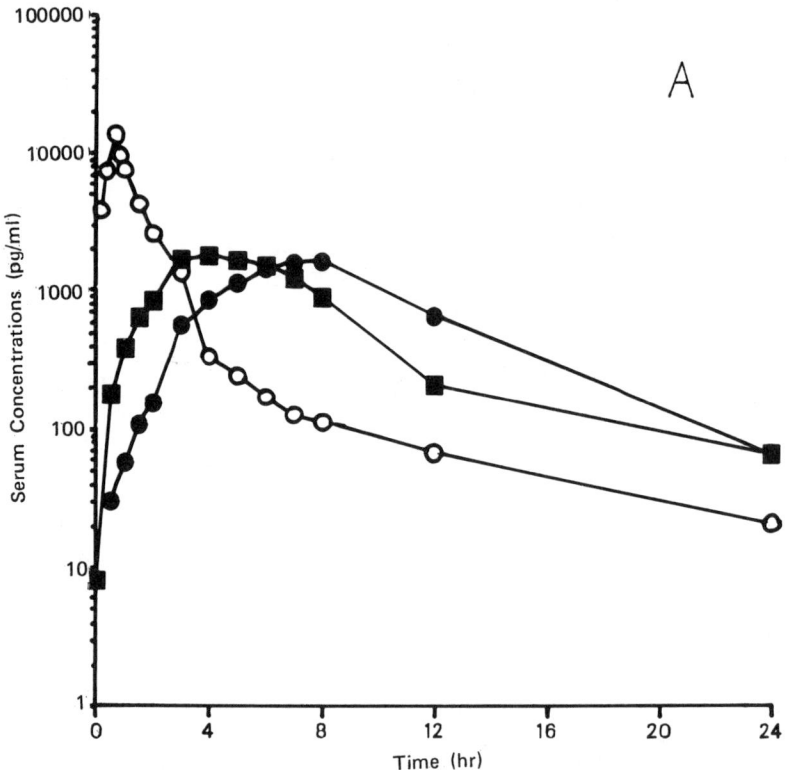

Figure 5 (A) Mean serum recombinant human interferon-a concentrations after a 36×10^6 IU dose given as a 40 min infusion (○), intramuscular injection (□), or subcutaneous injection (●). (B) Corresponding mean change in body temperature after infusion (○), intramuscular (□), or subcutaneous (○) injections (65).

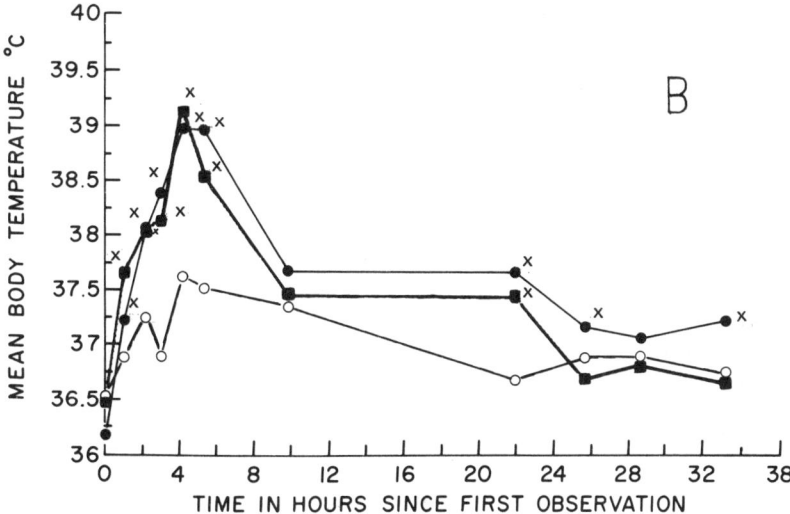

Figure 5 (Continued).

tolerated than intramuscular and subcutaneous injections (65,66). This was subsequently demonstrated for γ interferons as well. Recently, data from a preliminary study were presented that claimed improved tolerance after continuous subcutaneous infusion of interferon-α at doses up to 18×10^6 IU/day in patients with either hypernephroma or malignant melanoma (67).

Other routes of administration have been studied, including intrathecal (68), intraventricular (68-70), intralesional (71), and intranasal (72-74). Dosage regimens and routes of administration currently being evaluated in the clinic were selected empirically. As recently as 1985, phase I studies utilizing the newly available recombinant interferon-γ were geared toward assessing the merits of different routes of administration (75-77). Although many dosage regimens have been evaluated (59-61,66,78) in a variety of disease states, it is very clear that our understanding of the most favorable way of administering interferons is limited. This undoubtedly reflects our lack of knowledge of the inherent mechanisms of interferon action. The reader is referred to References 53 and 79, which provide greater detail in this area.

1. Absorption

The results have been similar to those seen in animals (Fig. 1). Intramuscular and subcutaneous administrations of interferon-α (65,66,80) and nonglycosylated interferon-γ (75) are well absorbed: >80% for interferon-α and 30-70% for interferon-γ. These routes exhibit protracted absorption, which results in maximum serum or plasma concentrations 1-8 hr postinjection followed by measurable concentrations through 4-24 hr for both α (65,66,80) and γ (75) interferons. Maximum serum concentrations following these routes of administration are at least an order of magnitude less than the highest concentration after an equal dose given intravenously. The absorption of interferon-β from muscle or skin has not been adequate enough to produce serum concentrations much above assay detection (28,69).

2. Distribution and Catabolism

Serum interferon concentrations decline rapidly in a biexponential, for interferon-α (28,65,66,80,81), or monoexponential, for interferon-γ (75-77), manner following intravenous administration. Initial interferon concentrations are known to fall several orders of magnitude over the measurable serum concentration-time course (Fig. 1). Terminal elimination half-lives range from 4 to 16 hr for α (66,66,80,81) and from 25 to 35 min for γ (75-77). Serum concentrations are generally measurable for 8-24 hr and up to 4 hr after injection of interferon-α (65,66,80,81) and interferon-γ (75-77), respectively. At this time, only preliminary data following intravenous administration of interferon-β to humans have been reported.

The volume of distribution is similar for both α and γ interferons, ranging from 12 to 40 liters (65,66,75,76,80). Although this volume is not physiologic it approximates 20-60% of body weight, which is similar to that observed in animals. Again, information regarding interferon-β has not been reported.

There has not been a great deal of research investigating the tissue distribution of interferons in humans. Most of this work was restricted to animals. One area that has been studied is that of penetration across the blood-brain barrier (68,81,83,84). Similar to that reported in animals, partially purified (68), natural (83), or recombinant (81,84) interferon-α does not readily cross the blood-brain barrier intact after intravenous, intramuscular, or subcutaneous administration (Table 1). These data must ultimately be reconciled with the occurrence of neurotoxicity, a common side effect of interferon therapy. Since the spinal fluid titers of interferon represent an average value, it is possible that CSF values do not faithfully mirror tissue concentrations at all sites. In the areas of the brain without a blood-brain barrier, particularly in parts of the hypothalamus and brain stem, interferon may reach high concentrations after systemic administration. To obtain data on the intraventricular route of administration, Smith et al. administered interferon-α via an Ommaya reservoir to patients with amyotrophic lateral sclerosis (68). A relatively high concentration in the CSF could be achieved (Table 2), and as expected, interferon was seen to wash out of the ventricles. It circulated freely as judged by its appearance in the lumbar CSF, where it could be detected at approximately 12 hr after dosing. As late as 24 hr after dosing, the lumbar CSF still contained interferon whereas the ventricular concentration was not measurable. It is assumed, but not proven, that intraventricularly administered interferon circulates over the hemispheres following the normal CSF pathway. Based on these studies, the estimated half-life of intraventricularly administered interferon-α is similar to that of systemically administered interferon at approximately 6 hr. When interferon was injected intrathetically, no measurable concentrations of interferon were detected in ventricular CSF.

Many studies have focused on the presence of natural interferon in a variety of diseases. Unfortunately, there is no good reference that collates this information. The point is that the presence of endogenous interferon has been detected in tissue and fluids of a wide variety of seemingly unrelated diseases. For example, interferon has been found in the brain (85) and CSF (86) of patients with multiple sclerosis, in the lesions of patients with recurrent herpes labialis (87) and psoriasis (88), and in the synovial fluid of patients with rheumatoid arthritis (89). The clinical relevance of these findings has yet to be determined.

Table 1 Titers in Serum and CSF After Intravenous Infusion of rIFN-αA

	rIFN-αA dose[b]			
	18×10^6 U		50×10^6 U	
Time	Serum (pg/ml)	Ventricular CSF (pg/ml)	Serum (pg/ml)	Ventricular CSF (pg/ml)
0	<23[b]	<15	<15	<15
5 min	5440 ± 775	—	21,000 ± 940	—
10 min	9340 ± 945	—	38,000 ± 2150	—
15 min	5260 ± 1050	—	35,100 ± 3290	—
30 min	2570 ± 1050	<15	18,900 ± 2240	<15
60 min	1150 ± 400	<15	9,900 ± 870	50
2 hr	430 ± 190	<15	3,210 ± 250	45
4 hr	170 ± 60	<15	595 ± 155	35
8 hr	55 ± 35	<15	165 ± 60	20
12 hr	35 ± 20	<15	95 ± 60	15
24 hr	—[c]	<15	30 ± 20	20
48 hr	—[c]	<15	—[c]	<15

[a]Data are $\bar{X}$ ± SE.
[b]One subject had elevated baseline serum rIFN-αA titers.
[c]An average was not computed when rILF-αA levels were undetectable in one or more subjects.
Source: From Reference 81.

Table 2 Cerebrospinal Concentrations (IU/ml) of Interferon-a After Intraventricular Administration

Time (hr)	Dose IU[a]				
	250,000	500,000		1,000,000	
	V	V	L	V	L
0	0	0		0	
2	<20	3900		3000	
4	3500	1400		2000	
8	1925	7500		350	350
12	<20	<20	350	35	200
24	<20	<20		<20	
48	<20	<20		<20	

[a]Ventricular (V) and lumbar (L).
Source: From Reference 68.

IV. CONCLUSION

As a result of technical advances, pharmacokinetic and clinical studies are now conducted with sensitive assays and highly purified interferons. To date, clinical success with interferons, albeit modest, has mostly been a matter of trial and error. Although clinical insight and perhaps fortune may continue to influence the outcome of clinical trials, there is reason to believe that the pharmacokinetic behavior of interferons is an important treatment variable—one that may not be fully appreciated in the case of neurologic disorders. As these and other considerations shape treatment strategies, it is likely that biomodulators will assume a respected place in the therapy of neurologic diseases that are incurable at present.

REFERENCES

1. Wagner, J. G. In: *Fundamentals of Clinical Pharmacokinetics.* Drug Intelligence Publications, Hamilton, Illinois (1975).

2. Rowland, M., and Tozer, T. N. In: *Clinical Pharmacokinetics.* Lea and Febiger, Philadelphia (1980).

3. Gibaldi, M., and Perrier, D. In: *Pharmacokinetics,* 2nd ed., Marcel Dekker, New York (1982).

4. Benet, L. F., Massoud, N., and Gambertoglio, J. G. (eds). In: *Pharmacokinetic Basis for Drug Treatment.* Raven Press, New York (1984).

5. Food and Drug Administration, *Fed. Regis. 42*:1638 (1977).

6. Goeddel, D. V., Yelverton, E., Ullrick, A., Heynecker, H. L., Miozzari, G., Holmes, R., Seeburg, P. H., Tabor, J. M., Gross, M., Familleti, P. C., and Pestka, S. Human leukocyte interferon produced by *E. coli* is biologically active. *Nature 287*:411-416 (1980).

7. Stewart, W. E., II. In: *The Interferon System.* Springer-Verlag, New York (1981).

8. Stringfellow, D. A. (ed.). In: *Interferon and Interferon Inducers.* Marcel Dekker, New York (1980).

9. Baron, S., Dianzani, F., and Stanton, G. J. (eds.). In: *The Interferon System: A Review to 1982—Parts I and II.* University of Texas Medical Branch, Galveston (1982).

10. Gibson, D. M., Cotler, S., Speigel, H. E., and Colburn, W. A. Pharmacokinetics of recombinant leukocyte A interferon following various routes of and modes of administration to the dog. *J. Interferon Res. 5*:403-408 (1985).

11. Wills, R. J., Spiegel, H. E., and Soike, K. F. Pharmacokinetics of recombinant leukocyte A interferon following iv infusion and bolus, im, and po administration to African green monkeys. *J. Interferon Res. 4*:399-409 (1984).

12. Yoshikawa, H., Takada, K., Satoh, Y., Naruse, N., and Muranishi, S.

Potentiation of enteral absorption of human interferon alpha and selective transfer into lymphatics in rats. *Pharm. Res. 2*:249-250 (1985).

13. Yoshikawa, H., Takada, K., Muranishi, S., Satoh, Y., and Naruse, N. A method to potentiate enteral absorption of interferon and selective delivery into lymphatics. *J. Pharm. Dyn. 7*:59-62 (1984).

14. Bocci, V., Corradeschi, F., Naldini, A., and Lencioni, E. Enteric absorption of human interferon α and β in the rat. *Int. J. Pharm. 34*:111-114 (1986).

15. Sarkar, F. H. Pharmacokinetic comparison of leukocyte and *Escheria coli*-derived human interferon type alpha. *Antiviral Res. 2*:103-106 (1982).

16. Naito, S., Tanaka, S., Mizuno, M., and Kawashima, H. Concentrations of human interferons α and β in rabbit body fluids. *Int. J. Pharm. 18*: 117-125 (1984).

17. Habif, D. V., Lipton, R., and Cantell, K. Interferon crosses blood-cerebrospinal fluid barrier in monkeys. *Proc. Soc Exp. Biol. Med. 149*:287-289 (1975).

18. Collins, J. M., Riccardi, R., Trown, P., O'Neill, D., and Poplack, D. G. Plasma and cerebrospinal fluid pharmacokinetics of recombinant interferon alpha A in monkeys: Comparison of intravenous, intramuscular and intraventricular delivery. *Cancer Drug Delivery 2*:247-253 (1985).

19. Cantell, K., Fiers, W., Hirvonen, S., and Pyhala, L. Circulating interferon in rabbits after simultaneous intramuscular administration of human alpha and gamma interferon. *J. Interferon Res. 4*:291-292 (1984).

20. Heremans, H., Billiau, A., and DeSorner, P. Interferon in experimental viral infection in mice: Tissue interferon levels resulting from virus infection and from exogenous interferon therapy. *Infect. Immun. 30*: 513-522 (1980).

21. Bocci, V., Muscettola, M., and Naldini, A. The lymphatic route. IV. Pharmacokinetics of human recombinant interferon α_2 and natural interferon β administered intradermally in rabbits. *Int. J. Pharm. 32*: 103-110 (1986).

22. Bocci, V., Muscettola, M., Naldini, A., Bianchi, E., and Segre, G. The lymphatic route. II. Pharmacokinetics of human recombinant interferon-α_2 injected with albumin as a retarder in rabbits. *Gen. Pharmacol. 17*:93-96 (1986).

23. Satoh, Y., Kasama, K., Kajita, A., Shinizer, H., and Ida, N. Different

pharmacokinetics between natural and recombinant human interferon beta in rabbits. *J. Interferon Res.* 4:411-422 (1984).

24. Gomi, K., Morimoto, M., Inoue, A., Kobayashi, H., Deguchi, T., Hara, T. and Nakamizo, N. Pharmacokinetics of human recombinant interferon-β in monkeys and rabbits. *Gann* 75:292-300 (1984).

25. Abreu, S. L. Pharmacokinetics of rat fibroblast interferon. *J Pharmacol. Exp. Ther.* 226:197-220 (1983).

26. Hilfenhaus, J., Damm, H., Hofstaetter, T., Mauler, R., Ronneberger, H., and Weinmann, E. Pharmacokinetics of human interferon-beta in monkeys. *J. Interferon Res.* 1:427-436 (1981).

27. Billiau, A., Heremans, H., Ververken, D., Van Damme, J., Carton, H., and de Somer, P. Tissue distribution of human interferon after exogenous administration in rabbits, monkeys and mice. *Arch. Virol.* 68:19-25 (1981).

28. Billiau, A., de Somer, P., Edy, V. G., de Clercq E., and Heremans, H. Human fibroblast interferon for clinical trials: Pharmacokinetics and tolerability in experimental animals and humans. *Antimicrob. Agents Chemother.* 16:56-63 (1979).

29. Maitani, Y., Igawa, T., Machida, Y., and Nagai, T. Intranasal administration of β-interferon in rabbits. *Drug Design Delivery* 1:65-70 (1986).

30. Cantell, K., Hirvonen, S., Pyhala, L., De Reus, A., and Schellekens, H. Circulating interferon in rabbit and monkeys after administration of human gamma interferon by different routes. *J. Gen. Virol.* 64:1823-1826 (1983).

31. Weck, P. K., Shalaby, M. R., Apperson, S., Gray, P. W., and Goeddel, D. V. Comparative biological properties of human alpha, beta and gamma IFN's derived from bacteria. Abstracts of the Third International Congress for Interferon Research, Miami, Florida (1982).

32. Bohoslawec, O., Trown, P. W., and Wills, R. J. Pharmacokinetics and tissue distribution of recombinant human A, D., A/D (Bgl) and I interferons and mouse alpha-interferon in mice. *J. Interferon Res.* 6:207-213 (1986).

33. Bocci, V., Pessina, G. P., Pacini, A., Paulesu, L., Muscettola, M., Naldini, A. and Lunghetti, G. Pharmacokinetics of human lymphoblastoid interferon in rabbits. *Gen. Pharmacol.* 16:277-279 (1985).

34. Bocci, V., Pacini, A., Pessina, G. P., Paulesu, L., Muscettola, M. and

Lunghetti, G. Catobolic sites of human interferon-γ. *J. Gen. Virol. 66*: 887-891 (1985).

35. Tokazewski-Chen, S. A., Marafino, B. J., Jr., and Stebbing, N. Effects of nephrectomy on the pharmacokinetics of various cloned human interferons in rats. *J. Pharmacol. Exp. Ther. 227*:9-15 (1983).

36. Jablecki, C. K., Poplack, D., Howell, S., Kingsbury, D., and Cantell, K. High-dose intravenous infusions of interferon. *Neurology (N.Y.) 33*:141-142 (1983).

37. Billiau, A. Interferon therapy: Pharmacokinetic and pharmacological aspects. *Arch. Virol. 67*:121-133 (1981).

38. Smith, R. A., and Landel, C. P. In: *The Biology of the Interferon System 1986* (K. Cantell and H. Schellekens, eds.). Martinus Nijhoff, Dordricht, pp. 563-566 (1987).

39. Maack, T., Johnson, V., Kan, S. T., Figueiredo, J., and Sigulem, D. Renal filtration, transport and metabolism of low-molecular weight proteins: A review. *Kidney Int. 16*:251-270 (1979).

40. Ashwell, G., and Morell, A. G. In: *Advance in Enzymology* (A. Meister, ed.), Vol. 41. John Wiley & Sons, New York, pp. 99-128 (1974).

41. Bose, S., and Hickman, J. Role of the carbohydrate moiety in determining the survival of interferon in the circulation. *J. Biol. Chem. 252*:8336-8337 (1977).

42. Fishman, A. P., and Pietra, G. G. Handling of bioactive materials by the lung. *N. Engl. J. Med. 291*:884-890 (1974).

43. Bocci, V., Pacini, A., Muscettola, M., Pessina, G. P., Paulesu, L., and Bandinellim L. The kidney is the main site of interferon catabolism. *J. Interferon Res. 2*:309-314 (1982).

44. Bocci, V., Pacini, A., Muscettola, M., Paulesu, L., Pessina, G. P., Santiano, M., and Viano, I. Renal filtration absorption and catabolism of human alpha interferon. *J. Interferon Res. 1*:347-352 (1981).

45. Bocci, V., Pacini, A., Muscettola, M., Paulesu, L., and Pessina, G. P. Renal metabolism of rabbit serum interferon. *J. Gen. Virol. 55*:297-304 (1981).

46. Bino, T., Edery, H., Gertler, A., and Rosenberg, H. Involvement of the kidney in catabolism of human leukocyte interferon. *J. Gen. Virol. 59*: 39-45 (1982).

47. Bino, T., Madar, Z., Gertler, A., and Rosenberg, H. The kidney is the main site of interferon degradation. *J. Interferon Res.* 2:301-308 (1982).

48. Bocci, V., Maunsboch, A. B., and Mogensen, E. K. Autoradiographic demonstration of human ^{125}I-interferon alpha in lysosomes of rabbit proximal tubule cells. *J. Submiscrosc. Cytol.* 16:753-757 (1984).

49. Rosenberg, H., Madar, F., Gertler, A., Rubinstein, M., and Bino, T. The fate of ^{125}I-labeled human leukocyte-derived alpha interferon in the rat. *J. Interferon Res.* 5:121-127 (1985).

50. Bocci, V., Mogensen, K. E., Muscettola, M., Pacini, A., Paulesu, L., Pessina, G. P., and Skiftas, S. Degradation of human ^{125}I-interferon alpha by isolated perfused rabbit kidney and liver. *J. Lab. Clin. Med.* 101:857-863 (1983).

51. Bocci, V., Pacini, A., Bandinelli, L., Pessina, G. P., Muscettola, M., and Paulesu, L. The role of liver in the catabolism of human α- and β-interferon. *J. Gen. Virol.* 60:397-400 (1982).

52. Bocci, V., Di Francesco, P., Pacini, A., Pessina, G. P., Rossi, G. B., and Sorrentino, V. Renal metabolism of homologous serum interferon. *Antiviral Res.* 3:53-58 (1983).

53. Bocci, V. Distribution, catabolism, and pharmacokinetics of interferons. In: *In Vivo and Clinical Fluids* (N. B. Finter and R. K. Oldham, eds.), Vol. 4. Elsevier, New York, pp. 47-72 (1985).

54. Parkinson, A., Lasker, J., Kramer, M. L., Huang, M. T., Thomas, P. E., Ryan, D. E., Reik, L. M., Norman, R. L., Levin, W., and Conney, A. H. Effects of three recombinant human leukocyte interferons on drug metabolism in mice. *Drug Metab. Dispos.* 10:579-585 (1982).

55. Secor, J., and Schenker, S. Effect of recombinant α-interferon on in vivo and in vitro markers of drug metabolism in mice. *Hepatology* 4:1081 (1984).

56. Taylor, G., Marafino, B. J., Jr., Moore, J. A., Gurley, V., and Blaschke, T. F. Interferon reduces hepatic drug metabolism in vivo in mice. *Drug Metab. Dispos.* 13:459-463 (1985).

57. Gutterman, J. U., Fine, S., Quesada, J., Horning, S. J., Levine, J. F., Alexanian, R., Bernhardt, L., Kramer, M., Speigel, H., Colburn, W., Trown, P., Merrigan, T., and Dziewanowski, F. Recombinant leukocyte A interferon: Pharmacokinetics, single-dose tolerance, and biologic effects in cancer patients. *Ann. Intern. Med.* 96:549-556 (1982).

58. Sherwin, S. A., Knost, J. A., Fein, S., Abrams, P. G., Foon, K. A., Ochs,

J. J., Schoenberger, C., Mauluish, A. E., and Oldham, R. K. A multiple-dose phase I trial of recombinant leukocyte A interferon in cancer patients. *JAMA 248*:2461-2466 (1982).

59. Sherwin, S. A., Mayer, D., Ochs, J. J., Abrams, P. G., Knost, J. A., Foon, K. A., Fein, S., and Oldham, R. K. Recombinant leukocyte A interferon in advanced breast cancer. *Ann. Intern. Med. 98*:598-602 (1983).

60. Quesada, J. R., and Gutterman, J. U. Clinical study of recombinant DNA-produced leukocyte interferon (Clone A) in an intermittent schedule in cancer patients. *JNCI 70*:1041-1046 (1983).

61. Krown, S. E., Real, F. X., Cunningham-Rundles, S., Myskowski, P. L., Koziner, B., Fein, S., Mittleman, A., Oettgen, H. F., and Safai, B. Preliminary observations on the effect of recombinant leukocyte A interferon in homosexual mean with Kaposi's sarcoma. *N. Engl. J. Med. 308*:1071-1076 (1983).

62. Smith, C. I., Weissberg, J., Bernhardt, L., Gregory, P. B., Robinson, W. S., and Merigan, T. C. Acute dane particle suppression with recombinant leukocyte A interferon in chronic hepatitis β virus infection. *J. Infect. Dis. 148*:907-913 (1983).

63. Hawkins, M. J., Borden, E. C., Merritt, J. A., Edwards, B. S., Ball, L. A., Grossbard, E., and Simon, K. J. Comparison of the biological effects of two recombinant human interferon alpha (rA and rD) in humans. *J. Clin. Oncol. 2*:221-226 (1984).

64. Nethersell, A., Smedley, H., Katrak, M., Wheeler, T., and Sikora, K. Recombinant interferon in advanced breast cancer. *Br. J. Cancer 49*: 615-620 (1984).

65. Wills, R. J., Dennis, S., Spiegel, H. E., Gibson, D. M., and Nadler, P. I. Interferon kinetics and adverse reactions after intravenous, intramuscular and subcutaneous injection. *Clin. Pharmacol. Ther. 35*:722-727 (1984).

66. Shah, I., Bond, J., Samson, M., Young, J., Robinson, R., Bailey, R., Lerner, A. M., and Prasad, A. S. Pharmacokinetics and tolerance of intravenous and intramuscular recombinant alpha-2 interferon in patients with malignancies. *Am. J. Hematol. 17*:363-371 (1984).

67. Ludwig, C. U., Stoll, H. R., Obrist, R., Sutter, C., and Obrecht, J. P. Improved tolerance of interferon by continuous subcutaneous infusion. *Proc. Am. Soc. Clin. Oncol. 5*:234 (1986).

68. Smith, R. A., Kingsbury, D., Alksne, J., James, H., and Cantell, K. Distribution of interferon in cerebrospinal fluid after systemic, intrathecal, and intraventricular administration. *Ann. Neurol. 12*:81 (1982).

69. Quesada, J. R., Gutterman, J. U., and Hersh, E. M. Clinical and immunological study of beta interferon by intramuscular route in patients with metastatic breast cancer. *J. Interferon Res.* 2:593-599 (1982).

70. Jacobs, L., Herndon, R., Freeman, A., Cuetter, A., Smith, W. A., Salazar, A. H., Reese, P. A., Jose Fowica, R., Husain, F., Ekes, R., and O'Malley, J. A. Multicenter double-blind study of effect of intrathecally administered natural human fibroblast interferon on exacerbations of multiple sclerosis. *Lancet* 2:1411-1413 (1986).

71. Green, J. R., Klein, R. J., and Friedman-Kien, A. E. Intralesional administration of large doses of human leukocyte interferon for the treatment of condylomata acuminata. *J. Infect. Dis.* 150:612-615 (1984).

72. Davies, H. W., Scott, G. M., Robinson, J. A., Higgins, P. G., Wooten, R., and Tyrrell, D. A. J. Comparative intranasal pharmacokinetics of interferon using two spray systems. *J. Interferon Res.* 3:443-449 (1983).

73. Phillpotts, R. J., Davies, H. W., Willman, J., Tyrrell, D. A. J., and Higgins, P. G. Pharmacokinetics of intranasally applied medication during a cold. *Aniviral. Res.* 4:71-79 (1984).

74. Samo, T. C., Greenberg, S. B., Palmer, J. M., Couch, R. B., Harmon, M. W., and Johnson, P. E. Intranasally applied recombinant leukocyte A interferon in normal volunteers. II. Determination of minmal effective and tolerable dose. *J. Infect. Dis.* 150:181-188 (1984).

75. Kurzrock, R., Rosenblum, M. G., Sherwin, S. A., Rios, A., Talpay, M., Quesada, J. R., and Gutterman, J. U. Pharmacokinetics, single-dose tolerance, and biological activity of recombinant γ-interferon in cancer patients. *Cancer Res.* 45:2866-2872 (1985).

76. Gutterman, J. U., Rosenblum, M. G., Rios, A., Fritsche, H. A., and Quesada, J. R. Pharmacokinetic study of partially pure γ-interferon in cancer patients. *Cancer Res.* 44:4164-4171 (1984).

77. Vadhan-Raj, S., Nathan, C. F., Sherwin, S. A., Oettgen, H. F., and Krown, S. E. Phase I trial of recombinant interferon gamma by 1-hour iv infusion. *Cancer Treat. Rep.* 70:609-614 (1986).

78. Groopman, J. E., Gottlieb, M. S., Goodman, J., Mitsuyasu, R. T., Conant, M. A., Prince, H., Fahey, J. L., Derezin, M., Weinstein, W. M., Casavante, C., Rothman, J., Rudnick, S. A., and Volberding, P. A. Recombinant alpha-2 interferon therapy for Kaposi's sarcoma associated with the acquired immunodeficiency syndrome. *Ann. Intern. Med. 100*: 671-676 (1984).

79. Bocci, V. Evaluation of routes of administration of interferon in cancer: A review and proposal. *Cancer Drug Delivery 1*:337-351 (1984).

80. Bornemann, L. D., Spiegel, H. E., Dziewanowska, Z. E., Krown, S. E., and Colburn, W. A. Intravenous and intramuscular pharmacokinetics of recombinant leukocyte A interferon. *Eur. J. Clin. Pharmacol. 28*:469-471 (1985).

81. Smith, R. A., Norris, F., Palmer, D., Bernhardt, and Wills, R. J. Distribution of alpha interferon in serum and cerebrospinal fluid after systemic administration. *Clin. Pharmacol. Ther. 37*:85-88 (1985).

82. Alexander McPherson, T., and Tan, Y. H. Phase I pharmacotoxicity study of human fibroblasts interferon in human cancers. *JNCI 65*:75-79 (1980).

83. Priestman, T. J., Johnston, M., and Whiteman, P. D. Preliminary observations on the pharmacokinetics of human lymphoblastoid interferon given by intramuscular injection. *Clin. Oncol. 8*:265-269 (1982).

84. Martino, S., and Singhakowinta, A. Serial interferon alpha-2 levels in serum and cerebrospinal fluid. *Cancer Treat. Rep. 68*:1057-1058 (1984).

85. Salonen, R. CSF serum interferon in multiple sclerosis: Longitudinal study. *Neurology (N.Y.) 33*:1604-1606 (1983).

86. Degre, M., Dahl, H., and Vandvik, B. Interferon in the serum and cerebrospinal fluid in patients with multiple sclerosis and other neurological disorders. *Acta. Neurol. Scand. 53*:152-160 (1976).

87. Overall, J. C., Jr., Spruance, S. L., and Green, J. H. Viral-induced leukocyte interferon in vesicle fluid from lesions of recurrent herpes labialis. *J. Infect. Dis. 143*:543-547 (1981).

88. Bjerke, J. R., Linden, J. K., Degre, M., and Matre, R. Interferon in suction blister fluid from psoriatic lesions. *Br. J. Dermatol. 108*:295-299 (1983).

89. Degre, M., Mellbye, O. J., and Clarke-Jensen, O. Immune interferon in serum and synovial fluid in rheumatoid arthritis and related disorders. *Ann.Rheum. Dis. 42*:672-676 (1983).

5
Neurotoxicity of Interferon Therapy

AMA Z. S. ROHATINER

St. Bartholomew's Hospital, London, England

MARKUS FÄRKKILÄ

University Hospital of Helsinki, Helsinki, Finland

I. INTRODUCTION

The systemic administration of interferon (IFN) is associated with symptoms analogous to those of influenza, regardless of dose, schedule, or the cellular origin of the interferon preparation (1-4). In the course of recent phase I and phase II studies in malignant disease, it has become apparent that in addition to these systemic effects, interferon therapy is associated with significant neurotoxicity. A number of different syndromes have been described; most are completely reversible on stopping treatment; some, although not all, are dose dependent.

II. CLINICAL TOXICITY

The acute effects of interferon comprise fever, chills, tachycardia, malaise, myalgia, and headache (1-4). These symptoms are associated with nonspecific fatigue and asthenia, which constitute the predominant dose-limiting toxicity of interferon therapy.

Patients complain of anorexia, weakness, tiredness, and absence of motivation. In the majority of patients a degree of adaptation occurs, allowing treatment to be continued for prolonged periods (5-7). Specific effects on the central nervous sytem have been described with high doses of interferon: somnolence, lethargy, confusion, loss of taste and smell, expressive dysphasia, and overall mental and motor slowing (8-10). Psychotic reactions, together with auditory and visual hallucinations, have occasionally been described in patients receiving $>20 \times 10^6$ U/m^2 per day (11-13). Seizures have also been reported (1,11,14).

Patients with multiple sclerosis receiving intrathecal IFN-a have experienced systemic symptoms (15). Adverse reactions were seen at cumulative doses of 1.0 and 3.0×10^6 U, and the authors concluded that a single dose of IFN-a should not exceed 0.3×10^6 U. In general, intraventricular therapy has been well tolerated. Systemic symptoms such as fever, malaise, and anorexia occur within 1-2 hr of treatment and subside over 24 hr. With chronic intraventricular treatment fatigue and anorexia are noted; if treatment is intermittent side effects are minimal but the dose must be individualized. If the dose is excessive, neurotoxic side effects occur (16).

Relatively small numbers of patients have hitherto received IFN-γ (17-19). To date, no significant neurologic toxicity has been reported at the doses used (1 μg to 2 mg IV twice or three times weekly), although patients have complained of headaches. On the basis of clinical examination, psychological testing, electroencephalography (EEG), and visual evoked potentials, Farkkila et al. (20) have concluded that IFN-γ is not neurotoxic.

A few patients have complained of symptoms suggestive of peripheral nervous system involvement (21,22). Paresthesias have been described most often in patients previously exposed to *Vinca* alkaloids and in patients receiving IFN-a in combination with vinblastine. In such patients, loss of tendon reflexes has been associated with minimal slowing of motor and sensory conduction velocities (16,22). Neuralgic amyotrophy and a polyradiculopathy have also been described in a patient with hairy cell leukemia receiving IFN-a_2 in increasing doses up to 30×10^6 U daily. A pre-existing polyneuropathy was also exacerbated (24).

III. NEUROPSYCHIATRIC MANIFESTATIONS

A number of studies have attempted to elucidate the nature of the neurologic symptoms by neuropsychiatric assessment. Adams et al. (25) studied patients with renal cell cancer receiving a relatively low dose of partially purified human leukocyte interferon, 3×10^6 U/day. During the first week of treatment, the majority of patients complained of intense fatigue and were found to have moderate to severe behavioral changes and mild to moderate cognitive, affective, and personality changes. The most notable finding was psychomotor retardation, with loss of cognitive, verbal, and motor spontaneity, incentive, and interest. The authors conclude on the basis of these findings that the fatigue so consistently described is a manifestation of a complex, diffuse toxic encephalopathy predominantly affecting the frontal lobes that results in reversible impairment of some higher mental functions.

Following an initial report describing the neurotoxicity associated with the administration of high doses of IFN-a by continuous intravenous (IV) infusion, (23) Mattson et al. subsequently compared the high dose regimen with a lower dosage in terms of psychometric monitoring. (26) Patients received either 800×10^6/U over 5 days followed by 6×10^6/U by intramuscular injection thrice weekly or 6×10^6/U daily. Both regimens resulted in progressive mental and motor slowing that was associated with marked dysfunction on testing of memory. The memory loss was accompanied by changes in visuoconstructional function, slowing of finger-tapping speed, and changes in psychomotor behavior. The degree of dysfunction was influenced by IFN dose. The two dosages induced the same kind of psychometric change but with a different time course. The greatest change was seen between 8 and 10 days in the patients receiving high-dose IFN and between the third and fourth weeks in patients receiving low doses. On discontinuation of IFN, the clinical and psychometric abnormalities disappeared within 2 weeks.

Behavioral changes have also been reported in five patients with amyotrophic sclerosis receiving high doses of partially purified human leukocyte interferon for 6 days (100×10^6/U/day, days 1 and 2, 200×10^6/U/day, days 3–6, by continuous IV infusion)

(27). Marked but reversible dysfunction was noted in short-term memory, coordination of hand movements, and drawing. Micrographia, motor perseveration, and slowing of behavior were also observed. The changes appeared 4–12 days after starting treatment, with the signs most marked on days 6–8. Recovery was almost complete by day 15.

IV. EEG CHANGES

EEG changes were originally described in patients receiving high doses of interferon (8,23), but it subsequently became apparent that similar effects were present in a proportion of patients receiving "conventional" doses (28). Clinical evaluation of human lymphoblastoid IFN (IFN-a) and subsequently recombinant DNA interferon (IFN-a_2) commenced at St. Bartholomew's Hospital in 1980 to establish whether interferons play a role in the treatment of leukemia. A phase I study was performed in patients with hematologic malignancy who had either failed to respond to conventional therapy or had relapsed following such therapy. A maximum tolerated dose (MTD) of 100×10^6 U/m^2 per day was established for IFN-a, administered by continuous intravenous infusion for 7 days (1). Clinical central nervous system (CNS) toxicity precluded the use of doses higher than the MTD and prompted a formal study of the electroencephalographic changes associated with the administration of lymphoblastoid IFN-a and recombinant IFN-a_2 (8).

A characteristic sequence of abnormalities evolved, reaching a peak between days 6 and 11 and returning toward normal by 3 weeks. The following changes were observed, even in patients who had no clinical evidence of CNS toxicity: slowing of the alpha rhythm with gradual loss of attenuation on eye opening and the appearance of diffuse slow waves (theta, then delta). Initially, these could be blocked by eye opening or auditory stimuli until monorhythmic frontal delta bursts became the prominent feature. Lambda waves also showed a transient increase in number, voltage, and duration. These changes were seen in all 11 patients investigated, but the EEG findings did not correlate with the extent of clinical dysfunction. Of the 11 patients, 7 became drowsy 24–72 hr after commencing the IFN infusion, and on questioning 3 were found to be disoriented for time and place. No focal neurologic signs were elicited. Slowing of background activity has also been described in patients receiving high doses of leukocyte IFN-α (23, 29). On spectral analysis a decrease in peak alpha frequency correlated best with the cumulative dose of IFN (29).

The EEG changes are suggestive of an encephalopathy and are similar to those described by Obrecht et al. (30) in toxic confusional states. Slowing of the alpha rhythm has also been reported in patients receiving conventional cytotoxic agents (31). Pattern-reversal visual evoked potentials have been shown to increase in amplitude and latency during high-dose interferon therapy (29). Auditory evoked brain stem potentials also show an increase in latency (32).

The mechanism accounting for these changes remains unclear, although there are data to support the concept that interferon does have widespread neurochemical activities. Incubating interferon with cat or rat cerebral cortex enhances spontaneous neuronal activity and evoked responses (33). Interferon is known to compete for membrane receptors with neurotropic hormones, such as thyrotropin (34). Intracerebral injection of leukocyte interferon into mice has been reported to produce endorphinlike effects, including decreased motor activity and catalepsy reversible with naloxone (35). However, interferon does not share structural homology with endorphin and neither interferon nor pepsin digests of interferon cross-react in an endorphin radioimmunoassay (36).

It has been demonstrated that IFN enhances the excitability of cultured neurons (37), and higher than normal levels of p67K kinase, an IFN-induced enzyme, have been demonstrated in the brains of mice treated with IFN (38). Adams et al. (25) have shown that both metoclopramide, a dopamine antagonist, and methylphenidate, a dopamine agonist, can reverse some of the neuropsychiatric effects of leukocyte interferon. Although this effect is not consistent, it points toward the involvement of central neurotransmitters. The authors suggest that hypersomnia reflects the effect of interferon on the reticular activating system (RAS) or interference with the frontal lobes' extensive RAS connections.

V. CONCLUSION

Neurologic dysfunction has been described in patients receiving both partially purified IFN-α or highly purified recombinant preparations, suggesting that the effects are due to interferon itself, not to impurities in the interferon preparations. Overall, the data are based on small numbers of patients, most of whom have received interferon in the context of advanced malignant disease. The administration of interferon is associated with dose-dependent, reversible neurologic toxicity, the mechanism of which has yet to be elucidated. These side effects represent the major dose-limiting toxicity of interferon therapy.

REFERENCES

1. Rohatiner, A. Z. S., Balkwill, F. R., Griffin, D. B., Malpas, J. S., and Lister, T. A. A phase I study of human lymphoblastoid Interferon administered by continuous intravenous infusion. *Cancer Chemother. Pharmacol.* 9:97 (1982).

2. Priestman, T. J. Initial evaluation of human lymphoblastoid interferon in patients with advanced malignant disease. *Lancet* 2:113 (1980).

3. Sherwin, S. A., Knost, J. A., Fein, S., Abrams, P. G., Foon, K. A., Ochs, J. J., Schoenberger, C., Maluish, A. E., and Oldham, R. K. A multiple-dose phase I trial of recombinant leukocyte A interferon in cancer patients. *JAMA* 248:2461 (1982).

4. McPherson, T. A., and Yott, T. Phase I study of human fibroblast interferon in human malignancy. *Proc. Am. Assoc. Cancer Res.* 20:378 (1979).

5. Quesada, J. R., Gutterman, J. U., Swanson, D., et al. Renal cell carcinoma: Antitumor effects of leukocyte interferon. *Cancer Res.* 43:940-945 (1983).

6. Talpaz, M., McCredie, K. B., Mavligit, G. M., et al. Leukocyte interferon

induced myeloid cytoreduction in chronic myelogenous leukemia. *Blood* 62:689-692 (1983).

7. Quesada, J. R., Reuben, J., Manning, J., et al. Alpha interferon for induction of remission in hairy cell leukemia. *N. Engl. J. Med.* 310:15-18 (1984).

8. Rohatiner, A. Z. S., Prior, P. F., Burton, A. C., et al. Central nervous system toxicity of interferon. *Br. J. Cancer* 47:419-422 (1983).

9. Smedley, H., Katrak, M., Sikora,K., et al. Neurological effects of recombinant human interferon. *Br. Med. J.* 286:262-264 (1983).

10. Mattson, K., Niiranen, A., Livanainen, M., et al. Neurotoxicity of interferon. *Cancer Treat. Rep.* 67:958-961 (1983).

11. Kirkwood, J. M., Ernstoff, M. S., Davis, C. A., et al. Comparison of intramuscular and intravenous recombinant alpha-2 interferon in melanoma and other cancers. 103:32-36 (1985).

12. Creagan, E. T., Ahmann, D. L., Green, S. J., et al. Phase II study of recombinant leukocyte A interferon (rIFN A) in disseminated malignant melanoma. *Cancer* 54:2844-2849 (1984).

13. Eggermont, A. M., Weimar, W., Marquet, R. L., et al. Phase II trial of high-dose recombinant leukocyte alpha-2 interferon for metastatic colorectal cancer without previous systemic treatment. *Cancer Treat. Rep.* 69:185-187 (1985).

14. Dierckx, R. A., Michotte, A., Schmedding, E., Ebinger, G., Degeeter, T., and van Camp, B. Unilateral seizures in a patient with hairy cell leukemia treated with interferon. *Clin. Neurol. Neurosurg.* 87-3 (1985).

15. Ruutianinen, J., Panelius, M., and Cantell, K. Toxic effects of interferon administered intrathecally. *Br. Med. J.* 268:940 (1983).

16. Salazar, A. M., Gibbs, C. U., Jr., Gajdusek, D. C., and Smith, R. A. Clinical use of interferons: Central nervous system disorders. In: *The Handbook of Experimental Pharmacology* Vol. 71, (P. E. Came and W. A. Carter, eds.). Springer-Verlag, Berlin (1984).

17. Quesada, J. R., Talpaz, M., Rios, A., Kurzrock, R., and Gutterman, J. Clinical toxicity of interferons in cancer patients. *J. Clin. Oncol.* 4:234-243 (1986).

18. Panitch, H. S., Haley, A. S., Hirsch, R. L., and Johnson, K. P. A trial of gamma interferon in multiple sclerosis. *Neurology (N.Y.)* 36:285 (1986).

19. Mattson, K., Niiranen, A., Farkkila, M., Hartel, G., Larsen, Holsti, L. R., Standertskiold-Nordenstam, C.-G., and Cantell, K. Comparison of clinical toxicity of natural and recombinant interferon. Results of phase II trials in lung cancer. In: *The Biology of the Interferon System*. (To be published 1987).

20. Farkkila, M., Niiranen, A., Mattson, K., Salmi, T., Iivanainen, M., and Cantell, K. Neurotoxicity of high or low-dose natural IFN- and of recombinant IFN- in patients with lung cancer. In: *The Biology of Interferon Systems*. (1986).

21. Gutterman, J. U., Fein, S., Quesada, J. R., et al. Recombinant leukocyte A interferon: Pharmacokinetics, single-dose tolerance, and biologic effects in cancer patients. *Ann. Intern. Med.* 96:549 (1982).

22. Quesada, J. R., and Gutterman, J. U. Clinical study of recombinant DNA produced leukocyte interferon in an intermittent schedule in cancer patients. *JNCI* 70:1041-1046 (1983).

23. Mattson, K., Niiranen, A., Iivanainen, M., Farkkila, M., Bergstrom, L., Holsti, L. R., Kauppinen, H.-L., and Cantell, K. Neurotoxicity of interferon. *Cancer Treat. Rep.* 67:958-961 (1983).

24. Bernsen, P. L. J. A., Wong-Chung, R. E., and Janssen, J. T. P. Neuralgic amyotrophy and polyradiculopathy during interferon therapy. *Lancet* 50 (1985).

25. Adams, F., Quesada, J. R., Jordan, U., and Gutterman, J. U. Neuropsychiatric manifestations of human leukocyte interferon therapy in patients with cancer. *JAMA* 252:938-941 (1984).

26. Mattson, K., Niiranen, A., Laaksonen, R., and Cantell, K. Psychometric monitoring of interferon neurotoxicity. *Lancet* 275-276 (1984).

27. Iivanainen, M., Laaksonen, R., Niemi, M. L., Farkkila, M., Bergstrom, L., Mattson, K., Niiranen, A., and Cantell, K. Memory and psychomotor impairment following high dose interferon treatment in amyotrophic lateral sclerosis. *Acta Neurol. Scand.* 72:475-480 (1985).

28. Smedley, H., Katrak, M., Sikora, K., and Wheeler, T. Neurological side effects of recombinants human interferon. *Br. Med. J.* 286:262-264 (1983).

29. Farkkila, M., Iivanainen, M., Laukkanen, R., Sainio, K., Bergstrom, L., and Cantell, K. Neurological and neurophysiological side effects of high-dose interferon treatment in amyotrophic lateral sclerosis. In: *The Biology of the Interferon System* (1985).

30. Obrecht, R., Okhomina, F. O. A., and Scott, D. F. Value of EEG in acute confusional state. *J. Neurol. Neurosurg. Psychiatry* 4:75 (1979).

31. Schaffler, I., Imbach, P., Rudeberg, A., Vassler, F., and Karbowski, K. Conventional and spectral EEG analysis in children treated with cytotoxic agents. *Eur. J. Cancer Clin. Oncol.* 18:827 (1982).

32. Farkkila, M., Iivanainen, M., Roine, R., Bergstrom, L., Laaksonen, R., Niemi, M.-L., and Cantell, K. Neurotoxic and other side effects of high-dose interferon in amyotrophic lateral sclerosis. *Acta Neurol Scand.* 69: 42-46 (1984).

33. Calvet, M. C., and Gresser, I. Interferon enhances the excitability of cultured neurons. *Nature* 178:558-560 (1979).

34. Maheshware, R. K., Lazo, P. S., and Friedman, R. M. Enhancement of interferon activity by a membrane glycoprotein related to the thyrotropin receptor. In: *Interferon: Properties and Clinical Uses.* pp. 387-396 (1979).

35. Blalock, J. E., and Smith, E. M. Human leukocyte interferon: Potent endorphin-like opioid activity. *Biochem. Biophys. Res. Commun.* 101: 472-478 (1981).

36. Wetzel, R., Levine, H. L., Hagman, J., and Ramachandran, J. *Biochem. Biophys. Res. Commun.* 104:944-949 (1982).

37. Calvet, M. L., and Gresser, I. Interferon enhances the excitability of cultured neurones. *Nature* 278:558 (1979).

38. Krust, B., Riviere, Y., and Hovanessian, A. G. p67K kinase in different tissues and plasma of control and interferon treated mice. *Virology* 120: 240 (1982).

6
Interferon Treatment of Herpes Simplex and Varicella-Zoster Virus Infections of the Nervous System

GEORGE J. PAZIN

School of Medicine and Graduate School of Public Health,
University of Pittsburgh, Pittsburgh, Pennsylvania

I. INTRODUCTION

Natural or recombinant interferon treatment in relation to herpes simplex virus (HSV) and varicella-zoster virus (VZV) infections of the nervous system has been the subject of numerous laboratory, animal, and human clinical investigations. The goals have been to determine the biologic effects of interferon on viral latency as well as replication and, in turn, the potential clinical benefits on the natural course of herpesvirus infections. Although the most serious and life-threatening aspect of HSV and VZV infections is the development of herpetic encephalitis, this aspect of herpesvirus infections has not been studied with respect to interferon. Likewise, HSV has been shown to infect autonomic ganglia (1), but that aspect of nervous system infections has also not been studied with respect to interferon. This chapter touches briefly on laboratory and animal studies and reviews the effects of interferon upon cutaneous HSV and VZV infections and presumably upon the associated sensorineural ganglionic infections that occur with these viruses.

II. LABORATORY AND ANIMAL STUDIES: HERPES SIMPLEX VIRUS INFECTIONS

In vitro studies of interferon in relation to herpes simplex virus and varicella-zoster virus have indicated that these viruses are not intrinsically very sensitive to interferon (2). In addition, the dose-response curve of human leukocyte interferon against HSV does not result in complete inhibition of HSV at the highest interferon concentrations (3). The relative insensitivity of HSV and VZV and the persistence of a resistant fraction suggest that interferon may not be able to eradiate persistent or latent HSV infections in humans.

Despite the in vitro findings, Cantell and Tomila (4) showed an effect of interferon in HSV infections in rabbit eyes, and exogenous interferon and interferon inducers were shown by Olsen and colleagues (5) to protect against death or delay death in mice inoculated intraperitoneally or intravaginally with HSV-2. However, the effect of interferon or inducers on central nervous system infections (encephalitis) in mice was less apparent since the time to death was increased but death was not prevented when intranasal inoculation was used (5,6). Catalano and Baron (7) were also not able to suppress HSV encephalitis in mice in earlier studies.

The partial success revealed in animal studies prompted clinical investigations of non-life-threatening manifestations of HSV and VZV infections in humans. Development of methods to produce natural human leukocyte interferon in sufficient quantities enabled investigators to extend these studies to appropriate clinical settings in humans. The subsequent development of recombinant human interferons has largely eliminated supply problems, but the toxicity of interferon in high dosages remains a deterrent to clinical usage.

III. CLINICAL HERPES SIMPLEX VIRUS STUDIES

A. Orolabial HSV Infections

Recurrent orolabial herpetic lesions, the most common manifestations of HSV infection of the trigeminal ganglia, are bothersome but of relatively little clinical importance. Nevertheless, the observation that recurrent herpes labialis and/or asymptomatic oropharyngeal shedding of HSV was a highly predictable occurrence in HSV-infected patients following microvascular decompression of the trigeminal sensory root (8) enabled Pazin et al. to investigate the efficacy of pooled human leukocyte interferon (Cantell variety) in a placebo-controlled, double-blinded prospective clinical trial (9). A group of 37 patients who had a prior history of herpes labialis and underwent the operation to relieve trigeminal neuralgia were treated with 70,000 U interferon per kilogram body weight administered intramuscularly in two divided doses beginning approximately 12 hr before surgery and continuing for a total of 5 days. Control patients received equivalent volumes of human serum albumin, the vehicle for the interferon, on an identical schedule. The interferon was generally well tolerated. Daily examinations and throat wash cultures on all patients revealed that overall reactivation detected in 15 of 18 (83%) of placebo-treated patients was reduced to 9 of 19 (47%) in interferon-treated patients ($p < 0.05$). In addition, the number and size of herpetic lesions were reduced in the interferon group. Finally, the total number of culture-positive days was reduced to a highly significant degree [53 of 127 (42%) versus 12 of 134 (9%); $p < 0.001$]. The culture-positive days for the interferon-treated patients is compared with those for the placebo-treated patients in Figure 1. This study clearly indicated that human leukocyte interferon administered before and after a highly potent mechanical stimulus to reactivation of latent HSV within the trigeminal ganglion was able to markedly suppress development of herpetic labial lesions and viral shedding in the mouth. A follow-up telephone survey study by Haverkos et al. (10) showed that the single course of interferon did not eradicate latency since patients who received interferon experienced recurrences of herpes labialis during the subsequent year.

As usual, several additional questions remained unanswered. Was the interferon administered before the operative stimulus, preventing reactivation of latent HSV within the ganglia, or was the interferon administered postoperatively, reducing the manifestations of HSV peripherally in a therapeutic rather than prophylactic sense? A second study was done in which interferon was only administered before or after surgery with placebo injections to

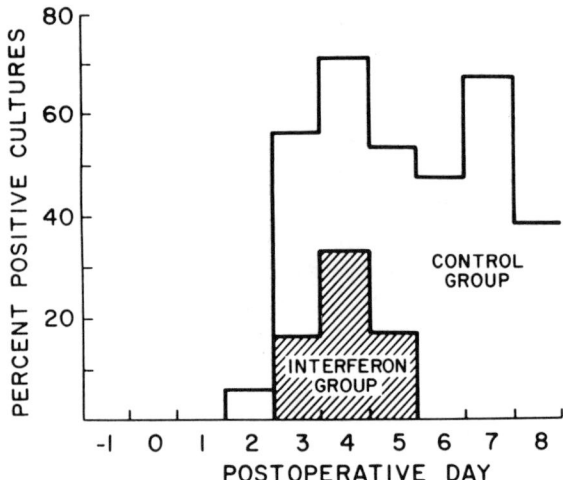

Figure 1 Percentage of positive throat wash cultures for HSV related to postoperative day. Hatched area represents interferon-treated patients, and clear area represents placebo-treated patients. (From Pazin et al., *N. Engl. J. Med.*, Ref. 9.)

maintain clinical blinding. The results of the second study were less conclusive but indicated that interferon only before the operation seemed to enhance reactivation, perhaps through its fever-producing properties, and interferon administered only after the surgical stimulus to reactivation was not able to suppress reactivation below that observed in patients who had received placebo injections before and after surgery (11). Therefore, it appears that interferon is needed before and after the stimulus to reactivation if it is to exert a statistically significant effect; the site of action of interferon, whether central or peripheral, remains uncertain and may be partially at both sites.

These studies of interferon in relation to reactivation of HSV-1 following neurosurgery on the trigeminal sensory root were very exciting from a biologic perspective but offered little promise in a therapuetic sense since the therapy required daily intramuscular injections before and after surgery and the clinical response was moderate. Nevertheless, these studies provided a biologic and clinical basis for studying interferon in the treatment of genital herpes.

A controlled clinical trial of human leukocyte interferon administered prophylactically for 6 weeks in renal transplant recipients was conducted by Cheeseman and her colleagues (12). Interferon-treated patients showed a reduction in excretion of cytomegalovirus, viremia, and clinical syndromes, but interferon administered as 3 million U twice a week did not alter the frequency of herpes labialis lesions or HSV excretion in oropharyngeal secretions.

B. Genital HSV Infections

Major advances have been made in the treatment of genital herpes with antiviral nucleoside analogs, in particular topical, intravenous, and most recently oral acyclovir (Zovirax). However, acyclovir does not prevent the establishment of ganglionic latency with HSV nor does it affect HSV present latently in sacral ganglia even though it is able to suppress overt recurrences of genital herpes to a highly significant, albeit incomplete, degree. Studies on the effect of interferon upon first episodes of genital herpes in nonpregnant women, initiated before the remarkable effects of acyclovir on genital herpes were reported, are being reported now.

The main objectives of the Pazin et al. study of human leukocyte interferon on genital herpes (13) were (a) to assess the clinical effect upon the natural course of first episode genital herpes and (b) to determine whether interferon treatment early in the episode might prevent or decrease the extent of establishment of HSV latency in sacral ganglia. It seemed likely that if interferon were able to prevent establishment of latency in sacral ganglia, it should be administered as early as possible. Within 3 days of the development of lesions was chosen as a clinically reasonable entrance criterion. Patients were randomly assigned to intramuscular treatment with pooled human leukocyte interferon (Cantell variety), 50,000 U/kg twice on the first day, then once daily for days 2–8 and 10, 12, and 14. Control patients received equivalent volumes of human serum albumin, the interferon vehicle.

Broad ranges for the duration of positive viral cultures and time to healing of lesions in both control patients and interferon-treated patients tended to obscure the effects of interferon treatment on mean values. However, analysis of survival curves revealed significant shortening of both duration of positive virus cultures and time to healing by interferon treatment. The survival curve for positive viral cultures in interferon- and placebo-treated patients is presented in Figure 2. Analysis of the size of lesions and quantities of virus recovered showed less progression of the disease in interferon-treated patients during therapy. Despite the statistically significant therapeutic effects on cultures and healing, no statistically beneficial effect upon pain could be demonstrated. Thus, beneficial biologic effects could be shown on the natural course of first-episode genital herpes, but the effects were generally less than responses to acyclovir therapy. The need for a series of intramuscular injections and the side effects of moderate fever and moderate neutropenia are important factors limiting the

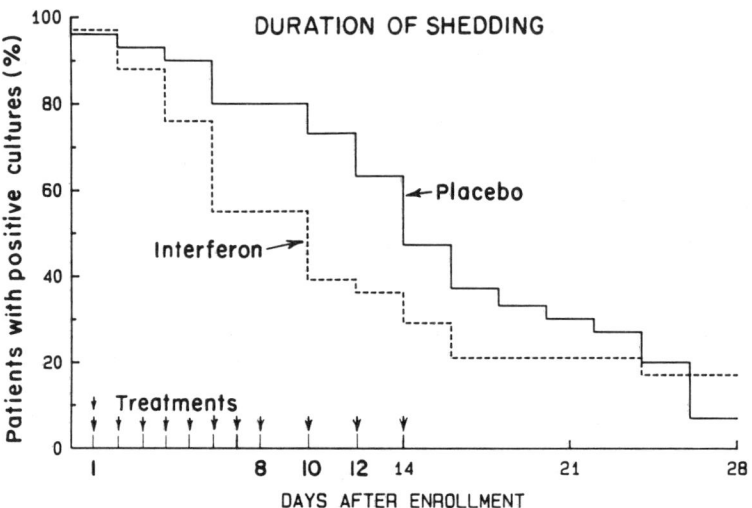

Figure 2 Duration of HSV shedding presented as the percentage of interferon-treated and placebo-treated patients with positive genital cultures for HSV related to days after enrollment with treatments indicated by arrows along x axis. (Modified from *J. Infect. Dis.* article by Pazin et al., Ref. 13.)

clinical usefulness of interferon unless it were to show significant effects upon establishment of latency.

Establishment of latency of HSV in sacral ganglia was assessed by comparing the recurrence rates in interferon- and placebo-treated patients. Approximately 35% of the patients experienced first-episode genital herpes due to HSV-1, and as has been previously shown, recurrences were rare even in placebo-treated patients with genital herpes due to HSV-1. Naturally, interferon-treated patients with first-episode genital herpes due to HSV-1 also showed few recurrences. The most disappointing aspect of the study was that the time to first recurrence and frequency of recurrences during 1 year of intensive follow-up in patients with genital herpes due to HSV-2 was not affected by the 2 week course of interferon therapy during the initial infection. It appears that latency of HSV in sacral ganglia becomes established during the incubation phase or proceeds during the initial stage of the infection despite interferon treatment.

Mendelson et al. have also studied the effect of recombinant interferon-a_2 on initial genital herpes (14), but they used a different approach. They enrolled patients up to 5 days into their first episode, and they followed an initial 5 day course of treatment with a maintenance phase of thrice weekly treatment for 3 months. They were not able to show beneficial effects of interferon during the initial episode, and recurrences occurred both in interferon-treated and control patients during the maintenance therapy phase. Although recurrences in men healed faster and duration of virus sheddding was shorter, the modest benefits to recurrences during maintenance treatment do not appear to be sufficient to warrant clinical usage during recurrences.

Kuhls et al. also studied recombinant interferon-a_2, but in an effort to suppress recurrences (15). Prophylactic administration of 3 million U of recombinant interferon-a_2 three times a week produced statistically significant reductions in virus shedding, healing time, and numbers of recurrences.

It is apparent from all these studies of interferon and genital herpes that interferon exerts a beneficial clinical effect on the natural course of initial and recurrent genital herpes, but owing to practical considerations of administration, side effects, and efficacy, it is not likely to replace oral acyclovir in clinical usage.

IV. CLINICAL VARICELLA-ZOSTER VIRUS STUDIES

A. Varicella Infections (Chickenpox)

Primary infection with varicella-zoster virus is principally an infection of childhood, but occasional patients acquire chickenpox as adults. Although primary infections with VZV are usually self-limited in normal children, the disease is a life-threatening infection in children with cancer and is occasionally responsible for fatalities in immunocompromised adult patients. The former situation occurs with sufficient frequency to permit controlled, prospective studies of human leukocyte interferon. The sporadic occurrence of primary VZV infections in adults has not permitted controlled studies in normal or immunocompromised patients, but recurrent VZV infections (shingles) in immunocompromised patients have been studied.

Arvin et al. at Stanford conducted relatively large placebo-controlled studies of the interferon treatment of varicella infection in children with cancer from 1974 to 1977 and from 1978 to 1981 (16). Importantly, children were enrolled within 72 hr of onset of lesions and were treated with 4.2×10^4 to 2.5×10^5 U interferon per kilogram body weight per day in the earlier trial and 3.5×10^5 U/kg for 2 days then 1.75×10^5 U/kg per day for 3 days in the latter trial. In the earlier trial, therapy was continued until no new vesicles were observed for 24 hr. Treatment varied from 3 to 11 days and averaged 6.4 days.

The cumulative results in 23 interferon-treated patients and 21 placebo recipients revealed significant reductions in days of new lesion formation [3.8 ± 1.89 ($\pm$ SD) versus 5.3 ± 2.56; $p < 0.05$] and greater proportions of patients free of new lesions for 24 hr at 7 or 6 days in interferon recipients. Unfortunately, three placebo recipients died of progressive varicella and two interferon recipients died after 2–3 weeks, including one patient with recurrent viremia upon completion of therapy. Similarly, life-threatening dissemination was reduced in survivors who received interferon (none of 21) compared with 3 of 18 survivors who received placebo. Comparison of interferon recipients with placebo recipients failed to demonstrate important toxicity. Thus, in this special group of patients, primary infection (varicella) in children with cancer, interferon was reasonably well tolerated and moderately efficacious and reduced serious morbidity in survivors but was not able to completely prevent fatalities in the most susceptible children. A precise comparison with acyclovir is not available as of mid-1988.

B. Zoster Infections (Shingles)

Although varicella does not occur commonly enough in adult immunocompromised patients to enable controlled studies to be carried out at one institution, the effect of natural interferon on recurrent varicella-zoster infections in 90 immunocompromised adults has been carefully studied in a series of clinical investigations at Stanford (17). Three dosage levels were studied: 4.2×10^4, 1.7×10^5, and 5.1×10^5 U/kg per day. Interferon at the lowest dosage level was much less efficacious, but at the higher levels, progression within the primary dermatome and distal cutaneous spread were significantly reduced. Treated patients also showed trends toward less acute pain and diminished severity of postherpetic neuralgia. Visceral complications were also less frequent in interferon-treated patients. However, in a subsequent study, short-term (2 day) interferon treatment of shingles in adult patients with cancer was not effective (18).

The availability of recombinant leukocyte interferon in the 1980s led to a multicentered trial by Winston et al. (19) of even higher dosages of interferon in immunocompromised patients with varicella-zoster. A dosage of 68 million U/day had to be discontinued owing to the excessive side effects. Fever, chills, headaches, myalgias, fatigue, and gastrointestinal irritability were also common at the 36 million U/day level, but dissemination of the zoster was significantly reduced in the interferon recipients [14 of 24 (58%) of placebo patients showed dissemination versus only 4 of 24 (17%) interferon-treated patients]. Thus interferon clearly modified varicella-zoster reactivation in immunocompromised adults, but side effects were frequent and interferon is unlikely to displace acyclovir or other nucleotide analogs in this treatment area.

V. SUMMARY

In vitro studies of leukocyte interferon and HSV and VZV suggested that interferon may be able to modify the natural course of HSV and VZV infections but may not be able to affect virus latent on sensory ganglia. Animal studies seemed to confirm partially beneficial effects if the interferon was administered before or very soon after challenge, but no effect upon established or latent virus. Well-designed, placebo-controlled, double-blinded trials of interferon in non–life-threatening infections with HSV, including postneurosurgical reactivation of HSV-1, and first and recurrent episodes of genital herpes due to HSV-1 or HSV-2, and primary varicella (chickenpox) in children with cancer, as well as zoster (shingles) in immunosuppressed adults, have all documented statistically significant beneficial clinical responses. However, since interferon must be administered parenterally and is associated with clinically significant side effects, interferon is not likely to challenge nucleoside analogs, such as acyclovir, in the treatment of HSV or VZV infections.

REFERENCES

1. Warren, K. G., Brown, S. M., Wroblewska, Z., Gilden, D., Koprowski, H., and Subak-Sharpe, J. Isolation of latent herpes simplex virus from the superior cervical and vagus ganglions of human beings. *N. Engl. J. Med.* 298:1068–1069 (1978).

2. Rasmussen, L., and Farley, L. B. Inhibition of *Herpesvirus hominis* replication by human interferon. *Infect. Immun.* 12:104–108 (1975).

3. Lazar, R., Breinig, M. K., Armstrong, J. A., and Ho, M. Response to cloned progeny of clinical isolates of herpes simplex virus to human leukocyte interferon. *Infect. Immun.* 28:708–712 (1980).

4. Cantell, K., and Tomila, E. Effect of interferon on experimental vaccinia and herpes-simplex virus infections in rabbits' eyes. *Lancet* 2:682-684 (1960).

5. Olsen, G. A., Kern, E. R., Overall, J. C., Jr., and Glasgow, L. A. Effect of treatment with exogenous interferon, polyriboinosinic-polyribocytidylic acid, or polyriboinosinic-polyribocytidylic acid-poly-L-Lysine complex on *Herpesvirus hominis* infections in mice. *J. Infect. Dis.* 137:428 (1978).

6. Kern, E. R., Overall, J. C., Jr., and Glasgow, L. A. *Herpesvirus hominis* infection in newborn mice: Treatment with interferon inducer polyinosinic-polycytidylic acid. *Antimicrob. Agents Chemother.* 7:793-800 (1975).

7. Catalano, L. W., Jr., and Baron, S. Protection against herpes virus and encephalomyocarditis virus encephalitis with double stranded RNA inducer of interferon. *Proc. Soc. Exp. Biol. Med.* 133:684-687 (1970).

8. Pazin, G. J., Ho, M., and Jannetta, P. J. Reactivation of herpes simplex virus after decompression of the trigeminal nerve root. *J. Infect. Dis.* 138:405-409 (1978).

9. Pazin, G. J., Armstrong, J. A., Lam, M. T., Tarr, G. C., Jannetta, P. J., and Ho, M. Prevention of reactivated herpes simplex infection by human leukocyte interferon after operation on the trigeminal root. *N. Engl. J. Med.* 301:225-230 (1979).

10. Haverkos, H. W., Pazin, G. J., Armstrong, J. A., and Ho, M. Follow-up of interferon treatment of herpes simplex. *N. Engl. J. Med.* 303:699-700 (1980).

11. Ho, M., Pazin, G. J., Armstrong, J. A., Haverkos, H. W., Dummer, J. S., and Jannetta, P. J. Paradoxical effects of interferon on reactivation of oral infection with herpes simplex virus after microvascular decompression for trigeminal neuralgia. *J. Infect. Dis.* 150:867-872 (1984).

12. Cheeseman, S. H., Rubin, R. H., Steward, J. A., Tolkoff-Ruben, N. E., Cosimi, A. B., Cantell, K., Gilbert, J., Winkle, S., Herrin, J. T., Black, P. H., Russell, P. S., and Hirsch, M. S. Controlled clinical trial of prophylactic human-leukocyte interferon in renal transplantation. Effects on cytomegalovirus and herpes simplex virus infections. *N. Engl. J. Med.* 300:1345-1349 (1979).

13. Pazin, G. J., Harger, J. H., Armstrong, J. A., Breinig, M. K., Caplan, R. J., Cantell, K., and Ho, M. Leukocyte interferon for treating first episodes of genital herpes in women. *J. Infect. Dis.* 156:891-898 (1987).

14. Mendelson, J., Clecner, B., and Eiley, S. Effect of recombinant interferon alpha 2 on clinical course of first episode genital herpes infection and subsequent recurrences. *Genitourin. Med. 62*:97-101 (1986).

15. Kuhls, T. L., Sacher, J., Pineda, E., Santomauro, D., Wiesmeier, E., Growdon, W. A., and Bryson, Y. J. Suppression of recurrent genital herpes simplex virus infection with recombinant alpha 2 interferon. *J. Infect. Dis. 154*:437-442 (1986).

16. Arvin, A. M., Kushner, J. H., Feldman, S., Baehner, R. L., Hammond, D., and Merigan, T. C. Human leukocyte interferon for the treatment of varicella in children with cancer. *N. Engl. J. Med. 306*:761-765 (1982).

17. Merigan, T. C., Rand, K. H., Pollard, R. B., Abdallah, P. S., Jordan, G. W., and Fried, R. P. Human leukocyte interferon for the treatment of herpes zoster in patients with cancer. *N. Engl. J. Med. 298*:981-987 (1978).

18. Merigan, T. C., Gallagher, J. G., Pollard, R. B., and Arvin, A. M. Short-course human leukocyte interferon in treatment of herpes zoster in patients with cancer. *Antimicrob. Agents Chemother. 19*:193-195 (1981).

19. Winston, D. J., Eron, L. J., Ho, M., Pazin, G. J., Kessler, H., Pottage, J. C., Jr., Gallagher, J., Sartiano, G., Ho, W. G., Champlin, R. E., Bernhardt, L., Bigley, J., Kanitra, L., Nadler, P. I., and the Hoffman LaRoche Herpes Zoster Study Group. Treatment of herpes zoster in immunocompromised cancer patients with recombinant A interferon (IFN-A). Abstract 462, 25th Interscience Conference on Antimicrobial Agents and Chemotherapy, Minneapolis, Minnesota, 1985.

7
Production and Action of Interferon in Rabies Virus Infection

ARA G. HOVANESSIAN, RUGIMAR MARCOVISTZ,
YVES RIVIÈRE, JEAN-CLAUDE GUILLON, and
HENRI TSIANG

Pasteur Institute, Paris, France

I. INTRODUCTION

The production of interferon is a routine consequence of viral infection (1). Accordingly, certain viral infections may be controlled immediately by interferon produced early during infection. In such cases, interferon can be effective if a viral infection does not trigger the evolution of other pathologic manifestations leading to the appearance of symptoms. In most infections with potentially lethal viruses, the host organism can stop the spread of virus by its primary defense mechanisms whereby endogenous interferon, referred to as physiologic interferon, may play an important role (2-4).

Rabies virus is usually transmitted by animal bites. From the site of the bite it migrates through the peripheral nerves to reach the central nervous system, where the virus starts to replicate (5,6). This infection is associated with such clinical symptoms as excessive salivation, biting, hydrophobia, extreme fear, and anxiety. The disease usually progresses toward paralysis, coma, and death. Thus rabies virus infection takes over in spite of the presence of physiologic interferon and in spite of the production of interferon soon after virus inoculation. This is perhaps because the concentration of physiologic interferon and the amount of interferon produced after virus infection are not high enough to stop the virus. For this reason, exogenous interferon has been suggested as a therapeutic agent to treat rabies virus infection (7-20). In various animal species, it has been shown that rabies disease can be prevented by exogenous interferon or by inducers of interferon. Here we discuss the results of experiments carried out in animal models in which interferon has been used alone or in conjunction with rabies vaccine to protect animals against rabies infection. We then discuss our own results, obtained in mice, to show the production and action of interferon produced during rabies virus infection. The effect of exogenous interferon in immunocompetent and immunosuppressed mice is also reported.

II. EFFECT OF INTERFERON ON RABIES INFECTION OF ANIMALS

Before migration by the peripheral nervous routes, rabies virus has an incubation period varying between 1 or 2 days in experimental animal models to several weeks or months in humans. Thus an antiviral treatment may be effective if the drug is administered before the virus starts its migration up the peripheral nerves.

A. Rabies Prophylaxis with Interferon

Kaplan et al. (10) reported the first rabies prophylaxis with interferon in guinea pigs but with a very slight effect. Other workers then reported that administration of interferon failed to protect mice against rabies whereas there was some protection in rabbits (11,12). The route of injection of interferon was considered important, since intramuscular administration of interferon was effective in rabies prophylaxis in mice compared with intracerebral injection of interferon (13). Postic and Fenje (14) reported that interferon at 10^6 U per rabbit protected against rabies if administered simultaneously with the virus. However, when interferon was given 24 hr after virus inoculation, only a prolonged incubation period was noted. In another study in rabbits, Ho et al. (15) emphasized the route of administration of interferon. Daily intramuscular or intravenous injections of 10^6 U of interferon for up to 3 weeks gave less favorable results than when 10^6 U of interferon was given both intramuscularly and intravenously at the time of rabies virus challenge.

Cynomolgus monkeys infected with rabies virus were protected by repeated intramuscular administration of human leukocyte interferon beginning 24 hr after virus inoculation (16-18). Administration of interferon after the eappearance of clinical symptoms did not influence the progress of the disease (16). In these experiments, rabies virus-infected monkeys died 20 days postinfection with symptoms several days before death. All the different interferon treatments started 24 hr postinfection. Daily intramuscular administration of human interferon near the site of virus inoculation protected 7 of 10 monkeys (18). Intralumbar administration of interferon (i.e., into the cerebrospinal fluid) on days 3, 5, 7, 9, and 11 postinfection protected only 5 out of 10 monkeys. When interferon was injected only once through the intralumbar route, 11 days after infection, the survival rate was 4 of 10 monkeys. The most successful treatment (8 survivors of 10 monkeys) was achieved by a combined intramuscular and intralumbar interferon injection (18).

Interferon inducers have also been used instead of interferon in rabies prophylaxis. For example, statolon gave slight protection in mice (20), whereas poly(I)·poly(C) resulted in moderate protection in mice but efficient protection in rabbits (21-24). In another study, administration of tilorone hydrochloride completely protected mice against either subcutaneous or intracerabral challenge with low doses of rabies virus (25). A potent interferon inducer formed by complexing poly-L-lysine to poly(I)·poly(C) (26) was found to be very effective in protecting monkeys infected with rabies virus (26). The site of poly(I)·poly(C) injection was also investigated in rabies virus-infected animals (27,28). Injection of the double-stranded RNA at the same intramuscular site as the rabies virus was more effective than injection in the opposite leg (28).

All these results illustrate that the action of interferon is variable in rabies prophylaxis. These discrepancies are probably due to the fact that in the different studies reported here, the preparations of rabies virus strains used in these experiments and the dose of virus inoculated are not always identical. Furthermore, the incubation period of rabies virus are not always comparable in the different experiments. Finally, it may also be possible that the pathogenesis of rabies virus infection is slightly different in different species.

B. Rabies Vaccine and Interferon

It has been suggested that the efficiency of a particular rabies vaccine is correlated with its capacity to induce interferon (29–36). Several authors have shown the presence of circulating interferon in hamsters and in mice injected with rabies vaccine. Wiktor and his colleagues (37) found that rhesus monkeys could be protected against rabies by the administration of a human diploid cell-derived rabies virus vaccine injected several hours after rabies virus inoculation and that this protective effect is related to the induction of interferon. Diluted preparations of the same vaccine were unable to induce interferon and were only partially protective. In these experiments, the level of virus-neutralizing antibody titers stimulated by the concentrated and diluted vaccines was not correlated with the protective effect. Thus a vaccine administered after exposure to rabies virus can either be effective or ineffective depending on its capacity to induce interferon and often irrespective of whether neutralizing antibody to rabies virus is produced (5,6). These suggestions were confirmed by Baer et al. (36) in rabies virus-infected mice using two different preparations of rabies vaccine which were injected 24 hr postinfection. Vaccine prepared from hamster BHK cell substrate resulted in the production of serum interferon and neutralizing antibody, whereas vaccine prepared from a human diploid cell substrate gave rise to neutralizing antibody but no interferon. Interestingly enough, only the vaccine capable of inducing interferon was effective in reducing mortality. In other studies in mice and monkeys, the addition of poly(I)·poly(C) to rabies virus vaccine resulted in a significant decrease in mortality rate compared with vaccine or poly(I)·poly(C) treatment alone (7,9,35). Locally administered poly(I)·poly(C) induced high levels of interferon, which seemed to be critical for the protective effect.

A dramatic field trial in humans has indicated that vaccination alone is not sufficient to confer protection against rabies virus exposure. However, a combined treatment of antiserum to rabies virus and vaccine provides efficient protection (38). Such treatment in addition to human leukocyte interferon has been recently administered successfully to a patient transplanted with a cornea taken from a donor whose death was found to be due to rabies encephalities (39).

III. PRODUCTION AND ACTION OF INTERFERON DURING RABIES VIRUS INFECTION IN MICE

Several investigators have suggested the induction of interferon in rabies virus infection (13,29,40). Interferon has also been studied for its potential value in postexposure rabies treatment (1,8,9) and for its induction and role during rabies vaccination (8,31,32,34, 41). However, little is known about the production and action of interferon produced during rabies virus infeciton. For this reason we investigated the production and action of interferon in the pathogenesis of rabies virus infection in mice in parallel with the induction of two interferon-induced, double-stranded (ds) RNA-dependent enzyme activities, $pppA(2'p5'A)n$ synthetase (2-5A synthetase) and a specific protein kinase that manifests by the phosphorylation of a 65,000–68,000 molecular weight protein (42,43). The protein kinase interferes with the initiation of protein synthesis by phosphorylating the initiation factor eIF2, whereas 2-5A activates a latent endonuclease that degrades both cellular and viral RNAs.

The 2-5A synthetase and the protein kinase are detectable in different tissues of mice. In accord with in vitro studies in cell cultures, the level of these enzymes is enhanced severalfold on injection of mice with interferon or inducers of interferon, such as virus or double-stranded RNA (44,45). The levels of these enzymes in different tissues of mouse have been successfully used as convenient markers to show the presence and action of circulating interferon (44–46).

A. Production of Interferon by Rabies Virus

The pathogenesis of rabies virus infection in mice inoculated with the challenge virus strain (CVS)-fixed rabies virus (injected into the footpad) is characterized by paralysis of the posterior limbs on day 5 or 6. This infection is lethal for all mice by day 7 or 8. Virus becomes detectable in the brain by immunofluorescence by day 4.

Two peaks of circulating interferon are detectable during rabies virus infection: an early peak 24–48 hr after inoculation followed by another peak on day 6 of infection. Production of the first peak of interferon is due to the response of mice to rabies virus at the site of inoculation, whereas the second peak of interferon is due to the production of high levels of interferon in the brain in response to rabies virus replication (47,48). Interferon in the brain and in the circulation of rabies virus-infected mice is resistant to treatment at pH 2 and is completely neutralized by antimouse α or β interferon serum, but not by antimouse interferon-γ serum. These results therefore confirm that interferon produced during rabies virus infection in mice is of the α-β type. Titration of organ extracts of rabies virus-infected mice for interferon activity showed the presence of interferon in the brain but not in the spleen or the lung (47). This is probably because rabies virus replication occurs mainly in the brain (49,50). Interferon in rabies virus-infected mice is active in the induction of 2-5A synthetase and protein kinase in the brain and other organs (47).

B. Role of Interferon Produced During Rabies Virus Infection

Antibodies against mouse α and β interferon have been used to demonstrate the role of interferon in the pathogenesis of several acute virus diseases in mice (51–57). In order to investigate the role of the early production of interferon in the pathogenesis of rabies virus infection, mice were administered (intravenously) antimouse α and β interferon globulin at 1, 10, and 40 hr after virus inoculation (47). In such mice, the circulating interferon activity became detectable only on day 4 of infection and increased until death. Thus, infected mice that were injected with anti-interferon globulin showed only one peak of interferon activity starting 2 days earlier than the corresponding second peak of interferon in control infected mice. This was probably because the development of rabies disease was accelerated by neutralizing the first peak of interferon.

Neutralization of the first peak of interferon blocked the induction of splenic 2-5A synthetase and accelerated the development of the disease (48). Infected mice that received antimouse interferon globulin had a morbidity period that was significantly less than that for the control infected mice. These results indicate that interferon produced early during the course of the disease may play a role in the onset of the infection. This effect probably occurs soon after virus inoculation and during the extraneuronal phase of the disease. The activity of antibody against rabies virus in the plasma and infectivity of virus in the brain were similar for both groups.

In an attempt to neutralize the second peak of interferon, infected mice were treated with the antibody on days 3, 4, and 5 after virus inoculation. However, in these experiments, only 20% of the circulating interferon activity was neutralized. It should be noted that very high levels of interferon are produced during the replication of rabies virus in the brain, which may account for this failure.

C. Distribution of Rabies Virus, Interferon, and Interferon-Mediated Enzymes in the Brains of Virus-Infected Rats

The CVS-fixed strain of rabies virus passaged in mouse brain was used to inoculate Wistar rats. After the onset of paralysis, the rats were killed and the brains were dissected (58,59). Tissue extracts of the different brain regions were assayed for the level of 2-5A synthetase and protein kinase activities, rabies virus infectivity in mice, and interferon activity on rat cells (60).

Table 1 gives the infectivity of rabies virus per milligram protein for different regions of the brain assayed in parallel with the level of interferon per milligram protein. These were found to be unrelated. The highest level of interferon was detected in the brain stem (60,000 U/mg protein). For the distribution of virus, the brain stem, the cortex, and the striatum showed much higher viral infectivity than the crebellum and the hippocampus. There was little correlation in each of these regions between the level of interferon and the virus infectivity. For example, there were comparable virus titers in the brain stem and cortex but the level of interferon in the cortex was one-third that in the brain stem. Similarly, the hippocampus and cerebellum showed comparable virus infectivities but the level of interferon was sixfold higher in the latter. Thus, there was a lack of correlation between the level of interferon and virus infectivity. It is conceivable, therefore, that neurons differ in the yield of virus and their production of

Table 1 Virus Titers and Levels of Interferon in Different Regions of the Brain of Rabies Virus-Infected Rats[a]

Brain region	Virus titer[b] (LD_{50}/mg $\times 10^{-2}$)	Interferon[c] (U/mg $\times 10^{-3}$)
Brain stem	70	60
Cerebellum	5	42
Cortex	63	24
Hippocampus	6	7
Striatum	28	3

[a]For details, see Reference 60.

[b]The infectivity of rabies virus in tissue extracts of the different brain regions was titrated in mice.

[c]Rat interferon activity was measured by inhibition of cytopathic effect of VSV on NRK-49F cells.

Table 2 Levels of 2-5A Synthetase and Protein Kinase in Different Regions of the Brain of Rabies Virus-Infected Rats[a]

Brain regions	2-5A synthetase[b] (nmol/mg per hr)		Protein kinase[b] ($_{32}$P cpm/mg per assay)		
	Control	Infected	Control	Infected	C/I
Brain stem	<0.5	71.5	90	622	6.9
Cerebellum	<0.5	52.6	187	1375	7.3
Cortex	<0.6	9.3	1005	2865	2.8
Hippocampus	<0.6	18.5	2125	3125	1.5
Striatum	<0.5	5.0	727	1850	2.5

[a]For details, see Reference 60.
[b]Enzyme levels were assayed after partial purification on poly(I)·ply(C)-Sepharose (47,73).

interferon. It should also be noted that interferon may diffuse from one section of brain to the other and give misleading results. Thus, the levels of interferon and virus infectivity should be considered representative values rather than evidence.

The interferon-mediated protein kinase activity in rat cells, as in mouse cells, is manifested by the phosphorylation of an endogenous 67,000 molecular weight protein. This phosphorylation was enhanced significantly in protein kinase preparations from the brain of rabies virus-infected rats. Similarly, the level of 2-5A synthetase in the brains of infected rats was enhanced more than 30-fold compared with control rats. The basal level of protein kinase activity was variable in different brain regions of normal uninfected rats (Table 2). However, regardless of this basal level, there was a severalfold enhancement in individual brain regions in the presence of interferon. This effect became apparent when the ratio was calculated of values obtained in enzyme fractions from the different brain regions of infected rats to values observed in the corresponding controls. Extracts of the individual brain regions from normal rats showed a very low level of 2-5A synthetase. In infected brains, the level of 2-5A synthetase in each region correlated well with the distribution of interferon. As for interferon activity (Table 1), the highest levels of 2-5A synthetase were found in the brain stem and the lowest were in the striatum (Table 2).

The presence of interferon in the brain of rabies virus-infected rats is most probably due to the replication of virus in susceptible neurons. This is in accordance with the results obtained in cell culture: neurons are the predominant cells supporting rabies virus replication when compared with fibroblasts and glial cells (61,62). Furthermore, rabies virus infection of neuroblastoma cells results in the production of high levels of interferon (unpublished results).

D. Synthesis of 2-5A During Rabies Virus Infection

Under routine experimental conditions, the level of 2-5A synthetase is measured in an in vitro assay in the presence of optimal amounts of dsRNA (43,63). Results obtained in such assays, although valuable, are of limited significance since they show neither the in vivo activity of 2-5A synthetase nor the actual concentrations of 2-5A. Little is known about the intracellular concentrations of these compounds. The synthesis of 2-5A has been detected in cultured cells treated with interferon in response to virus infections (64).

In the experiments discussed here we investigated the changes in intracellular 2-5A concentrations in rabies virus-infected mice since such mice produce interferon. Concentrations of 2-5A increased exponentially up to day 5 after infection to reach values equal to 300 and 500% of the control values for spleens and brains, respectively (65). In the brain, the concentration of 2-5A started to increase dramatically 4 days after infection at a time when rabies virus had already reached the brain and started to replicate (66). In the spleen, the levels of 2-5A increased 2 days after infection. On day 5 of infection, the mean values for 2-5A in livers, spleens, and brains were 250, 20, and 27 pmol/g wet weight of the respective tissues (65). However, in the noninfected mice, the levels of 2-5A were very low or nondetectable.

The enhanced concentrations of 2-5A in rabies virus-infected mice imply the activation of 2-5A synthetase, probably by a factor accumulated during virus infection. The observation that injection of mice with interferon and poly(I)·poly(C) leads to the activation of 2-5A synthetase (i.e., to synthetize 2-5A in vivo) suggests that the formation of a viral double-stranded RNA replicative intermediate is responsible for the activation of 2-5A synthetase in virus-infected mice (66,67). An intriguing observation is the activation of 2-5A synthetase in organs other than the brain since it is well established that rabies virus replicates in the brain and virus is not detectable in other organs. Virus infection may therefore stimulate the accumulation of agents (double-stranded RNA or other factors) that activate the 2-5A synthetase.

The role of 2-5A [$P \times A2'p5')nA, 2 \leqslant X, 2 \geqslant n$] is to activate a latent endoribonuclease capable of degrading RNA. This endocrinuclease loses activity once it is degraded by a phosphatase to nonphosphorylated 2′,5′-adenyladenosine oligonucleotides [$(A2'p5')nA, 1 \leqslant n < 10$] or by a 2′-phosphodiesterase to give rise to AMP and ATP (68,69). It is well established that not all the 5′-phosphorylated adenyladenosine oligonucleotides synthetized by 2-5A synthetase are able to activate the 2-5A-dependent nuclease; only di- and triphosphate trimers and oligomers of greater length are effective at the concentrations found intracellularly (64). It was therefore essential to analyze the oligonucleotide composition in the different organs of rabies virus-infected mice by high-performance liquid chromatographic (HPLC) fractionation. The results indicated that the 2-5A present in organs of infected mice consisted primarily of dimers [pppA2′p5′A] that, it should be recalled, are not able to activate the 2-5A-dependent nuclease. In contrast, organs of mice treated with the combination of interferon and poly(I)·poly(C) contained all the phosphorylated oligomers ranging in size from dimer to pentamer. This difference between the two situations does not seem to be due to an intrinsic inability of the virus-induced 2-5A synthetase to catalyze the formation of oligomers of greater length since the enzyme catalyzes the formation of the higher oligomers in broken cell preparations; the explanation may lie in an incomplete or very transitory activation of 2-5A synthetase, which, in this case, synthesizes mostly pppA2'p5'A.

Rabies virus-infected mice die in the presence of very high levels of interferon activity in the circulation and the brain (47,48). This interferon seems to be ineffective in inhibiting replication of virus, since infected mice do not survive. The absence of 2-5A molecules that activate the 2-5A-dependent nuclease in virus-infected mice may well be one of the reasons that the interferon system is ineffective during rabies virus infection.

IV. ACTION OF EXOGENOUS INTERFERON ON THE PROPHYLAXIS OF RABIES INFECTION IN MICE

Rabies virus-infected mice die in spite of interferon produced during this infection. Thus, it may be that interferon is produced in insufficient amounts or is produced too late in the infection to exert an efficient antiviral effect on the brain. It should also be emphasized that the development of rabies depends on many interacting factors, such as the host immune response. For example, the occurrence of paralysis is dependent on the efficiency of an immune response, as has been shown by experiments using athymic nude mice (55) or cyclophosphamide-treated mice (70). In order to dissociate the specific role of interferon from that of the overall immune response, we investigated the action of exogenous interferon in immunocompetent, immunosuppressed, and immunodeficient athymic mice. Before performing these experiments, we first demonstrated that interferon is capable of inducing an antiviral response in neuroblastoma cell cultures against infection with rabies virus, and second, we could show that interferon in the circulation crosses the blood-brain barrier.

A. Protection Against Rabies Virus Infection in Cell Cultures Treated with Interferon

Treatment of a mouse neuroblastoma cell line with mouse interferon resulted in a dose-dependent increase in the level of 2-5A synthetase and the protein kinase. Thus indicating that these cells respond to interferon. Accordingly, treatment of mouse neuroblastoma cells with 10^3 and 10^4 U/ml of mouse a and β interferon resulted in a 100- and a 10,000-fold reduction of rabies virus yield, respectively (71).

B. Response of Normal Mice to Exogenous Interferon Treatment

The level of 2-5A synthetase and the double-stranded RNA-dependent protein kinase provides a convenient and efficient marker to assess the response of different tissues to interferon, and thus they indirectly show the presence of interferon in a particular tissue (3,44,48). This is of great interest since circulating interferon has a very short half-life and, in some cases, the level of interferon produced is too low to be detectable in an antiviral assay in vitro (2). In contrast, enhanced levels of 2-5A synthetase and the protein kinase last several hours and it is possible to assay efficiently any modification in the level of these enzymes (72,73). Using these enzymes, we therefore investigated the response of the brain of normal mouse to exogenous a and β interferon administered by different routes: intravenous (IV), intraperitoneal (IP), subcutaneous (SC) and intracerebral (IC). Table 3 gives the levels of 2-5A synthetase and the protein kinase in the spleen and brain of normal mice injected with interferon (5×10^4 U) by four different routes. All the different treatments resulted in enhanced levels of enzymes in both the brain and spleen. These enhanced enzyme levels were comparable in the spleen of mice in response to interferon treatment by different routes. On the other hand, there was a better response in the brain when interferon was administered intracerebrally (71). These results illustrate two

Table 3 Enhancement of 2-5A Synthetase and Protein Kinase in Mouse Treated with Interferon[a]

Organ	Route of injection	2-5A Synthetase[b] (nmol/mg per hr)	Protein kinase[b] (^{32}P cpm/mg per hr)
Spleen	No treatment	183	5,220
	IFN IV	345	11,695
	IP	375	12,373
	SC	396	10,342
	IC	335	12,025
Brain	No treatment	0.1	3,266
	IFN IV	2.1	9,555
	IP	1.9	9,287
	SC	1.8	7,525
	IC	4.5	15,860

[a]IFN: mouse $\alpha + \beta$ interferon (5×10^8 U/mg protein), 5×10^4 units.

[b]The 2-5A synthetase and the protein kinase were assayed after partial purification on poly (I)·poly(C)-Sepharose (for details, see Ref. 71).

major points: (1) interferon injected IV, IP, or SC crosses the blood-brain barrier to enhance the level of 2-5A synthetase and the protein kinase in the brain; (2) interferon injected IC passes into the circulation to cause the induction of these enzymes in the spleen.

C. Action of Exogenous Interferon in Rabies Virus-Infected, Immunocompetent Mice

In these experiments, mice were infected with two different strains of rabies virus: (1) CVS-fixed rabies virus, which has a short incubation period; and (2) street rabies virus, which has a longer incubation period. Mice aged 2 months (C3H/He Pasteur Institute) were inoculated with rabies virus into the footpad (71). Interferon was produced by mouse C-243 cells infected with Newcastle disease virus. The purified interferon had a specific activity of 10^9 U/mg of protein (45). In all cases, treatment with interferon started 1-2 hr after virus inoculation and continued every day until the appearance of paralysis; 100,000 U interferon was administered intraperitoneally.

Treatment of rabies virus-infected mice with interferon resulted in a delay of the onset of paralysis, but in general it did not rescue mice from death. These results emphasize that interferon may play a role early after infection by delaying progression of the disease (see also results given in Tables 4 and 5).

1. Action of Exogenous Interferon in Rabies Virus-Infected Mice: Immunocompetent or Immunosuppressed

It has been reported that suppression of the immune response by cyclophosphamide in rabies virus-infected mice both increased the overall mortality rate and delayed onset of disease signs and death for 1-2 weeks (70). Therefore, it was of interest to study the action of interferon on the outcome of rabies virus infection in a host in which the immune response is suppressed and in which the onset of disease signs is delayed. Cyclophosamide has the capacity to suppress in a nonselective manner both cellular and humoral immune responses (74). Cyclophosphamides does not seem to interfere with the production of interferon during rabies virus infection in mice. Similarly, the action of interferon in normal mice immunosuppressed by cyclophosamide is comparable to that observed in immunocompetent mice, at least for the induction of 2-5A synthetase and the protein kinase in the lung and spleen.

In immunocompetent mice, paralysis of the inoculated limb is the first symptom that is characteristic of rabies infection before weight loss and general prostration leading to death. Paralysis of hind limbs does not occur in immunosuppressed mice in which the first sign of onset of rabies disease is shaggy hair accompanied by an incoordination of both hind limbs before weight loss and general prostration. Mice infected either with fixed rabies virus or

Table 4 Action of Exogenous Interferon on Fixed Rabies Virus-Infected Immunocompetent or Immunosuppressed Mice

Treatment	Day of onset of disease[a]	Day of death[a]	Mortality
None	6.0 ± 0.0	7.4 ± 0.7	10/10
IFN[b]	8.1 ± 0.6	10.4 ± 1.1	9/10
Cy[c]	7.1 ± 0.9	8.5 ± 1.1	10/10
IFN and Cy	7.9 ± 0.9	9.1 ± 1.0	10/10

[a]Arithmetic mean ± standard deviation.

[b]IFN: 10^5 U of interferon injected IP 1 hr after virus inoculation and every day until paralysis.

[c]Cy: A single 150/mg/kg dose of cyclophosphamide given 7 hr after virus inoculation.

Table 5 Action of Exogenous Interferon on Street Rabies Virus-Infected Immunocompetent or Immunosuppressed Mice

Treatment	Day of onset of disease[a]	Day of death[a]	Mortality
None	10.3 ± 1.5	15.2 ± 5.4	10/15
IFN[b]	13.7 ± 6.0	19.7 ± 5.3	7/14
Cy[c]	11.8 ± 2.8	15.8 ± 2.4	14/14
IFN and Cy	13.8 ± 2.6	16.2 ± 1.6	15/15

[a]Arithmetic mean ± standard deviation.

[b]IFN: 10^5 U of interferon injected IP 1 hr after virus inoculation and every day until paralysis.

[c]Cy: A single 150/mg/kg dose of cyclophosphamide given 7 hr after virus inoculation and once a week at 75/mg/kg doses.

street rabies virus were treated with interferon in the absence or presence of the immunosuppressor, cyclophosphamide. The results of this experiment (71) are summarized in Tables 4 and 5. In immunocompetent mice infected with either type of rabies virus, interferon treatment did not prevent the appearance of paralysis. There was a very slight protection by interferon: 1 of 10 mice survived fixed rabies virus infection whereas in the group of mice infected with street rabies virus, 7 of 14 survived compared with 10 of 15 in the untreated infected mice. All immunosuppressed mice treated or not with interferon died of rabies. The day of onset disease signs and the day of death varied individually for the mice of each group. The most pronounced effect of interferon treatment was observed in immunocompetent mice on the day of onset of paralysis (Tables 4 and 5). In both types of infections (fixed or street rabies virus), interferon treatment resulted in a significant delay in the first clinical signs ($p < 0.01$).

2. Effect of Exogenous Interferon on Antibody Synthesis
   Against Rabies Virus in Immunocompetent and in
   Immunosuppressed Mice

Interferon treatment of immunocompetent mice infected with fixed or street rabies virus resulted in a 10-fold reduction of rabies virus production in the brain. On the other hand, there was a significant increase ($p < 0.02$) in antibody synthesis against rabies virus in response to treatment with interferon (Table 6). This is therefore a good example of interferon treatment triggering enhanced antibody synthesis. This is one of the properties of interferon that was reported previously by several workers (76-79).

As expected, antibody synthesis in immunosuppressed mice was almost not detectable. However, in mice treated with interferon and cyclophosphamide there was still a significant antibody synthesis against rabies virus (Table 6). These antibodies were of the IgM class. The mechanism by which interferon somehow bypasses the inhibitory action of cyclophosphamide on the antibody synthesis remains to be clarified. It should be noted that there was no apparent difference in the clinical symptoms observed in immunosuppressed mice treated or not with interferon.

Table 6 Action of Interferon on Virus and Antibody Titers in Rabies Virus-Infected Immunocompetant or Immunosuppressed Mice

Virus	Treatment[a]	Virus titer[b] (DL_{50}/ml)	Antibody titer[c] (IU)
Fixed rabies	None	$10^{7.3}$	18.4 ± 8.6
	IFN	$10^{6.2}$	23.8 ± 8.9
	Cy	10^{7}	0.4 ± 0.1
	IFN and Cy	10^{6}	4.2 ± 0.9
Street rabies	None	$10^{3.2}$	25.4 ± 8.6
	IFN	10^{2}	36.8 ± 8.5
	Cy	$10^{4.2}$	0.5 ± 0.1
	IFN and Cy	$10^{4.2}$	11.7 ± 8.6

[a]The different treatments were as in Tables 5 and 6.

[b]Titrated in Swiss mice; the average from two mice.

[c]Antibody production against rabies virus was titrated by the fluorescent focus reduction test (75).

D. Action of Exogenous Interferon in Rabies Virus Infection of Nude Mice

Athymic nude mice provide a useful experimental animal model to investigate the role of T cells in the development of clinical signs and pathogenesis during a viral infection (80). For example, paralysis of hind limbs of mice during street rabies virus infection is considered a consequence of events in which T cells seem to play a major role. Athymic nude mice infected with street rabies virus become cachectic but do not show paralysis, which is the routine clinical symptom observed in normal mice (55).

1. Infection with Street Rabies Virus

Homozygous nude (background Swiss; nu/nu) mice inoculated with street rabies virus become cachectic without symptoms of paralysis. Such infected mice started to lose weight significantly 15 days after virus inoculation. This loss of weight increased progressively until the death of all animals (8 of 8) between days 22 and 30 of infection (71). Interferon (10^5 U) administered 1 hr after virus inoculation and every 24 hr up to 30 days protected nude mice against rabies infection. A month after the end of interferon treatment (i.e., 60 days after virus inoculation), one mouse developed rabies and died a few days later. In this mouse, diagnosis of rabies virus was made by immunofluorescence study of brain sections. The rest of the interferon-treated mice (7 of 8) remained healthy until the end of the experiment, 90 days after virus inoculation (71).

Treatment of homozygous (nu/nu) mice with interferon protected against street rabies virus infection. On the other hand, treatment of heterozygous ($nu/+$) normal mice with interferon did not at all affect street rabies virus infection.

2. Infection with CVS-Fixed Rabies Virus

Athymic nude mice inoculated with fixed rabies developed a paralysis of the inoculated limb on day 6 of infection. This was a genuine paralysis (Fig. 1), which is routinely observed in normal mice infected with fixed or street rabies virus. All mice (8 of 8) died between days 7 and 8 of infection. Treatment of fixed rabies-infected nude mice with interferon (as in Sec. IV. D. 1) did not modify the day of paralysis and death. These results indicated that the pathogenesis of rabies virus and the action of interferon are variable according to the type of virus inoculated. The presence of paralysis in fixed rabies virus-infected nude mice is very intriguing and suggests that other factors besides T cells must participate for the establishment of paralysis. It may also be possible that different virus strains trigger different mechanisms leading to paralysis. Whatever the situation, further investigation of such experimental models should provide more information concerning the mechanism(s) involved in the pathogenesis of rabies virus infection.

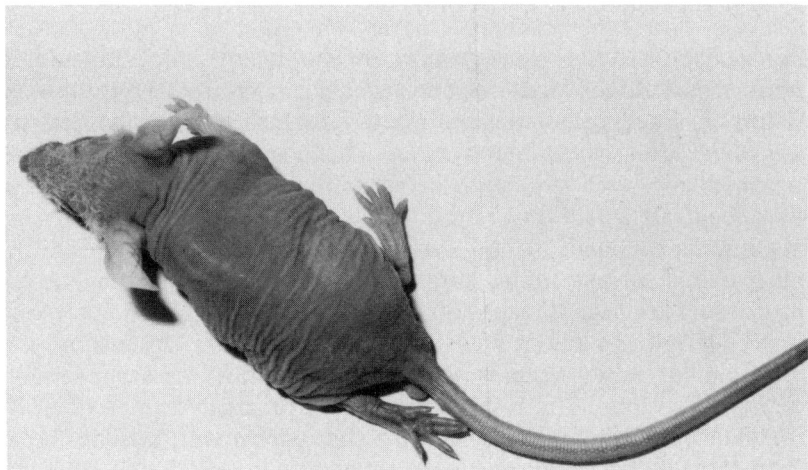

Figure 1 Paralysis of the inoculated limb of an athymic nude mouse infected with CVS-fixed strain of rabies virus.

Paralysis is not observed in fixed rabies virus-infected normal mice injected with cyclophosphamide (Table 4). In view of this, fixed rabies virus-infected nude mice were injected with cyclophosphamide 7 hr after virus inoculation and then once every week (as in Table 4). These immunosuppressed nude mice became cachectic and showed general prostration before death. Thus, paralysis did not occur in fixed rabies virus-infected nude mice injected with cyclophosphamide (71).

V. CONCLUSIONS

Evidence has been accumulated during the last 15 years to suggest that rabies disease can be prevented by treatment with interferon or interferon inducers. Some data are controversial, however, with reports of partial protection by interferon or no protection at all. It has now become evident that interferon treatment is useless once the replication of rabies virus has started in the central nervous system. Interferon administered during the incubation period of rabies virus protects monkeys and rabbits but in mouse seems to be ineffective. Whatever the situation, there is no doubt that early administration of interferon leads to a significant delay in the appearance of the first clinical symptoms that accompany rabies infection. In the future, interferon will probably be used as has been reported recently (39), in conjunction with the administration of rabies vaccine and antirabies serum.

During rabies virus infection in mice, interferon is produced. This interferon induces enhanced levels of 2-5A synthetase and double-stranded RNA-dependent protein kinase and causes a delay in the onset of disease signs. The 2-5A synthetase becomes activated during rabies virus infection, but unfortunately the 2-5A synthesized is of dimer form, which does not activate the endonuclease. In spite of in vitro and in vivo evidence that (1) treatment of mouse neuroblastoma cells with interferon provides protection against eventual infection with rabies virus, and (2) interferon in the circulation crosses the blood-brain barrier, treatment of mice infected with either fixed or street rabies virus does not prevent the development of rabies disease (Table 7). Interferon treatment stimulates a significant enhancement in the level of antibodies against rabies and causes a delay in the appearance of the first signs of paralysis and death. However, although interferon may be functional during the incubation period of rabies virus, the evolution of rabies disease depends on other mechanisms related to the immune response of the host. For this reason we investigated the action of interferon in rabies virus-infected mice during immunosuppression by cyclophosphamide. This substance is capable of suppressing in a nonselective way both cellular and humoral immune responses of the host. Cyclophosphamide-administered mice died irrespective of interferon treatment (Table 7). However, an intriguing observation was the enhancement of antirabies antibodies in immunosuppressed mice in response to treatment with interferon.

The pathogenesis of CVS-fixed rabies virus seems to be different from that of street rabies virus. This was illustrated by experiments carried out in immunodeficient (nude) mice infected with either fixed or street rabies virus. Both viral infections are lethal in

Table 7 Action of Interferon on Paralysis and Mortality in Immunocompetent, Immunosuppressed, or Immunodeficient Mice Infected with CVS-Fixed or Street Rabies Virus[a]

Virus	Disease	Immunocompetent mice		Immunosuppressed mice		Immunodeficient mice	
		Control	IFN	Control	IFN	Control	IFN
CVS-Fixed	Paralysis	+	+	−	−	+	+
	Mortality (%)	100	90	100	100	100	100
Street	Paralysis	+	+	−	−	−	−
	Mortality (%)	66.6	50	100	100	100	12.5

[a] +, paralysis; −, lack of paralysis. For details, see Tables 4 and 5 and Section IV.

mice. However, paralysis does not occur in mice infected with street rabies virus in contrast to infection with fixed rabies virus. In this latter infection, cyclophosphamide inhibits the development of paralysis (Table 7). These results suggest that paralysis observed during fixed rabies virus infection in the nude mice is not due to mechanisms dependent on the T-cell system.

The efficacy of the interferon treatment was illustrated by using nude mice infected with street rabies virus. It is therefore tempting to suggest that a combination of interferon treatment with a specific T-cell suppressor may be efficiently used in the postexposure prophylaxis of rabies.

There is growing evidence that in rabies virus infection the mechanisms of pathogenesis may be related to functional alterations in the nervous system. This hypothesis has been substantiated by neuropharmacologic studies showing impairment at the level of receptors to neurotransmitters (81) and by neurophysiologic studies showing electroencephalographic disturbancies and sleep alterations (82) during experimental rabies infection. Since interferon may also have some activity in neural functions (83), the eventual role of interferon in the modulatory effect of brain function alterations during rabies virus infection cannot be ruled out.

REFERENCES

1. Stewart, W. E., II. *The Interferon System.* Springer-Verlag, Wien (1979).

2. Bocci, V. Production and role of interferon in physiological conditions. *Biol. Rev. 56*:49–85 (1981).

3. Galabru, J., Robert, N., Buffet-Jnvresse, C., Riviere, Y., and Hovanessian, A. G. Continuous production of interferon in normal mice: Effect of anti-interferon globulin, sex, age, strain and environment on the levels of 2-5A synthetase and p67K kinase. *J. Gen. Virol. 66*:711–718 (1985).

4. Bellardelli, F., Bignaux, F., Proietti, E., and Gresser, I. Injection of mice with antibody to interferon renders peritoneal machrophages permissive for vesicular stomatitis virus and encephalomyocarditis virus. *Proc. Natl. Acad. Sci. USA 81*:602–606.

5. Baer, G. M., Shanthaveerappa, T. R., and Bourne, G. H. Studies on the pathogenesis of fixed rabies virus in rats. *Bull WHO* 33:783-784 (1965).

6. Baer, G. M., Shantha, T. R., and Bourne, G. H. The pathogenesis of street rabies virus in rats. *Bull. WHO* 38:119-125 (1968).

7. Wiktor, T. J., Postic, B., Ho, M., and Koprowski, H. Role of interferon induction in the protective activity of rabies vaccine. *J. Infect. Dis.* 126:408-418 (1972).

8. Baer, G. M. Antiviral action of interferon in animal systems: Effect of interferon on rabies infections of animals. *Tex. Rep. Biol. Med.* 35:461-471 (1977).

9. Baer, G. M. The effect of interferon on rabies infection of animals. *Tex. Rep. Biol. Med.* 41:526-531 (1981-1982).

10. Kaplan, M. M., Cohen, D., Koprowski, H., Deam, D., and Ferrigan, L., Studies on the local treatment of wounds for the prevention of rabies. *Bull. WHO* 26:765-775 (1962).

11. Finter, N. B. Interferon in mice: Protection against small doses of virus. *J. Gen. Virol.* 1:395-397 (1967).

12. Vieuchange, J. Role d:un interféron dans le phénomène de l'interférence entre le virus vaccinal et le virus rabique fixe. *C.R. Acad. Sci. (Paris)* D264:426-428 (1967).

13. Karakuyumchan, M. K., and Bektemirova, M. S. Production and effect of interferon in experimental infection with fixed rabies virus. *Vopros. Virusol.* 13:596-599 (1968).

14. Postic, B., and Fenje, P. Effect of administered interferon on rabies in rabbits. *Appl. Microbiol.* 22:428-431 (1971).

15. Ho, m., Nash, C., Morgan, C. W., Armstrong, J. A., Carroll, R. G., and Postic, B. Interferon administered in the cerebrospinal space and its effect on rabies in rabbits. *Infect. Immun.* 9:268-293 (1974).

16. Hilfenhaus, J., Karges, H. E., Weinmann, E., and Barth, R. Effect of administered leukocyte interferon on experimental rabies in monkeys. *Infect. Immun.* 11:1156-1162 (1975).

17. Hilfenhaus, J., Weinmann, E., Majer,M., Barth, R., and Jaeger, J. Post-exposure administration of human interferon to rabies infected monkeys. *J. Infect. Dis.* 135:846-851 (1977).

18. Weinmann, E., Majer, M., and Hilfenhaus, J. Intramuscular and/or

intralumbar postexposure treatment of rabies virus infected cynomolgus monkeys with human interferon. *Infect. Immun.* 24:24-31 (1979).

19. Atanasiu, P., Barroeta, M., Tsiang, H., and Favie, S. Inhibition in vivo de la multiplication du virus rabique par un interferon endogène. *Ann. Virol.* (Inst. Pasteur) 119:767-777 (1979).

20. Soave, O. A. Influence of statolon-induced interferon on rabies virus infection in mice. *Am. J. Vet. Res.* 29:1507-1508 (1968).

21. Nemes, M. M., Tytell, A. A., Lampson, G. P., Field, A. K., and Hilleman, M. R. Inducers of interferon and host resistance. VII. Antiviral efficacy of poly I:C in animal models. *Proc. Soc. Exp. Biol. Med.* 132:776-783 (1969).

22. Hemes, M. M., Tytell, A. A., Lampson, G. P., Field, A. K., and Hilleman, M. R. Inducers of interferon and host resistance. VI. Antiviral efficacy of double-stranded RNA of natural origin. *Proc.Soc. Exp. Biol. Med.* 132: 784-789 (1969).

23. Harmon, M. W., Jamis, B., and Levy, M. Post-exposure prophylaxis of murine rabies with polyinosinic-polycytidylic acid and chlorite-oxidized amylose. *Antimicrob. Agents Chemother.* G:507-511 (1974).

24. Fenje, P., and Postic, B. Protection of rabbits against experimental rabies by poly(I)·poly(C). *Nature* 226:171-172 (1970).

25. Fornosi, F., Talas, M., and Weizfeller, G. Effect of tilorone hydrochloride on the experimental rabies of mice. *Acta Microbiol. Acad. Sci Hung.* 18: 327-331 (1971).

26. Levy, H. B., Baer, G., Baron, S., Buckler, C. E., Gibbs, C. J., Iabarola, M. J., London, W. T., and Rice, J. A. A modified polyriboinosinic-polyribocytidylic acid complex that induces interferon in primates. *J. Infect. Dis.* 132:434-439 (1975).

27. Janis, B., and Habel, K. Rabies in rabbits and mice: Protective effect of polyriboinosinic-polyribocytidylic acid. *J. Infect. Dis.* 125:345-353 (1972).

28. Harmon, M. W., and Janis, B. Therapy of murine rabies after exposure: Efficacy of polyinosinic-polyribocytidylic acid alone and in combination with three rabies vaccines. *J. Infect. Dis.* 132:241-247 (1975).

29. Stewart, W. E., II, and Sulkin, S. E. Evaluating the role of interferon in rabies infection. *Bacteriol. Proc. 23* (1968).

30. Wiktor, T. J., Koprowski, H., Mitchell, J. R., and Merigan, T. C. Role

of interferon in prophylaxis of rabies after exposure. *J. Infect. Dis. 133*: A260-A266.

31. Nozaki, J., and Atanasiu, P. Evaluation du pouvoir inducteur d'interféron des vaccins antirabiques. *Ann. Microbiol.* (Inst. Pasteur) *126B*:381-388 (1975).

32. Baer, G. M., and Cleary, W. F. A model in mice for the pathogenesis and treatment of rabies. *J. Infect. Dis. 125*:520-527 (1972).

33. Turner, G. S. Rabies vaccines and interferon. *J. Hyg. (Camb.)* 70:445-453 (1972).

34. Nicholson, K. G., Harrison, P., Kuwert, E. K., and Werner, J. Cell culture rabies vaccines and their protective effect in man. In: (E. K. Kuwert, T. J. Wiktor, and H. Koprowski, eds.). International Green Gross, Geneva (1981).

35. Baer, G. M., Shaddock, J. H., Moore, S. A., Yage, P. A., Baron, S. S., and Levy, H. B. Successful rabies prophylaxis of mice and rhesus monkeys with the interferon system and vaccine. *J. Infect. Dis. 136*:58-62 (1977).

36. Baer, G. M., and Yager, P. A. A mouse model for post-exposure rabies prophylaxis: The comparative efficacy of two vaccines and of antiserum administration. *J. Gen. Virol. 36*:1-8 (1977).

37. Wiktor, T. J., Sokol, F., Kuwert, E., and Korprowski, H. Immunogenicity of concentrated and purified rabies vaccine of tissue culture origin. *Proc. Soc. Exp. Biol. Med. 131*:799-805 (1969).

38. Baltazard, M., and Bahmanyar, M. Practical trial of antirabies serum in those bitten by rabid wolves. *Bull. WHO 13*:747-772 (1955).

39. Sureau, P., Portnoi, D., Rollin, P., Lapresle, C., and Chaoni-Berbich, A. Prevention de la transmission inter-humaine de la rage après greffe de cornée. *C.R. Acad. Sci (Paris) t293*:689-692 (1981).

40. Wiktor, T. J., Koprowski, H., and Rorke, L. B. Localized rabies interferon in mice. *Proc. Soc. Exp. Biol. Med. 140*:759-764 (1972).

41. Atanasiu, P. Rôle de l'interféron dans l'immunité antirabique. *Comp. Immunol. Microbiol. Infect. Dis. 5*:123-127 (1982).

42. Hovanessian, A. G. Intracellular events in interferon-treated cells. *Differentiation 15*:139-151 (1979).

43. Hovanessian, A. G. Interferon: Direct effects upon virus replication. In: *Approaches to Antiviral Agents* (M. R. Harnden, ed.). Macmillan, New York pp. 217-260 (1985).

44. Hovanessian, A. G., and Rivière, Y. Interferon-mediated induction of 2-5A synthetase and proteinkinase in the liver and spleen of mice infected with Newcastle disease virus or injected with poly(I)·poly(C). *Ann. Virol.* (Inst. Pasteur) *131E*:501-516 (1980).

45. Krust, B., Rivière, and Hovanessian, A. G. p67 kinase in different tissues and plasma of control and interferon-treated mice. *Virology 120*:240-246 (1982).

46. Saron, M. F., Rivière, Hovanessian, A. G., and Guillon, J. C. Chronic production of interferon in carrier mice congenitally infected with lymphocytic choriomeningitis virus. *Virology 117*:253-256 (1982).

47. Marcovistz, R., Tsiang, H., and Hovanessian, A. G. Production and action of interferon in mice infected with rabies virus. *Ann Virol.* (Inst. Pasteur), *135E*:19-33 (1984).

48. Marcovistz, R., Galabru, J., Tsiang, H., and Hovanessian, A. G. Neutralization of interferon produced during rabies virus infection in mice. *J. Gen. Virol. 67*:387-390 (1986).

49. Debbie, J. G., and Trimarchi, C. V. Pantropism of rabies virus in free-ranging rabid red fox, *Vulpes fulva. J. Wildlife Dis. 6*:500-506 (1970).

50. Murphy, F. A., Harrison, A. K., Winn, W. C., and Baner, S. P. Comparative pathogenesis of rabies and rabies-like viruses. *Lab Invest. 29*:1-16 (1973).

51. Fauconnier, B. Augmentation de la pathogénécité virale par l'emploi de sérum anti-interféron in vivo. *C.R. Acad. Sci. (Paris) 271*:1464-1466 (1970).

52. Gresser, I., Tovey, M. G., Bandu, M. T., Maury, C., and Brouty-Boye, D. Role of interferon in the pathogenesis of virus diseases in mice as demonstrated by the use of anti-interferon serum. I. Rapid evolution of encephalomyocarditis virus infection. *J. Exp. Med. 144*:1305-1315 (1976).

53. Gresser, I., Tovey, M. G., Maury, C., and Bandu, M. T. Role of interferon in the pathogenesis of viral diseases in mice as demonstrated by the use of anti-interferon serum. II. Studies with herpes simplex, Moloney, sarcoma, vesicular stomatitis, Newcastle disease and influenza viruses. *J. Exp. Med. 144*:1316-1323 (1976).

54. Gresser, I., Maury, C., Kress, C., Blangy, D., and Maunoury, M. T. Role of interferon in the pathogenesis of virus disease in mice as demonstrated by the use of anti-interferon serum. VI. Polyoma virus infection. *Int. J. Cancer 24*:178-183 (1979).

55. Guillon J. C., and Tsiang, H. Rôle de l'interféron et du thymus dans la pathogènése de l'infection rabique chez la souris. *Ann. Virol. 131E*:229-245 (1980).

56. Rivière, Y., Gresser, I., Guillon, J. C., and Rovey, M. G. Inhibition by anti-interferon serum of lymphocytic choriomeningitis disease in suckling mice. *Proc. Natl. Acad. Sci. USA 74*:2135-2139 (1977).

57. Saron, M. F., Rivière, I., Gresser, and Guillon, J. C. Prévention par les globulines anti-interféron de la mortalité des souris infectées par le virus de la chorioméningite lymphocytaire. I. Lésions histologiques, titres sériques du virus et de l'infection. *Ann, Virol. 133E*:241-253 (1982).

58. Koning, J. F. R., and Klippel, R. A. *The Rat Brain: A Stereotaxic Atlas.* R. E. Krieger, New York (1967).

59. Tsiang, H. Neuronal function impairment in rabies-infected rat brain. *61*: 277-281 (1982).

60. Marcovistz, R., Hovanessian, A. G., and Tsiang, H. Distribution of rabies virus, interferon and interferon-mediated enzymes in the brains of virus-infected rats. *J. Gen. Virol. 65*:995-997 (1984).

61. Matsumoto, S. Electron microscopy of nerve cells infected with street rabies virus. *Virology 17*:198-202 (1962).

62. Tsiang, H., Koulakoff, A., Bizzini, B., and Berwald-Netter, Y. Neurotropism of rabies virus: An in vitro study. *J. Neuropathol. 42*:439-452 (1983).

63. Hovanessian, A. G., and Kerr, I. M. The $(2'-5')$ oligoadenylate $(pppA2'p5'A2'p5A)$ synthetase and protein kinases(s) from interferon-treated cells. *Eur. J. Biochem. 93*:515-526 (1969).

64. Kerr, I. M., Cayley, P. J., Roberts, W. K., Rice, A., Reid, A., Hersh, C., Stark, G. R., Laurent, L., Cailla, H., Marti, J., Wells, V., and Malluci, L. Molecular mechanisms of interferon action and the possible wider significance of the 2-5A system. In: *The Biology of the Interferon System 1983* (E. De Maeyer and H. Schellekens, eds.). Elsevier, Amsterdam, pp. 213-222 (1983).

65. Laurence, L., Roux, D., Cailla, H., Riviére, Marcovistz, R., and Hovanessian, A. G. Comparison of the effects of rabies virus infection and of combined interferon and poly(I)·poly(C) treatment on the levels of $2'$-$5'$-adenyladenosine oligonucleotides in different organs of mice. *Virology 143*:290-299 (1985).

66. Johnson, R. T., and Mercier, H. E. The development of fixed rabies virus in mouse brain. *Aust. J. Exp. Biol. Med. Sci.* 42:449–456 (1964).

67. Laurence. L., Trujillo, M., Samuel, D., Kaplan, S., Roux, R., Hovanessian, A. G., Marti, J., and Cailla, H. Immunological approach of intracellular 2'-5'-linked adenyladenosine oligonucleotides. In: *The 2-5A System: Molecular and Clinical Aspects of the Interferon-Regulated Pathway* (R. H. Silverman and B. R. G. Williams, eds.). pp. 3–10 (1985).

68. Nilsen, T. W., Maroney, P. A., and Baglioni, C. Synthesis of (2'-5') oligoadenylated and activation of an endoribonuclease in interferon-treated HeLa cells infected with reovirus. *J. Virol.* 42:1039–1045 (1982).

69. Schmidt, A., Chernajovsky, Y., Shulman, L., Federman, P., Verissi, H., and Revel, M. An interferon-induced phosphodiesterase degradation (2'-5') oligoisoadenylate and C-C-A terminus of tRNA. *Proc. Natl. Acad. Sci. USA* 76:4788–4792 (1979).

70. Smith, J. S., McClelland, C. L., Reid, F. L., and Baer, G. M. Dual role of the immune response in street rabies virus infection in mice. *Infect. Immun.* 35:213–221 (1982).

71. Marcovistz, R. Etude de l'action de l'interferon endogène et exogène au cours de l'infection de la souris par le virus rabique. Thèse de Doctorat d'Etat, ès Sciences Naturelles, Université Paris VII (1985).

72. Hovanessian, A. G., Rivière, Y., Robert, N., Svab, S., Chamaret, S., Guillon, J. C., and Montagnier, L. Protein kinase in plasma and tissues of mice with high levels of circulating interferon. *Ann. Virol.* 132E:175–188 (1981).

73. Hovanessian, A. G., Rivière, and Krust, B. Assay of interferon-mediated protein kinase activity from plasma and tissue extracts. Ann. Biochem. 129:349–356 (1983).

74. Bach, J. F. The mode of action of immunosuppressive agents. In: *Frontiers of Biology*, Vol. 41 (A. Neuberger and E. L. Tatum, eds.). pp. 173–225 (1975).

75. Sureau, P., Rollin, P. E., and Zeller, H. Correlation entre l'épreuve immunoenzymatique, la séroneutralisation et la réduction de foyers fluorescents pour le titrage des anticorps rabique. *Comp. Immunol. Microbiol. Infect. Dis.* 5:143–150 (1982).

76. De Mayer, E., Interferon and the immune system: A review. In: *The Biology of the Interferon System* (E. De Maeyer, G. Galasso, and H.

Schellekens, eds.). Elsevier/North-Holland Biomedical Press, Amsterdam, pp. 203-209 (1981).

77. Gresser, I., Commentary: On the varied biologic effects of interferon. *Cell. Immun.* *34*:406-415 (1977).

78. Epstein, L. B. The effects of interferons on the immune response in vitro and in vivo. In: *Interferon and Their Actions* (W. Stewart, II, ed.). CRC Press, Cleveland, pp. 91-132 (1977).

79. Nakamura, M., Manser, T., Pearson, G. D. N., Daley, M. J., and Gefter, M. L. Effect of IFN- on the immune response in vivo and on gene expression in vitro. *Nature* *307*:381-382 (1984).

80. Iwasaki, Y. Experimental virus infections in nude mice. In: *The Nude Mouse in Experimental and Clinical Research* (J. Fogh and B. C. Grovanella, eds.). Academic Press, New York, pp. 457-475 (1978).

81. Koschek, K., and Munzel, M. Inhibition of opiate receptor-mediated signal transmission by rabies virus in persistently infected NG-108-15 mouse neuroblastoma-rat glioma hybrid cells. *Proc. Natl. Acad. Sci. USA* *81*:950-954 (1984).

82. Gourmelon, P., Briet, D., Court, L., and Tsiang, H. Electrophysiological and sleep alterations in experimental mouse rabies. *Brain Res.* In press (1986).

83. Smedley, H., Katrack, M., Sikora, K., and Wheeler, T. Neurological effect of recombinant human interferon. *Br. Med. J.* *286*:262-264 (1983).

8
Treatment of Subacute Sclerosing Panencephalitis with Interferon

HILLEL S. PANITCH

*University of Maryland School of Medicine and
Veterans Administration Medical Center, Baltimore, Maryland*

I. INTRODUCTION

Subacute sclerosing panencephalitis (SSPE) is a progressive and fatal central nervous system (CNS) disease of children caused by persistent infection with measles (rubeola) virus. The clinical and pathological features were described by Dawson in 1933 (1), and more recently several comprehensive reviews have appeared (2-4). Clinical symptoms appear at a mean age of 7-8 years and typically progress inexorably over a period of 1-3 years. The clinical course has been divided into three (5) or four (6) stages, with the latter the most commonly used classification. Stage I is marked by subtle behavioral changes and deterioration in school performance. Stage II is characterized by development of generalized or multifocal myoclonic jerks, seizures, akinetic phenomena, and focal motor deficits. In state III, the child is comatose or semicomatose with generalized spasticity, decorticate or decerebrate rigidity, and autonomic insufficiency. In stage IV, there is hypotonia, mutism, and loss of all cortical function leading ultimately to death. In approximately 10% of patients, the course may be more fulminant; in others (estimated at 10% but possibly more) the course is prolonged by periods of stabilization or even definite clinical remission (2,7-9). The diagnosis is confirmed by a burst suppression pattern on the electroencephalogram (EEG) consisting of periodic sharp and slow wave complexes superimposed on a low-voltage background. Computed tomographic (CT) scans demonstrate cortical atrophy, ventricular dilation, and low-density areas in the periventricular white matter (10a) with occasional contrast enhancement secondary to blood-brain barrier damage (10b). Early in the disease the CT scan is often normal, and the radiographic abnormalities appear with progressive clinical deterioration. Lesions in subcortical and periventricular white matter have also been described by magnetic resonance imaging (11).

Distinctive cerebrospinal fluid (CSF) findings are also present, consisting of elevated levels of IgG, oligoclonal IgG bands on agarose electrophoresis, and high titers of antibodies to measles virus (2-4). Serum antibody titers are also elevated, often to extremely high levels. However, the blood-brain barrier remains relatively intact, and the excess IgG is produced within the CNS, probably as a result of continuous antigenic stimulation. Studies in which the serum and CSF were absorbed with measles virus antigen and then eluted and subjected to electrophoresis have shown that the oligoclonal bands consist largely of antibodies to measles virus proteins (12). More recently, measles-specific antibody in the CSF was shown to account for most, but not all, of the oligoclonal IgG synthesized within the CNS (13). Other investigators have found antibody activity to myelin basic protein in the CSF of SSPE patients (14); however, this finding has not been confirmed and its significance is uncertain.

II. ETIOLOGY AND PATHOGENESIS

Pathologically, SSPE affects both gray and white matter and is characterized by variable degrees of neuronal loss, inflammation, and demyelination. Retinal lesions are sometimes seen and can be useful as an aid to early diagnosis (15). The most distinctive hallmark is the presence of intranuclear and intracytoplasmic inclusion bodies, which are found in neurons, astrocytes, and, most strikingly, in oligodendrocytes (16). Immunofluorescent staining shows extensive intracellular measles antigen, and on electron-microscopy the inclusion bodies are shown to be composed of paramyxovirus nucleocapsids. No free virus is present in the CNS; however, measles virus can be isolated by cocultivation of brain tissue with permissive cell lines in vitro (17;18).

Numerous theories have been proposed to account for the cell-associated state and for the pathogenesis of the disease. At present, the factors that determine susceptibility are still incompletely understood. Most investigators believe that children with SSPE are immunologically normal (2,19), but because the disease typically occurs in children with a history of measles infection early in life, usually below 2 years of age, it may be that immaturity of the immune system and of the CNS permit the virus to establish itself (3,20). The presence of antibody may result in attenuation of the acute measles infection but lead to modulation of surface antigens of infected cells and to subsequent persistent CNS infection (21). This phenomenon can be demonstrated in animal models (22-24) and has been postulated as the mechanism of at least one case of human SSPE (25). A recent report of measles virus RNA detected by in situ hybridization showed genomic material in 70-90% of peripheral blood mononuclear cells from patients with SSPE (26). This finding raises new questions about the locus of viral persistence and also about the existence of subtle immunologic defects in the infected cells (27).

Several studies have shown that SSPE patients fail to produce antibody to the matrix (M) protein of measles virus (20,28). This is not the result of an immunologic defect but probably of a deficit in production of the M protein itself in infected brain cells (29,30). This protein is necessary for assembly of the virus and release of infectious particles, and its absence could account for the cell-associated nature of the measles virus infection. However, the origin and mechanism of this defect are still unclear. Recently M protein-specific RNA has been detected in SSPE tissue (31), although the protein itself was not detectable, suggesting a defect in translation. In another study, however, M protein antigen could be detected by immunofluorescence in fresh autopsy and biopsy tissue (32). There appears to be considerable variation among patients in expression of the M protein. Variations in production of the measles hemagglutinin or H protein have also been reported, possibly related to increasing maturity of brain cells (33). Haase et al. reported that expression of the NP protein was also reduced (34) and postulated that early repression of both transcription and translation of the entire measles virus genome was responsible for the resistance of infected cells to attack by the immune response and that, later in the infection as the various viral proteins accumulated, only a relative defect in M protein translation remained, accounting for the persistent cell-associated state. Obviously the last word on the mechanism of viral persistence in SSPE has not yet been written.

III. CHANGING CLINICAL COURSE OF SSPE

SSPE has nearly disappeared from the United States since the introduction of an effective measles vaccination program in the mid-1960s (4,35). Approximately five new cases are reported per year in unvaccinated children or, rarely, in a recipient of the live virus vaccine. In other parts of the world, such as Latin America, the Middle East, and Eastern Europe, the incidence is considerably higher (36). SSPE in these areas is, in fact, a major pediatric neurologic problem for which no effective treatment exists. In such countries, the clinical course of SSPE seems to be more variable than previously reported, with a larger proportion of cases experiencing stabilization or remission (7,8,37). Among 118 cases from the Middle East, Risk and Haddad (7) found that 53% experienced improvement, remission, or stabilization. A study of malnourished Haitian children showed a high incidence of early measles infection associated with low levels of antibody (38). Malnutrition or other factors that alter the immunologic status of children in underdeveloped nations may play a role not only in the increased incidence of SSPE but also in its clinical expression.

The natural history of the disease has also changed, to some extent, in the United States (39). DuRant and colleagues (40,41) divided cases into rapidly and slowly developing types, with the former progressing to severe disability or death within 1 year and the latter experiencing a prolonged course, often 5–10 years in duration, in some cases with sustained remissions. In their series, the chronic form accounted for up to 20% of cases. Nevertheless, the disease ultimately results in severe disability and death, even in those patients who undergo clinical remissions.

IV. TREATMENT OF SSPE

A. Antiviral and Immunomodulatory Agents Other Than Interferon

The rarity of SSPE and the necessity for conducting clinical trials over long periods of time to allow spontaneous stabilization or remission have made the evaluation of therapy difficult. Numerous modes of treatment have been attempted with minimal success. Immunostimulatory agents, particularly transfer factor (42,43), have been used because of suggestive evidence for a defect in the immune response to measles virus but have generally proved to be ineffective. Reports of a circulating inhibitor of cell-mediated cytotoxicity (44) and more recent evidence for circulating immune complexes (45,46) have led to clinical trials of plasmapheresis, also with negative results (47). In a trial of the synthetic antiviral agent amantadine (48), prolonged remissions occurred in four of eight treated patients but not in untreated controls.

Isoprinosine (Inosiplex), a drug with both antiviral and immunomodulatory properties, has undergone more extensive testing in SSPE than any other single agent (40,41,49-54). It is practically free of side effects and can be given safely for years. Its mechanism of action in vivo has not been thoroughly investigated, and the possibility that it may act as an interferon inducer has not been addressed. Nevertheless, in each of two separate clinical trials (49,52), isoprinosine was reported to induce significant remissions or stabilization in 10 of 15 patients. In some cases the remissions were quite dramatic (49). In the largest study to date, Jones et al. (53) found that isoprinosine improved survival in 98 treated patients in comparison with 590 untreated controls. Others, however, have found isoprinosine to be ineffective (50,51) and have concluded that the occasional remissions seen in treated patients could be accounted for by the variable natural history of the disease. DuRant and Dyken divided patients into slowly and rapidly progressive groups and showed by life table analysis that isoprinosine was effective only in the slowly progressive type (41). In those patients in whom serum and CSF IgG and measles antibody titers have been reported, there were no significant changes during clinical remissions induced by isoprinosine. Because of its partial effectiveness and low risk, isoprinosine may prove useful as an adjunct to other modes of therapy for SSPE.

B. Rationale for Treatment with Interferon

For a variety of reasons, interferon should be regarded as a logical candidate for therapy of SSPE. This previously rare and expensive material is now generally available in synthetic form. With the advent of recombinant DNA technology, the production of interferon is accelerating along with a reduction in its cost. The subtypes of α, as well as β and γ interferons, have been cloned, and many of these are now available for clinical trials. Interferon can be safely administered intrathecally and intraventricularly (55-57). Thus, even though systemically administered interferon fails to cross the intact blood-brain barrier in significant amounts, it can be instilled directly into the cerebral ventricles or lumbar subarachnoid space so that it equilibrates with the extracellular fluid of the CNS (58). Another important consideration in a cell-associated infection like SSPE is that interferon acts directly on infected cells to prevent viral replication by interfering with the synthesis of viral RNA and the translation of RNA into viral protein (59). The antiviral effect does not depend on neutralization of free virus or on interference with viral attachment or penetration into cells.

Inteferon is also important in activation of natural killer (NK) cells (60,61), and measles-infected cells are susceptible to NK-mediated cytotoxicity (62). Although there is no evidence for defective NK activity in SSPE, augmentation of this system by interferon would theoretically help to eradicate the persistent infection. Joncas et al. (63) found interferon in CSF in three of eight patients with SSPE. There was no apparent correlation with clinical outcome, CSF abnormalities, or measles antibody titers, but the levels (200-800 U/ml) may not have been adequate to produce a therapeutic effect.

C. Pharmacokinetics and Neurotoxicity of Interferon

The pharmacokinetics and toxicity of interferon are discussed in more detail elsewhere in this volume, but several points should be mentioned briefly in considering the administration of interferon by intrathecal or intraventricular injection. Because interferon poorly crosses the intact blood-brain barrier, large systemic doses are necessary to produce measurable titers in CSF and presumably in CNS parenchyma. The serum-CSF concentration ratio is usually cited as 30:1 (64) but may be much greater. After intravenous infusion of 50 million units (MU) of natural interferon-α in patients with amyotrophic lateral sclerosis, Smith et al. (65) found ratios as high as 1100:1 between serum and ventricular CSF, indicating poor penetration of the blood-brain barrier. In order to attain 'therapeutic levels in CSF, extremely high systemic doses must be given, which can result in severe neurotoxic side effects. These have been reported primarily in patients receiving doses in excess of 100 MU of interferon per day by intravenous infusion (66-68). They include lethargy, confusion, somnolence, memory loss, weakness, and generalized slowing of EEG activity (69). The mechanism of these phenomena is unknown, but a direct neurotoxic effect has been postulated based on studies in vitro that showed that interferon could affect neuronal excitability (70). Although neurotoxic side effects are dose related and reversible, they could easily confuse the assessment of clinical change in neurologic diseases. Most studies of intrathecal and intraventricular interferon therapy have been carried out using much lower doses. These reports include patients with multiple sclerosis (71), amyotrophic lateral sclerosis (72), meningeal leukemia (73), meningeal gliomatosis (74), carcinomatosis (75), and viral encephalitides including rabies (75-77). Constitutional symptoms of fever, chills, headache, myalgia, and fatigue have occurred (78), and in some cases more severe reactions, including seizures (75), have been reported. In general, intrathecal and intraventricular interferon in doses of approximately 1 MU per injection have been well tolerated. Because many of the patients in these studies had far advanced malignancies or other terminal conditions, any statement about the efficacy of intrathecal or intraventricular interferon would be premature. However, the relative safety of these procedures should be emphasized. Despite repeated injections into the lumbar subarachnoid space or into subcutaneous reservoirs communicating with the cerebral ventricles, there were remarkably few instances of iatrogenic infection and no permanent sequelae of treatment in surviving patients.

D. Early Studies of Interferon and Interferon Inducers

Small numbers of SSPE patients have been treated with α or β interferon given systemically or intrathecally at several dose levels and for different lengths of time (Table 1). Reunanen et al. (79) reported apparent clinical improvement in a patient treated with 10 MU of human leukocyte interferon given intramuscularly every day for 4 weeks. Because this patient had previously undergone a 10 year spontaneous remission, the significance of this result is questionable. Behan (80) treated three patients with human leukocyte interferon by intramuscular injection of 3 MU/day for 20-90 days with no clinical improvement. One of the patients was also given 12 MU intrathecally over 3 days with no benefit. Bartram et al. (81) treated a patient with a total of 87 MU of human interferon β by a combination of intravenous and intraventricular routes over 21 days with no change in clinical status.

Clinical trials of interferon inducers have also been carried out in a few instances with disappointing results. A group of six children with SSPE showed no significant improvement after treatment with the synthetic ribonucleotide poly(I)·poly(C) (82), and in another study (83) there was no improvement in three patients treated with pyran copolymer, despite documentation of interferon induction.

E. Recent Trials of Intrathecal and Intraventricular Interferon

Bye et al. (84) treated six patients with human lymphoblastoid interferon (predominantly natural α) by a combination of intravenous and lumbar intrathecal routes. Over 6 days in succession, five patients received either 10 or 70 MU/m^2 intravenously and 1 MU/m^2 per day intrathecally. A single patient who received only

Table 1 Treatment of SSPE with Interferon[a]

Author	No. of patients	Stage	IFN	Route	Dose	Duration	Result
Reunanen et al. (79)	1	II	Natural α	IM	10 MU/day	4 weeks	Slight improvement
Behan (80)	2	II	Natural α	IM	3 MU/day	20-90 days	No change
	1	I	Natural α	IT	12 MU	3 days	No change
Bartram et al. (81)	1	II	Natural β	IV +IVT	3.5 MU/day 1 MU/day	21 days 14 days	No change
Bye et al. (84)	5	II	Lymphoblastoid	IV +IT	10-70 MU/mu^2 1 MU/m^2 per day	1-6 days 6 days	Worse
	1	II	Lymphoblastoid	IT	1 MU/m^2 per day	6 days	Slight improvement
Huttenlocher et al. (85)	5	III-IV	Natural α	IT	1 MU every other day	30 days	1/5 improved
Panitch et al. (86)	3	II-III	Natural α	IVT	1 MU twice weekly	6 months	3/3 improved
Smith et al. (87)	3	II	Natural α	IVT	0.5-1 MU twice weekly	9-18 months	2/3 improved

[a]Abbreviations: IFN, interferon; IM, intramuscular; IT, intrathecal (lumbar); IVT, intraventricular; MU, million international reference units. Staging on I-IV scale of Jabbour et al. (6). For studies in which this scale was not used, stage is estimated from clinical description of patients.

the six intrathecal injections was the only one to show clinical improvement, whereas the other five continued to deteriorate. Because the course of therapy was so brief, this probably was not an adequate trial from which to draw conclusions.

In a more extended study, Huttenlocher et al. (85) treated five patients with advanced (stage III-IV) slowly progressive SSPE with human leukocyte interferon. Every other day for 30 days, 1 million units were given by the lumbar subarachnoid route, and patients were followed for up to 24 months. All patients had previously been treated with isoprinosine, and two had experienced temporary remissions. Following interferon treatment two patients improved, one of them dramatically and one transiently. In the patient with marked clinical improvement, there was recovery of speech, ambulation, and bowel and bladder control. Myoclonus ceased and the EEG returned to normal. However, no consistent changes in CSF immunoglobulin levels, IgG synthesis, oligoclonal bands, or measles antibody titers were detected. The authors concluded that intrathecal interferon could be given safely and that further trials were warranted in less advanced SSPE.

Two recent clinical trials of intraventricular interferon have produced the most promising results to date (Table 2). Panitch et al. (86) treated three Latin American children with stage II or III SSPE by injection of natural interferon a into an Ommaya reservoir connected to a ventricular catheter. The dose was gradually increased from 250,000 U/week to 1 MU twice weekly and was maintained at that level for 6 months. None of the patients had previously been treated with antiviral or immunosuppressive agents, and all had rapidly progressive disease of 4-18 months' duration. Patient 1 improved from stage III to stage I during treatment but relapsed shortly after interferon was discontinued. A second course of treatment was ineffective. Patient 2 experienced gradual improvement that began during treatment and continued for 10 months thereafter. At that time there was a relapse that was successfully treated with a second course of interferon. The third patient improved briefly during treatment, then deteriorated while still receiving interferon. However, he later stabilized and regained some of the functions he had lost during the relapse. There was distinct improvement of the EEG in all

Table 2 Intraventricular Interferon in SSPE

Patients[a]	Age	Sex	Months of treatment	Stage[b] Before	Stage[b] After	Measles antibody[c] Before	Measles antibody[c] After	Relapse[d]	Effect of retreatment
1	11	F	6	III	I	1:64	1:16	+	None
2	12	M	6	III	I/II	1:64	1:16	+	Improved
3	11	M	6	II	I/II	1:128	1:32	+	NT[e]
4	12	F	18	I/II	I	1:32	1:16	−	NT
5	10	M	9	II	I	1:16	1:8	−	NT
6	9	M	12	II	II	1:64	1:64	−	NT

[a]Patients 1–3 from Panitch et al. (86); patients 4–6 from Smith et al. (87).
[b]Staging according to Jabbour et al. (6). "After" is stage at time of maximum improvement, during or following IFN.
[c]HI titer before treatment and at time of greatest decline in titer.
[d]Relapses occurred after cessation of treatment in patients 1 and 2 and during treatment in patient 3.
[e]Not treated.

three patients, and the intraventricular injection of interferon was remarkably well tolerated. Although side effects of fever and mild CSF pleocytosis were noted, there was no evidence of meningeal infection at any time during the trial. CSF IgG and measles antibody levels decreased with clinical improvement and increased with relapses, suggesting that interferon may have reduced the expression of measles virus antigens on cells within the CNS.

In a concurrent study, Smith et al. (87) treated three Palestinian patients in Israel using a similar protocol, although the doses of interferon and frequency of administration were more variable, and treatment was carried out for 9–18 months. All patients were in clinical stage II at the beginning of treatment, and two of them improved substantially. As in the previous study, the EEG returned toward normal and CSF measles antibody titers were reduced in conjunction with improvement in clinical status. Although the number of patients treated in these two studies is quite small, the occurrence of partial remissions in five of the six patients during interferon treatment is likely to be more than coincidental. Further clinical trials of intraventricular interferon seem to be indicated in patients with SSPE.

V. DIRECTIONS FOR FUTURE THERAPEUTIC TRIALS IN SSPE

Attempts at the therapy of SSPE have been partially successful at best. Reports of improvement with isoprinosine, interferon, or any other treatment must be viewed with skepticism against the background of the variable course of the disease, the frequent occurrence of spontaneous remissions, and the possibility that measles vaccination is not only reducing the incidence of SSPE but changing the clinical expression of those cases that do occur. The variety of interferons now available also presents a problem. Thus far, most clinical trials in SSPE have been conducted using natural interferon a, but cost and availability make recombinant interferons much more attractive candidates for future trials. Because of the rarity of SSPE in the United States, treatment trials in statistically meaningful numbers of patients must be performed elsewhere. Previous studies have shown that such trials can be carried out in the Middle East and Mexico without undue complications and with adequate data collection, as long as protocols are carefully designed and followed. In addition, care should be taken to incorporate virologic and immunologic studies into future therapeutic trials insofar as possible. Storage and processing of serum, CSF, and biopsy or autopsy tissue may be suboptimal unless great care is taken to coordinate efforts between the clinical and laboratory components of individual studies. We propose the following recommendations for conduct of future trials of interferon therapy in SSPE.

Treatment should be started early in the course of the disease, preferably during stages I or II, while patients are still intellectually and neurologically functional and before the signs of permanent CNS damage are apparent on CT scans.

Recombinant interferons should be used because of their advantages in terms of availability, cost, and safety. Recombinant interferon-α_2 was licensed for use in the treatment of certain types of leukemia in 1986 and would be the most logical candidate for initial studies. Other subtypes of α and β interferon are also available in quantity and should be considered. However interferon γ should probably not be used because it possesses no advantages over α or β as an antiviral agent and may possibly have adverse effects on the disease process (88).

The intraventricular route of administration seems to be the most promising at present and should be pursued. Installation of indwelling intraventricular catheters and subcutaneous reservoirs is quite feasible, and the incidence of bacterial infection is acceptably low, if careful aseptic technique is maintained. Moreover, relatively low doses of interferon induce high CSF titers yet are associated with only modest side effects. We also propose a trial of combination therapy with intraventricular interferon-α_2 and isoprinosine to determine whether the partial responses seen with these agents individually may be additive and lead to greater improvement and more sustained remissions in treated patients.

Every effort should be made to obtain as much clinical and experimental information as possible from these trials. Protocols must be carefully designed so that they are neither too simple nor too complex, and provisions must be incorporated for immunologic and virologic analysis at frequent intervals. Because the areas of the world in which SSPE is prevalent are often technologically and medically underdeveloped, the success of these efforts will depend, to a great extent, on meticulous organization and international cooperation.

REFERENCES

1. Dawson, J. R., Jr. Cellular inclusions in cerebral lesions of lethargic encephalitis. *Am. J. Pathol. 9*:7-15 (1933).
2. Agnarsdottir, G. Subacute sclerosing panencephalitis. In: *Recent Advances in Clinical Virology* (A. P. Waterson, ed.). Churchill Livingstone, Edinburgh, 1977, pp. 21-49.
3. Johnson, R. T. *Viral Infections of the Nervous System.* Raven Press, New York, 1982, pp. 244-252.
4. Graves, M. C. Subacute sclerosing panencephalitis. *Neurol. Clin. 2*:267-280 (1984).
5. Freeman, J. M. The clinical spectrum and early diagnosis of Dawson's encephalitis. *J. Pediatr. 75*:590-603 (1969).
6. Jabbour, J. T., Garcia, J. H., Lemmi, H., et al. Subacute sclerosing panencephalitis: A multidisciplinary study of eight cases. *JAMA 207*:2248-2254 (1969).
7. Risk, W. S., and Haddad, F. S. The variable natural history of subacute sclerosing panencephalitis: A study of 118 cases from the Middle East. *Arch. Neurol. 36*:610-614 (1979).
8. Risk, W. S., Haddad, F. S., and Chemali, R. Substanial spontaneous long-term improvement in subacute sclerosing panencephalitis: Six cases from the Middle East and a review of the literature. *Arch. Neurol. 35*:494-502 (1978).
9. Resnick, J. S., Engel, W. K., and Sever, J. L. Subacute sclerosing panencephalitis: Spontaneous improvement in a patient with elevated measles antibody in blood and spinal fluid. *N. Engl. J. Med. 279*:126-129 (1968).
10a. Duda, E., Petronas, N., and Huttenlocher, P. R. Computed axial tomography in subacute sclerosing panencephalitis. *AJNR 1*:35-38 (1980).

10 b. Krawiecki, N. S., Dyken, P. R., Gammal, T. E., et al. Computed tomography of the brain in subacute sclerosing panencephalitis. *Ann. Neurol.* 15:489-493 (1984).

11. Case records of the Massachusetts General Hospital, Case 25-1986. *N. Engl. J. Med.* 314:1689-1700 (1986).

12. Vandvik, B., Norrby, E., Nordal, H., et al. Oligoclonal measles virus specific IgG antibodies isolated by virus immunoabsorption of cerebrospinal fluids, brain extracts, and sera from patients with subacute sclerosing panencephalitis and multiple sclerosis. *Scand. J. Immunol.* 5: 979-992 (1976).

13. Tourtellotte, W. W., Ma, B. I., Brandes, D. B. et al. Quantification of de novo central nervous system IgG measles antibody synthesis in SSPE. *Ann. Neurol.* 9:551-556 (1981).

14. Panitch, H. S., Hooper, C. J., and Johnson, K. P. CSF antibody to myelin basic protein: Measurement in patients with multiple sclerosis and subacute sclerosing panencephalitis. *Arch. Neurol.* 37:206-209 (1980).

15. Robb, R. M., and Watters, G. V. Ophthalmic manifestations of subacute sclerosing panencephalitis. *Arch. Ophthalmol.* 83:426-435 (1970).

16. Johannes, R. S., and Sever, J. L. Subacute sclerosing panencephalitis. *Annu. Rev. Med.* 26:589-601 (1975).

17. Payne, F. E., Baublis, J. V., and Itabashi, H. H. Isolation of measles virus from cell cultures of brain from a patient with subacute sclerosing panencephalitis. *N. Engl. J. Med.* 281:585-589 (1969).

18. Horta-Barbosa, L., Fuccillo, D. A., Sever, J. L., et al. Subacute sclerosing panencephalitis: Isolation of measles virus from a brain biopsy. *Nature* 221:974 (1969).

19. Dhib-Jalbut, S. S., Abdelnoor, A. M., and Haddad, F. S. Cellular and humoral immunity in subacute sclerosing panencephalitis. *Infect. Immun.* 33:34-42 (1981).

20. Choppin, P. W. Measles virus and chronic neurological diseases. *Ann. Neurol.* 9:17-20 (1981).

21. Fujinami, R. S., and Oldstone, M. B. A. Antiviral antibody reacting on the plasma membrane alters measles virus expression inside the cell. *Nature* 279:529-530 (1979).

22. Rammohan, K. W., McFarland, H. F., and McFarlin, D. E. Induction of

subacute murine measles encephalitis by monoclonal antibody to virus haemagglutinin. *Nature 290*:588-589 (1981).

23. Johnson, K. P., and Norrby, E. Subacute sclerosing panencephalitis (SSPE) agent in hamsters. III. Induction of defective measles infection in hamster brain. *Exp. Mol. Biol. 21*:166-178 (1974).

24. Byington, D. P., and Johnson, K. P. Subacute sclerosing panencephalitis in the hamster: Correlation of age with chronic inclusion-cell encephalitis. *J. Infect. Dis. 126*:18-26 (1972).

25. Rammohan, K. W., McFarland, H. F., and McFarlin, D. E. Subacute sclerosing panencephalitis after passive immunization and natural measles infection: Role of antibody in persistence of measles virus. *Neurology 32*:390-394 (1982).

26. Fournier, J.-G., Tardieu, M., Lebon, P., et al. Detection of measles virus RNA in lymphocytes from peripheral-blood and brain perivascular infiltrates of patients with subacute sclerosing panencephalitis. *N. Engl. J. Med. 313*:910-915 (1985).

27. Gerson, K. L., and Haslam, R. H. A. Subtle immunologic abnormalities in four boys with subacute sclerosing panencephalitis. *N. Engl. J. Med. 285*: 78-82 (1971).

28. Hall, W. W., Lamb, R. A., and Choppin, P. W. Measles and subacute sclerosing panencephalitis virus proteins: Lack of antibodies to the M protein in patients with subacute sclerosing panencephalitis. *Proc. Natl. Acad. Sci. USA 76*:2047-2051 (1979).

29. Hall, W. W., and Choppin, P. W. Measles-virus in the brain tissue of patients with subacute sclerosing panencephalitis: Absence of the M-protein. *N. Engl. J. Med. 304*:1152-1155 (1981).

30. Johnson, K. P., Norrby, E., Swoveland, P., and Carrigan, D. R. Experimental subacute sclerosing panencephalitis: Selective disappearance of measles virus matrix protein from the central nervous system. *J. Infect. Dis. 144*:161-169 (1981).

31. Shapshak, P., Tourtellotte, W. W., Nakamura, S., et al. Subacute sclerosing panencephalitis: Measles virus matrix protein nucleic acid sequences detected by in situ hybridization. *Neurology 35*:1605-1609 (1985).

32. Norrby, E., Kristensson, K., Brzosko, W. J., et al. Measles virus matrix protein detected by immune fluorescence with monoclonal antibodies in the brain of patients with subacute sclerosing panencephaltisis. *J. Virol. 56*:337-340 (1985).

33. Swoveland, P. T., and Johnson, K. P. Age-related expression of measles virus hemagglutinin (H) in hamster brains. *Neurology* 35(Suppl. 1): 281 (1985).

34. Haase, A. T., Gantz, D., Eble, B., et al. Natural history of restricted synthesis and expression of measles virus genes in subacute sclerosing panencephalitis. *Proc. Natl. Acad. Sci. USA* 82:3020-3024 (1985).

35. Modlin, J. F., Jabbour, J. T., Witte, J. J., and Halsey, N. A. Epidemiologic studies of measles vaccine and subacute sclerosing panencephalitis. *Pediatrics* 59:505-512 (1977).

36. Modlin, J. F., Halsey, N. A., Eddins, D. L., et al. Epidemiology of subacute sclerosing panencephalitis. *J. Pediatr.* 94:231-236 (1979).

37. Toro, G., Roman, G., and Navarro de Roman, L. Subacute sclerosing panencephalitis (letter). *Arch. Neurol.* 36:453-454 (1979).

38. Halsey, N. A., Boulos, R., Mode, F., et al. Response to measles vaccine in Haitian infants 6 to 12 months old. Influence of maternal antibodies, malnutrition, and concurrent illnesses. *N. Engl. J. Med.* 313:544-549 (1985).

39. Dyken, P. R., Krawiecki, N. S., DuRant, R. H., et al. The changing clinical expression of subacute sclerosing panencephalitis in the United States (abstract). *Ann. Neurol.* 14:386-387 (1983).

40. DuRant, R. H., Dyken, P. R., and Swift, A. V. The influence of inosiplex treatment on the neurological disability of subacute sclerosing panencephalitis patients. *J. Pediatr.* 101:288-293 (1982).

41. DuRant, R. H., and Dyken, P. R. The effect of inosiplex on the survival of subacute sclerosing panencephalitis. *Neurology* 33:1053-1055 (1983).

42. Vandvik, B., Froland, S. S., Hoyeraal, H. M., et al. Immunological features in a case of subacute sclerosing panencephalitis treated with transfer factor. *Scand. J. Immunol.* 2:367-374 (1973).

43. Kackell, Y. M., Grob, P. J., Kreth, W. H., et al. Transfer factor therapy in patients with subacute sclerosing panencephalitis. *J. Neurol.* 211:39-49 (1975).

44. Sell, K. W., Ahmed, A., and Bailey, D. W. Attempts to remove an inhibitor of cellular immunity found in plasma and spinal fluid inpatients with SSPE. *Arch. Neurol.* 32:502-503 (1975).

45. Derakhshan, I., Massoud, A., Foroozanfar, N., et al. Subacute sclerosing

panencelphalitis: Clinical and immunologic study of 23 patients. *Neurology 31*:177-180 (1981).

46. Sotrel, A., Rosen, S., Ronthal, M., and Ross, D. B. Subacute sclerosing panencelphalitis: An immune complex disease? *Neurology 33*:885-890 (1983).

47. Rotteveel, J. J., Renier, W., Weemaes, C., et al. Plasmapheresis does not affect subacute sclerosing panencephalitis. *Ann. Neurol. 14*:491 (1983).

48. Robertson, W. C., Clark, D. B., and Markesbery, W. R. Review of 38 cases of subacute sclerosing panencephalitis: Effect of amantadine on the natural course of the disease. *Ann. Neurol. 8*:422-425 (1980).

49. Huttenlocher, P. R., and Mattson, R. H. Isoprinosine in subacute sclerosing panencephalitis. *Neurology 29*:763-771 (1979).

50. Silverberg, R., Brenner, T., and Abramsky, O. Inosiplex in the treatment of subacute sclerosing panencephalitis. *Arch. Neurol. 36*:374-375 (1979).

51. Haddad, F. S., and Risk, W. S. Isoprinosine treatment in 18 patients with subacute sclerosing panencephalitis: A controlled study. *Ann. Neurol. 7*: 185-188 (1980).

52. Dyken, P. R., Swift, A., and DuRant, R. H. Long-term follow-up of patients with subacute sclerosing panencephalitis treated with Inosiplex. *Ann. Neurol. 11*:359-364 (1982).

53. Jones, C. E., Dyken, P. R., Huttenlocher, P. R., et al. Inosiplex therapy in subacute sclerosing panencephalitis: A multicentre, non-randomized study in 98 patients. *Lancet 1*:1034-1037 (1982).

54. Streletz, L. J., Sethi, B. S., Graziani, L. J., Duckett, S. W. SSPE treated with isoprinosine: Immunopathological observations. *Ann. Neurol. 17*: 105-106 (1985).

55. Smith, R. A., Kingsbury, D., Alksne, J., et al. Distribution of interferon in cerebrospinal fluid after systemic, intrathecal, and intraventricular administration (abstract). *Ann. Neurol. 12*:81 (1982).

56. Smith, R. A., Norris, F., Bernhardt, L., and Cantell, K. Intravenous and intraventricular administration of interferon (abstract). *Ann. Neurol. 14*: 139 (1983).

57. Salazar, A. M., Gibbs, C. J., Gajdusek, D. C., and Smith, R. A. Clinical use of interferon: Central nervous system disorders. In *Handbook of*

Experimental Pharmacology (P. E. Came and W. A. Carter eds.). Springer-Verlag, Berlin, 1984, pp. 472-497.

58. Rennels, M. L., Gregory, T. F., Blaumanis, O. R., et al. Evidence for "paravascular" fluid circulation in the mammalian central nervous system, provided by the rapid distribution of tracer protein throughout the brain from the subarachnoid space. *Brain Res. 326*:47-63 (1985).

59. Friedman, R. M. *Interferons: A Primer.* Academic Press, New York, 1981, pp. 47-71.

60. Saksela, E. Interferon and natural killer cells. In: *Interferon 1981* (I. Gresser, ed.). Academic Press, London, 1981, pp. 45-63).

61. Huddlestone, J. R., Merigan, T. C., and Oldstone, M. B. A. Induction and kinetics of natural killer cells in humans following interferon therapy. *Nature 282*:417-419 (1979).

62. Ault, K. A., and Weiner, H. L. Natural killing of measles-infected cells by human lymphocytes. *J. Immunol. 122*:2611-2616 (1979).

63. Joncas, J. H., Robillard, L. R., Boudreault, A., et al. Interferon in serum and cerebrospinal fluid in subacute sclerosing panencephalitis. *Can Med. Assoc. J. 115*:309 (1976).

64. Habif, D. V., Lipton, R., and Cantell, K. Interferon crosses the blood-cerebrospinal fluid barrier in monkeys. *Proc. Soc. Exp. Biol. Med. 149*: 287-289 (1975).

65. Smith, R. A., Norris, F., Palmer, D., Bernhardt, L., and Wills, R. J. Distribution of alpha interferon in serum and cerebrospinal fluid after systemic administration. *Clin. Pharmacol. Ther. 37*:85-88 (1985).

66. Rohatiner, A. Z. S., Prior, P. F., Burton, A. C., et al. Central nervous system toxicity of interferon. *Br. J. Cancer 47*:419-422 (1983).

67. Smedley, H., Katrak, M., Sikora, K., et al. Neurological effects of recombinant human interferon. *Br. Med. J. 286*:262-264 (1983).

68. Farkilla, M., Iivanainen, M., Roine, R., et al. Neurotoxic and other side effects of high dose interferon in amyotrophic lateral sclerosis. *Acta Neurol. Scand. 69*:42-46 (1984).

69. Suter, C., Westmoreland, B. F., Sharbrough, F. W., et al. Electroencephalographic abnormalities in interferon encephalography: A preliminary report. *Mayo Clin. Proc. 59*:847-850 (1984).

70. Calvert, M. C., and Gresser, I. Interferon enhances the excitability of cultured neurons. *Nature 278*:558-560 (1979).

71. Jacobs, L., O'Malley, J., Freeman, A., and Ekes, R. Intrathecal interferon reduces exacerbations of multiple sclerosis. *Science* 214:1026–1028 (1981).

72. Mora, J. S., Munsat, T. L., Kao, K.-P., et al. Intrathecal administration of natural human interferon in amyotrophic lateral sclerosis. *Neurology* 36: 1137–1140 (1986).

73. Misset, J. L., Mathe, G., Horoszewicz, J. S. Intrathecal interferon in meningeal leukemia (letter). *N. Engl. J. Med.* 304:1544 (1981).

74. Slatkin, N. E., Jaeckle, K. A., Lukes, S. A., and Posner, J. B. Treatment of leptomeningeal gliomatosis with human leukocyte interferon: Results in two patients (abstract). *Neurology* 34(suppl. 1):151 (1984).

75. Jaeckle, K. A., Lukes, S. A., Krown, S. E., et al. Phase I study of intraventricularly administered human alpha interferon in patients with leptomeningeal tumor (abstract). *Ann. Neurol.* 14:138 (1983).

76. Prange, H., and Wismann, H. Intrathecal use of interferon in encephalitis (letter). *N. Engl. J. Med.* 305:1283 (1981).

77. Merigan, T. C., Baer, G. M., Winkler, W. G., et al. Human leukocyte interferon administration to patients with symptomatic and suspected rabies. *Ann. Neurol.* 16:82–87 (1984).

78. Ruutiainen, J., and Panelius, M. Toxic effects of interferon administered intrathecally. *Br. Med. J.* 286:940 (1983).

79. Reunanen, M., Ilonen, J., Cantell, K., et al. Treatment of an SSPE case undergoing a sudden relapse after a ten year remission. *Acta. Neurol. Scand.* 57(Suppl. 67):239–240 (1978).

80. Behan, P. O. Interferon in treatment of subacute sclerosing panencephalitis (letter). *Lancet 1*:1059–1060 (1981).

81. Bartram, C. R., Henke, J., Treuner, J., et al. Subacute sclerosing panencephalitis in a brother and sister. Therapeutic trial of fibroblast interferon. *Eur. J. Pediatr.* 138:187–190 (1982).

82. Guggenheim, M. A., and Baron, S. Clinical studies of an interferon inducer, polyriboinosinic-polyribocytidilic acid [Poly (I)-Poly (C)] in children. *J. Infect. Dis.* 136:50–58 (1977).

83. Freeman, J. M. Treatment of subacute sclerosing panencephalitis with 5-bromo-2-deoxyuridine and pyran copolymer. *Neurology* 18:176–180 (1968).

84. Bye, A., Balkwill, F., Brigden, D., and Wilson, J. Use of interferon in

the management of patients with subacute sclerosing panencephalitis. *Dev. Med. Child Neurol.* 27:170-175 (1985).

85. Huttenlocher, P. R., Picchietti, D. L., Roos, R. P., et al. Intrathecal interferon in subacute sclerosing panencephalitis. *Ann. Neurol.* 19: 303-305 (1986).

86. Panitch, H. S., Gomez-Plascencia, J., Norris, F. H., Cantell, K., and Smith, R. A. Remission of subacute sclerosing panencephalitis in patients treated with intraventricular interferon. *Neurology* 36:562-566 (1986).

87. Smith, R. A., Abramsky, O., Steiner, I., Panitch, H., and Cantell, K. The experimental treatment of subacute sclerosing panencephalitis with interferon. In: *The Biology of the Interferon System 1985* (W. E. Stewart and H. Schellekens, eds.). Elsevier Science Publishers, Amsterdam, 1986, pp. 505-510.

88. Vilcek, J., Gray, P. W., Rinderknecht, E., and Sevastopoulos, C. G. Interferon gamma: A lymphokine for all seasons. In: *Lymphokines*, Vol. 11 (E. Pick, ed.). Academic Press, New York, 1985, pp. 1-32.

9
Treatment of Multiple Sclerosis by Systemic Administration of Interferon

HILLEL S. PANITCH and KENNETH P. JOHNSON

University of Maryland School of Medicine and
Veterans Administration Medical Center, Baltimore, Maryland

I. INTRODUCTION

Despite a vast amount of information on the antiviral and immunologic effects of interferons, the rationale for their use in multiple sclerosis (MS) is highly speculative. Nevertheless, several clinical trials have been undertaken using different types of interferon given via the subcutaneous, intravenous, and intrathecal routes. In some studies interferon has been given as a potential antiviral agent and in others as an immunoregulatory mediator. To a certain extent it has been tested simply because of the widespread publicity it has received and because of the willingness of MS patients and clinical investigators to try a potential treatment that offers reasonable hope without undue risk of serious complications. The earliest clinical trials in MS were conducted with natural α and β interferons; however, the scarcity and cost of these preparations made large-scale studies prohibitively expensive. The recent introduction of recombinant interferons now provides purer, better standardized products with greatly increased availability and lower cost. Because of generally favorable, although not conclusive, results of the early trials, it is likely that further studies will be conducted using the recombinant agents. This review describes studies that have recently been completed or are in progress and attempts to provide a rational basis for the prediction that systemic administration of certain recombinant interferons may, in the future, have a scientifically proven place in the treatment of MS.

The most prevalent working hypothesis for the pathogenesis of MS is that of a virally induced immune-mediated disease occurring in a genetically susceptible host (1-3). It seems logical in this setting to consider interferons as possible therapeutic agents. Although hard evidence for a viral etiology of MS is lacking, viral infection has been a recurrent theme in the MS investigative story since the discovery of elevated measles antibody titers in serum and cerebrospinal fluid (CSF) of MS patients (4). The presence of oligoclonal IgG bands in CSF is reminiscent of findings in certain chronic neurovirologic infections (5), although efforts to determine the antigenic specificity of the bands have not been fruitful (6,7). Reports of increased or decreased cell-mediated immunity to viral antigens have appeared occasionally (8,9), and recently a specific T-cell-mediated defect in immunity to measles virus has been described (10). Measles virus RNA has been identified in brain cells of some MS patients (11), although it is also present, less commonly, in control brain tissue. Other viruses have been implicated from time to time by epidemiologic evidence, serologic testing, nucleic acid hybridization, or isolation from MS brain tissue. The epidemiologic data (12-14) suggest that an infectious agent, probably a virus, is directly involved in the etiology of MS, and canine distemper virus has been proposed as a likely candidate (15). However, at least a dozen other viruses have either been isolated from MS brain tissue or detected by other means (16). None of these reports has been adequately confirmed in independent testing. Recently a retrovirus, similar although not identical to HTLV-I and HTLV-III, has been implicated in some MS patients by serologic and hybridization techniques (17). Other investigators have failed to detect antibody to these viruses in their patient populations (18), and additional studies will be needed to confirm or disprove this association. A more general, but less specific, relationship of viral infection to exacerbations of MS was recently proposed by Sibley et al. (19), who found that a significant proportion (27%) of exacerbations were preceded by an identifiable viral illness. Prevention of upper respiratory and other common infections by interferon could conceivably reduce the incidence of MS exacerbations.

Several experimental animal models of virus-induced demyelinating disease have been described and studied for their potential relevance to mechanisms of inflammation and demyelination in MS (20). In some cases demyelination is associated with acute or persistent infection, whereas in others it is more probably related to a virus-induced autoimmune process. Thus far there have been no reports of inhibition of experimental virus-induced demyelinating disease by treatment with interferon. However, a few patients with subacute sclerosing panencephalitis (SSPE) have been treated with intraventricular (21,22) or intrathecal interferon (23) with encouraging results. If the antiviral rationale is invoked in MS, it would seem logical to administer interferon intrathecally or intraventricularly, since the central nervous system (CNS) is the most probable site of viral infection or persistence.

All interferons exert a wide variety of effects on the immune system, which are reviewed elsewhere in this volume. Although systemic interferon poorly crosses the blood-brain barrier and produces little or no detectable titer in the cerebrospinal fluid (CSF) (24), the inflammatory cells in active MS plaques are derived from the peripheral blood (25) and would presumably be exposed to and altered by circulating levels of interferon. Also, interferons could modulate systemic immunologic activity and, in so doing, decrease the likelihood of further attacks. Finally, lymphocytes could be exposed to systemic interferon in areas of the CNS in which the blood-brain barrier is damaged, as occurs frequently in acute exacerbations of MS (26).

During the past 10 years a voluminous literature has arisen describing numerous immunoregulatory defects in MS. These are systemic abnormalities in immune responsiveness that are detected in significant numbers, although by no means all, of MS patients in comparison with normal controls and subjects with other neurologic diseases. Several of these abnormalities have been reported to fluctuate in conjunction with MS exacerbations. Because they involve the peripheral immune system, they provide a rational basis for the systemic administration of interferon or other immunomodulatory agents via the intravenous. intramuscular, or subcutaneous routes. In the following discussion, an attempt is made to distinguish the effects of α, β, and γ interferons. This is of some importance because the studies cited each involve only one type of interferon, and the results from one study may not be generally applicable to other interferon trials. Whenever the term "interferon" is used alone, it should be understood to indicate α and/or β. Interferon-γ is so different from the others that it must be considered separately (27,28).

One of the most characteristic features of MS, recognized for over 40 years, is the increased concentration of IgG in the CSF (29). This is the result of elevated immunoglobulin synthesis within the CNS by plasma cells, which are present in much greater numbers in MS brain than in controls (30). These cells are thought to invade the CNS during periods of disease activity when vascular permeability is increased in the vicinity of MS plaques. Interferon-α has been shown to affect immunoglobulin synthesis via a direct effect on B cells (31) and could, therefore, induce or suppress IgG synthesis in MS lesions. Peripheral effects on B cells before they enter the CNS, on T-helper cells, or on antigen presenting cells, such as macrophages or endothelial cells, may also be important in regulating IgG synthesis and would be susceptible to systemically administered interferons.

Evidence has been reported from several laboratories that peripheral blood lymphocytes of MS patients produce subnormal levels of α (32) and γ interferons (33,34) in response to such inducers as viruses, T-cell mitogens, and poly(I)·poly(C). As is the case with most of the immunologic abnormalities described in MS, there is a lack of consensus about these findings. Some investigators have reported interferon production to be normal (35) or even (in the case of interferon-γ) elevated (36). Natural killer (NK) cell activity, which is partially interferon dependent, also appears to be reduced in most patients with MS. NK cells produce interferon-α and can be stimulated by it to exert cytotoxic activity against susceptible target cells in vitro. Whereas some investigators have reported a general depression of NK activity in MS (37,38), others have found normal activity (39) or depressed NK function only in patients with active or progressive disease (40). The addition of natural or recombinant interferon-α to NK cell cultures from MS patients or normal controls markedly enhances cytotoxicity (38,39), but treatment with interferon in vivo first augments then suppresses the NK effect (39,41). These findings suggest that NK cells from MS patients are probably normally responsive to interferon. Although the function of NK cells in MS is unknown, reduced levels of interferon and NK activity are thought to represent immunologic defects that ought to be susceptible to treatment with exogenous interferon.

Another immunoregulatory abnormality in MS, which may be affected by interferon treatment, is reduced T-suppressor cell activity during acute exacerbations (42,43). The basis of this apparent defect is unclear, and it has been attributed either to reduced numbers of suppressor cells or to inadequate suppressor cell function (44). Early reports of low numbers of suppressor T cells and of increased ratios of T-helper to suppressor cells as detected by monoclonal antibodies (45,46) have been confirmed in some laboratories (47) and contradicted in others (48,49). It is generally agreed that immunofluorescent surface markers are probably not an adequate indicator of suppressor activity. On the other hand, a defect in functional suppression, as measured in the concanavalin A (ConA)-activated T-suppressor cell assay, has been repeatedly confirmed and seems to correlate better with disease activity (50). In a murine system, T-suppressor activity could be increased by exposure of cells to interferon-β in vitro (51). Enhancement of T-suppressor activity by interferons in humans has not been well documented, although it has been reported to occur (52).

Additional evidence for the potential efficacy of systemic interferon comes from studies of experimental allergic encephalomyelitis (EAE), a useful animal model for some of the immunologic and pathologic features of MS. In rats with acute EAE induced by inoculation of myelin basic protein in complete Freund's adjuvant, rat interferon-β given by intravenous injection delayed or prevented the clinical disease and reduced the number and intensity of histologic lesions (53). Adoptive transfer of EAE with sensitized lymphocytes was abrogated by incubation of the cells with interferon-β before transfer (54,55). In contrast, intraventricular administration of interferon in this model system failed to have any effect on either primary induction or adoptive transfer of EAE (56). EAE is by no means an ideal model of MS; for example, there is little convincing evidence for autosensitization to myelin basic protein in the human disease. Nevertheless, the striking contrast reported between systemic and intraventricular interferon in EAE supports the concept of systemic treatment of immunologically mediated CNS disease.

II. CLINICAL TRIALS OF SYSTEMIC INTERFERONS IN MULTIPLE SCLEROSIS

A. Early Studies

By the late 1970s, sufficient evidence had accumulated on the immunoregulatory activity of interferons and the immunologic abnormalities of MS to justify a major clinical trial (Table 1). Previous small trials in Europe had shown no effect of either α or β interferon on the clinical course of chronic progressive MS. They had, however, demonstrated that systemic administration of relatively large doses of natural interferon (up to 5×10^6 units) was well tolerated by MS patients and resulted in no long-term side effects. Of the six patients treated by Fog (57) with intramuscular natural interferon-α, one became acutely worse during treatment, but the individual was undergoing a severe acute exacerbation at the time, which could have accounted for her clinical deterioration. The other five patients all had chronic progressive MS that continued to progress despite treatment for 5–15 months.

Ververken et al. (58) treated three patients with 5×10^4 U/kg body weight (approximately 3–4×10^6 U per patient) of fibroblast (β) interferon injected intramuscularly every other day for 2 weeks, and none showed any significant clinical improvement or stabilization during follow-up periods of 9–18 months. However, none of the patients became acutely worse or experienced unacceptable toxic side effects.

In another pilot study, Montezuma-de Carvalho (59) treated 12 patients with chronic stable MS with lymphoblastoid interferon (a mixture of natural α and β). They received 6×10^4 U/kg of body weight intramuscularly daily for 1 month, then every other day for 2 months. The patients also received ACTH, imipramine, 5-hydroxytryptophan, diazepam, antibiotics, psychotherapy, and physiotherapy. All patients were reported to have improved. Moreover, their CSF IgG levels decreased, and oligoclonal bands disappeared. Unfortunately, the administration of multiple concurrent medications renders this study essentially uninterpretable.

B. Systemic Natural α Interferon

In 1980, investigators at Stanford University, the University of California–San Francisco, and the Scripps Clinic in La Jolla, California, undertook a multicenter double-blind trial of human leukocyte (natural α) interferon in patients with relapsing clinically definite MS (60,61). Because of the scarcity and cost of the interferon, the study was limited to 24 patients and incorporated a crossover design so that each patient would receive both interferon and placebo in random order during the trial. Patients received either 5×10^6 U of interferon or placebo by subcutaneous injection daily for 6 months. Following a 6-month washout period, they were crossed over to the alternate treatment for 6 months and finally underwent a second 6-month washout. Neurologic testing, immunologic studies, and toxicity were evaluated at regular intervals, with the principal clinical objective the prevention of acute exacerbations. Analysis of the results was unexpectedly complicated by the crossover design and a marked placebo effect. Patients had fewer exacerbations during the study than during the preceding 2 years; however, the differences between exacerbation rates during interferon treatment and placebo treatment were not statistically significant (61). In addition, patients who received interferon after placebo had fewer exacerbations than those who received interferon first, possibly because of a learning effect based on side effects of interferon, such as fever, myalgia, and fatigue. After the crossover, most patients were able to guess correctly which treatment they were receiving. Accordingly, patients taking interferon after the crossover may have experienced a placebolike augmentation of their response to interferon. Conversely, patients receiving placebo after the crossover

Table 1 Clinical Trials, Completed or in Progress, of Systemic Interferon in Multiple Sclerosis[a]

Investigator	IFN	Dose	Route
Ververken et al. (58)	Natural β	5×10^4 IU/kg alternate days	IM
Fog (57)	Natural α	$2.5\text{-}5 \times 10^6$ IU/day	IM
Montezuma-de Carvalho (59)	Lymphoblastoid	6×10^4 IU/kg/day then alternate days	IM
Knobler et al. (61)	Natural α	5×10^6 IU/day	SC
Camenga et al. (73)	R α_2	2×10^6 IU 3X/week	SC
Panitch et al. (78,80)	R γ	$15 \times 10^3\text{-}15 \times 10^6$ IU, 2X/week	IV
Bever et al. (91)	Poly ICLC	20-100 μg/kg 1X/week-1X/month	IV
McLeod et al.	Natural α	3×10^6 IU 2X/week, then 1X/week	SC
Paty et al.	Lymphoblastoid	5×10^6 IU/day	SC
Multicenter	R β	$4.5\text{-}90 \times 10^6$ IU, 3X/week	SC

[a]Abbreviations: R, recombinant; IFN, interferon; IU, international units; IM, intramuscular; SC, subcutaneous; RR, relapsing-remitting; RP, relapsing-progressive; CP, chronic progressive; CS, chronic stable; DB, double blind; P, placebo; PC, placebo controlled.

Duration of Rx	No. of patients	Clinical type	Design	Result
2 weeks	3	CP	Open	No effect
15 months	6	CP	Open	No effect
3 months	12	CS	Open, with ACTH	All patients improved
6 months	24	15 RR 9 RP	DB, PC crossover	Reduced attacks in RR group; no effect on RP
12 months	98	72 RR 25 RP 1 CP	DB, PC	No difference between IFN and P
1 month	18	RR	Single-blind	Attacks in 7 patients during treatment
18 months	18	CP	Open	5 improved, 7 stabilized
12 months	225	RR CP	DB, PC	In progress
6 months	101	CP	DB, PC	In progress
24 months	30	RR	DB, PC	In progress

were aware of not having the side effects they had experienced earlier while taking interferon, which may have accounted for their placebo response being less pronounced than that of the patients who were given placebo first. A third complicating factor was failure to randomize patients according to subtype of MS; that is, there were 15 relapsing-remitting and 9 relapsing-progressive patients. The latter had acute exacerbations superimposed on chronic progressive deterioration and responded poorly to interferon, whereas the strictly relapsing-remitting patients responded well (Fig. 1). Patients with a history of clear cut exacerbations and remissions during the 2 years preceding treatment had only five attacks during administration of interferon and the subsequent washout period (0.34 exacerbations per year), none of which were severe. The same patients had 17 attacks (1.14 exacerbations per year) during placebo treatment and washout. This difference was not statistically significant ($P = 0.08$), although there was an obvious trend in favor of interferon. Relapsing-progressive patients failed to improve on interferon; in fact, they had more exacerbations than during placebo treatment, and the exacerbations tended to be more severe. Overall neurologic condition, as quantitated by the Kurtzke Disability Status Scale (DSS) and Scripps Neurological Rating Scale (NRS) scores (62,63), followed the same trends as exacerbation rates; that is, they remained unchanged or improved slightly in the relapsing-remitting group but deteriorated in the relapsing-progressive group. Side effects during interferon treatment, especially fever, fatigue, myalgias, headache, anorexia, and depression, were prominent, but serious hematologic toxicity was not encountered. Focal reactions at injection sites were a common occurrence and may have been related to the development of circulating immune complexes (64).

Additional immunologic testing during the trial was carried out at frequent intervals to identify correlates of disease activity and therapeutic effect (64,65). Unfortunately, none of these studies identified a satisfactory immunologic marker, and several gave unexpected results. For example, serum IgG increased with treatment, and in 50% of the patients treated there was increased synthesis of CSF IgG. In addition, patients developed a circulating antibody to a contaminant of the interferon preparation, which

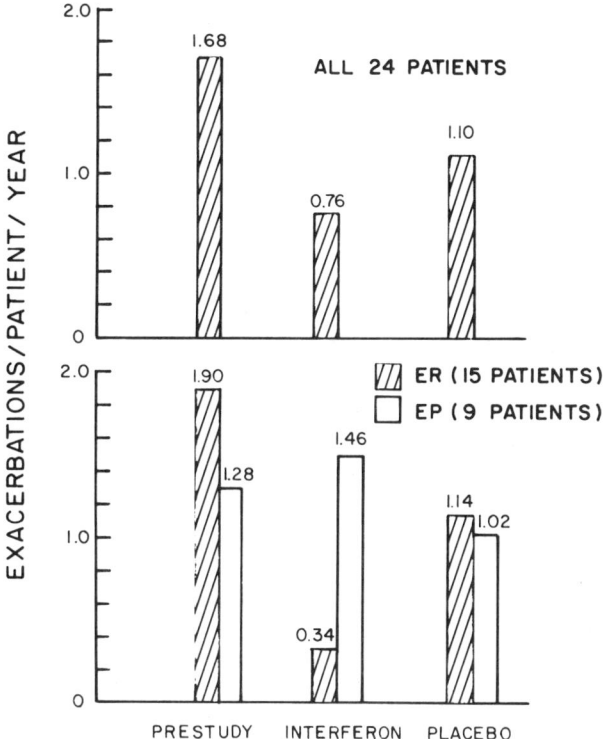

Figure 1 (Above) Exacerbation rates for all 24 patients before and during natural interferon-α trial, irrespective of order in which interferon and placebo were given. Duration of prestudy phase = 2 years; interferon phase = 6 months of interferon treatment plus 6 months washout; placebo phase = 6 months placebo plus 6 months washout. (Below) Exacerbation rates for ER and EP subgroups in prestudy, interferon, and placebo phases of the trial. For interferon versus placebo in 15 ER patients, $P = 0.08$ (two-tailed t-test). [Adapted from Knobler et al. (61).]

was identified as a protein derived from Sendai virus, used in manufacturing the interferon. It has been suggested that the immune response to impurities contained in the interferon may have been responsible for at least some of the findings described in these studies (66).

T-cell phenotypes and ratios of T-helper to suppressor cells, as determined by fluorescent staining with monoclonal antibodies, seemed to fluctuate randomly, in contrast to earlier reports of reduced numbers of T-suppressor cells and increased helper-suppressor ratios during acute exacerbations of MS. NK cell activity against K-562 target cells, which some investigators have found to be reduced in MS patients, was relatively normal before treatment in the patients tested (39). NK activity was transiently increased by administration of interferon but returned to baseline levels after 1 week and remained there during the treatment period, suggesting a partial loss of responsiveness to interferon. In other studies, peripheral blood leukocytes from interferon-treated patients lost their ability to synthesize interferon (67). Furthermore, these cells could not be primed to produce interferon by preincubation with small amounts of interferon in vitro, as they could be prior to treatment. Both of these defects and the reduction in NK activity are compatible with a generalized loss of responsiveness to interferon. Responsiveness to interferon-β was also reduced, even though the patients had only been exposed to α. Because α and β interferons share the same receptor (68), down-regulation of the receptor was thought to be the most probable mechanism for these effects (67). All the observed immunologic effects returned to prestudy levels once interferon administration was stopped (69). On the basis of these studies, the investigators suggested that a lower dose of interferon or less frequent administration may exert the same immunomodulatory effects while permitting cellular responsiveness to be retained and side effects to be reduced (70).

Long-term follow-up of 12 of these patients living in the San Francisco Bay area 2 years after completion of the trial (48–56 months after initiation of interferon treatment) disclosed that most continued to experience fewer exacerbations than they had during or prior to the study (71). The mean attack rate for this group was 0.92 per year during the 2 years of the clinical trial but only 0.47 per year for the subsequent 2 years. Of the 12, 3 stopped having attacks because they entered a chronic-progressive phase. Of the remaining 9 patients, 3 continued to have frequent severe exacerbations, 2 had infrequent mild exacerbations, and 4 had prolonged remissions. The latter 6 patients were able to work and to carry on other normal daily activities. The only two predictive factors that could be identified in retrospective analysis were duration of disease and pretreatment DSS score. The mean duration of MS in patients who did well was 4.8 years compared with 10.2 years for patients who either progressed or experienced frequent exacerbations during the follow-up period. In addition, patients with lower initial DSS scores tended to have a better long-term outcome. This follow-up study indicates, like the follow-up of patients treated with intrathecal interferon-β by Jacobs et al. (72), that there were no long-term complications of interferon treatment and that patients with multiple sclerosis of relatively short duration, who were classified as relapsing-remitting before treatment, may have sustained prolonged benefit from their course of interferon treatment.

C. Recombinant Interferon-a_2

Based on the results of the California study, a protocol was designed by investigators at the University of Maryland and Temple University in which the dosage and frequency of administration were reduced to prevent side effects, improve blinding, and possibly avoid the induction of hyporesponsiveness to interferon (73). To a group of 98 patients with clinically definite MS, 2 million units (MU) of recombinant a_2 interferon (Intron, Schering-Plough Corp.) or a placebo were given three times a week. There was no crossover in the design, and each patient was treated for 1 year with an additional 3 months of follow-up. Of 98 patients, 48 received interferon and 50 received placebo. Side effects were minimal, and those that did occur were mild and well tolerated. Exacerbations were reduced in both the interferon and placebo groups. When attacks were classified as mild, moderate, or severe, no difference was found between the two groups. The absence of any clinical difference between patients treated with interferon and those receiving placebo was confirmed at the end of the study when examining physicians, still blinded, were asked to select those patients who had improved during treatment or who had done well in terms of reduction of exacerbations: 29 patients were designated as improved, of whom 16 had received placebo and 13 interferon during the trial. The drop in exacerbation rates was also due in part to progression of disease requiring changes in classification of the patients from relapsing-remitting to relapsing-progressive or chronic progressive during the year of treatment. In contrast to the California interferon trial, there were no significant differences in exacerbation rates or clinical outcome between the relapsing-remitting and relapsing-progressive subgroups. Of the 29 patients who improved, 25 elected to continue interferon or placebo in a single-blind study for an additional 18 months in an effort to determine if the low dose had any long-term benefit.

Most of the immunologic studies performed during the trial did not correlate with disease activity. These included NK cell activity, T-cell and NK phenotypic markers, and lymphocyte proliferation in response to mitogens (41,74). ConA-induced suppressor activity was reduced during acute attacks and increased with recovery but was unaffected by interferon treatment. A curious and unexplained finding was the apparent change in NK activity induced by placebo (75). The pattern of NK enhancement and suppression was nearly identical in both the interferon- and placebo-treated groups, suggesting that the placebo effect was a genuine physiologic phenomenon that could alter immune responsiveness. Despite the low dose and reduced frequency of administration compared with the California trial, there was a loss of responsiveness by cells from interferon-treated patients. The addition of interferon to NK cell cultures failed to enhance the cytolytic activity of cells from interferon-treated patients as it did before treatment or in cells from the placebo-treated group (41).

In short there was no recognizable therapeutic or immunologic effect in this interferon-a_2 study, which could be directly attributable to interferon, suggesting that the dose may have been too low or that the preparation itself was ineffective. There was an overall reduction in new attacks in both groups, however, and the suggestion of a physiologic effect of placebo is of interest. The importance of the study, therefore, lies not in its clinical result, but in the demonstration that a large multicenter double-blind clinical trial of interferon can be carried out successfully with minimal discomfort and no substantial risk to patients in the early stages of MS. In addition, the results of serial immunologic studies performed during the trial suggest that many of the so-called immunoregulatory defects in MS do not correlate well with either disease activity or interferon therapy and are not suitable markers for evaluating future therapeutic agents.

D. Recombinant Interferon-γ

The rationale for conducting a clinical trial of interferon-γ in MS has both pro and con features. On the one hand, interferon-γ has many of the antiviral, antiproliferative, and immunomodulatory properties of other interferons; furthermore, several investigators have reported that production of interferon-γ is defective in MS patients. On the other hand, interferon-γ is a potent lymphokine, which is probably instrumental in the induction and augmentation of immune responses and as such would probably be contraindicated in an immunologically mediated disease. The only way to resolve this issue was to undertake a closely observed pilot study to assess the safety of interferon-γ administered to MS patients.

At least three groups have reported a defect in interferon-γ secretion by mitogen-stimulated peripheral blood leukocytes from patients with MS (33,34,76–78). These studies involve patients in different stages of disease, incubation of cells for various lengths of time under nonstandardized conditions, and different interferon assay systems. In contrast, Hirsch et al. (36), using a monoclonal antibody-based radioimmunoassay, recently reported increased interferon-γ synthesis in cultured peripheral blood leukocytes from relapsing-remitting MS patients who were in remission at the time of testing. They also found small amounts of interferon-γ in 30 CSF samples from MS patients but in only 4 sera from the same patients. Further work will be needed to understand the factors responsible for the production or suppression of interferon-γ in MS.

In the pilot trial of interferon-γ (78), 18 patients were randomly assigned to each of three groups and received either a low (1 μg), intermediate (30 μg), or high (1000 μg) dose of recombinant interferon-γ (Immuneron, Biogen Research Corp.) by intravenous infusion twice a week for 4 weeks. These doses corresponded to approximately 15,000, 450,000, and 15,000,000 U, respectively. All patients had clinically definite, laboratory-supported, relapsing-remitting MS (79) and were in remission at the initiation of treatment. Their mean prestudy exacerbation rate was 1.42 attacks per year. During the month of treatment, 7 of the 18 developed acute exacerbations, resulting in a rate of 4.67 attacks per year (Fig. 2), a significant increase (p < 0.01). The attacks

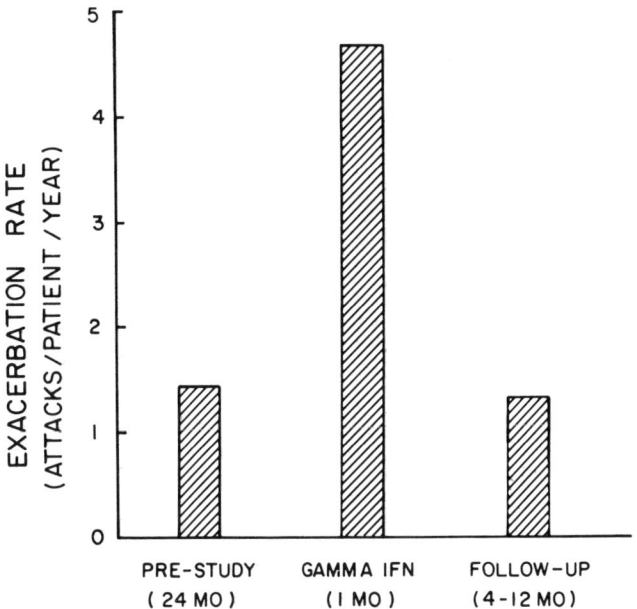

Figure 2 Exacerbation rates before, during, and following 1-month trial of intravenous interferon-β in 18 patients. For interferon phase versus prestudy or follow-up phases, P < 0.01 (chi-square analysis). [Adapted from Panitch et al. (78).]

were not dose related either in severity or time of onset after beginning treatment. They were mild or moderate in degree, and all resolved spontaneously within 1 week to 3 months. The patients then returned to their prestudy exacerbation rates and overall neurologic status. Side effects (fever, chills, myalgias, headache, and fatigue) occurred predominantly in the high-dose group and were not directly responsible for the exacerbations since some of the patients with severe side effects had no exacerbation and others receiving the lowest dose of interferon had exacerbations in the absence of clinical side effects.

Immunologic studies performed in conjunction with this trial (80) showed changes in NK cell activity different from those observed in the previous trials of natural and recombinant a interferons (39,74); that is, after an early peak of activity 1–3 days after the first dose of interferon, cytolytic activity fell somewhat but remained above baseline levels. Cells from treated patients did not lose their responsiveness to interferon-γ, as shown by augmentation of cytotoxicity when interferon was added to NK cell cultures. Cells from 8 of 10 patients tested produced normal levels of interferon-γ and continued to do so during treatment. Despite the administration of high doses to some patients, no interferon was detected by bioassay in the CSF 2 hr after intravenous infusions. A highly interesting finding that may have contributed to the increase in attacks was the induction of HLA-DR surface antigen on peripheral blood monocytes. Induction of class II MHC antigens (HLA-DR or Ia) is a well-recognized property of interferon-γ (81,82) and is thought to enable monocytes and macrophages to function as antigen presenting cells in the induction of T-cell-mediated immune responses (83). Interferon-γ has also been reported to induce Ia determinants on endothelial cells (84) and astrocytes (85,86), which may be important in the pathogenesis of autoimmune responses within the CNS. Although the evidence for such a process in this group of MS patients was only circumstantial, it remains that the administration of interferon-γ led to a definite increase in exacerbations during the month of treatment.

This study provides the first clear-cut demonstration that systemic administration of an interferon can produce a significant effect on disease activity within the CNS, despite that interferon levels in CSF were undetectable by conventional methods. It also indicates that endogenous interferon-γ may play an important role in the pathogenesis of acute exacerbations of MS and suggests that further clinical trials of this substance in MS patients are contraindicated. Alternatively, treatment with inhibitors of interferon-γ or of interferon-γ-mediated functions may prevent or modify MS exacerbations. Such agents include antibodies to interferon-γ or antibodies to Ia determinants. The latter have already been shown to prevent EAE in mice (87,88), but their application to humans may not be feasible. Another means of inhibiting γ-mediated effects on immune induction may simply be treatment with α or β interferons. Recent studies have shown that pretreatment of cell cultures with recombinant α or β interferons can inhibit subsequent induction of Ia antigen by interferon-γ (89,90). If α and β interferons are found to be effective in MS, this may be one of the mechanisms responsible for their therapeutic effect.

III. TREATMENT OF MS WITH AN INTERFERON INDUCER

Treatment of chronic progressive MS patients with the interferon inducer poly ICLC has recently been reported by Bever et al. (91). Poly ICLC induced high levels (50-500 U/ml) of interferon in serum, in some cases higher than those measured after systemic administration of α or γ interferons. Interferon induced by poly ICLC has been identified as a mixture of α and β subtypes. Fever and other side effects were pronounced, and several patients experienced transient but severe worsening of signs and symptoms after each infusion of the drug. Nevertheless, 12 of the 18 patients improved or stabilized during treatment, with the most striking results occurring in the more rapidly progressive patients. Several of these improved 1-3 points on the Kurtzke DSS; however, improvement was not maintained after treatment was discontinued. Although CSF interferon was not measured in this study, other reports indicate that high interferon titers may be reached in the CSF after systemic administration of poly ICLC (92). Poly ICLC may therefore be useful in patients with rapidly progressive MS unresponsive to other modes of therapy; however, it is probably too toxic for routine long-term clinical use outside the hospital setting, where patients can be carefully monitored. Further clinical trials have been suggested, although poly ICLC seems to offer little, if any, advantage over systemic treatment with recombinant α and β interferons, which are available in large quantity at relatively low cost and produce less severe toxic side effects.

IV. STUDIES IN PROGRESS

Paty and his colleagues at the University of British Columbia have treated approximately 50 early chronic progressive MS patients with lymphoblastoid interferon (Wellferon, Burroughs Wellcome) and 50 with placebo in a double-blind trial. Patients received 5×10^6 U of the preparation (consisting predominantly of natural interferon-α) daily by subcutaneous injection for 6 months after which they were followed for 2 years. Concurrent treatment with corticosteroids was permitted for acute exacerbations of MS. Preliminary evaluation (D. W. Paty, personal communication) indicates that there were significant side effects, including fever, fatigue, weakness, and other flulike symptoms, but that these were generally well tolerated, and few patients left the study because of interferon toxicity. In vitro studies of immunoglobulin synthesis were performed that showed a striking decrease in pokeweed mitogen-stimulated IgG production by peripheral blood leukocytes from interferon-treated patients (93). After completion of treatment, the patients returned to their original high synthesis rates. Clinical correlations with disease activity are not yet available, but there was a difference between interferon- and placebo-treated patients in the size of MS plaques, as determined by quantitative magnetic resonance imaging during the 6 months of treatment. This technique may prove to be a useful indicator of disease activity and effectiveness of treatment in future clinical trials.

In Australia, a multicenter study comparing natural interferon-α to placebo and to transfer factor has been undertaken by McLeod and coworkers. In this double-blind trial, 3×10^6 U of interferon are to be given subcutaneously twice a week for 2 months and then once a week for 10 months to relapsing-remitting and early progressive patients. Similar groups of up to 75 subjects each will be treated with placebo or with transfer factor, which has been used previously in MS with negative results (94). No preliminary data are currently available.

A trial of recombinant interferon-β (Betaseron, Triton Biosciences) has recently been undertaken in the United States. Betaseron is a variety of cloned interferon-β, produced in bacteria, that has been genetically engineered by substitution of a serine residue for cysteine at position 17 to improve stability. The antiviral, antiproliferative, and immunomodulatory activities of α and β interferons are similar, and they apparently share a common receptor. Furthermore, because there is only a single human interferon-β gene, the question of choosing among multiple subtypes of interferon-α may be avoided (95). A pilot study in 30 patients with relapsing-remitting MS is being conducted at the University of Maryland, Temple University, and Jefferson Medical College to evaluate toxicity and to select the appropriate dose for a more extensive effort. Subjects were randomized to receive 4.5, 22.5, 45, or 90 MU three times per week by subcutaneous injection. A fifth subgroup will receive placebo. If no major complications or toxic side effects occur, the maximum tolerated dose will then be administered to a larger group of patients in a multicenter placebo-controlled, double-blind clinical trial.

V. COMPLICATIONS OF STUDY DESIGNS

Although the results of the early trials of systemically administered interferons and interferon inducers have been only moderately successful, one must realize that they have been designed by using the small amount of information available from clinical trials of interferons in seriously ill patients with malignancies and acute viral infections. Preclinical data on interferons in relation to MS are grossly inadequate in part because the immunologic basis of the disease is so poorly understood and in part because there is no entirely satisfactory animal model or immunologic marker of disease activity. In EAE, the best available animal model of MS, only a handful of studies related to interferon have been done. Admittedly, interferons are highly species specific, and results in an animal model may not be directly applicable to human disease, but a better understanding of the role of interferons, especially interferon-γ, in EAE may well be of value in the design of future clinical trials in MS.

The following discussion indicates some areas of controversy that can only be addressed by well-designed clinical studies. There is, first of all, complete uncertainty about the proper dose of interferon for treatment of multiple sclerosis. The California natural a trial, for example, was designed according to the philosophy used for the treatment of cancer patients, namely, to give the largest amount of interferon possible under the existing limitations of availability, side effects, and cost. Patients treated with 5×10^6 U/day lost cellular sensitivity to interferon as measured by NK cell activity, the priming effect, and the ability of their cells to secrete interferon in response to conventional inducers. Nevertheless, the treatment did seem to exert a beneficial effect in some patients. In the subsequent recombinant a_2 trial, NK responsiveness was lost, even though the dose was reduced to a level that was apparently clinically ineffective. In the interferon-γ trial, NK function and responsiveness to interferon were preserved; however, the interferon had other immunologic effects that apparently induced acute attacks. Future trials of a and $β$ interferons must begin with an attempt to assess the appropriate dose of the particular preparation being tested. Very high doses have the additional potential complication of inducing neurologic side effects, including encephalopathy and worsening of MS symptoms (96–98).

The frequency of interferon administration is another unsettled issue. Subcutaneous, intramuscular, and intraventricular routes all give different blood levels that may or may not correlate with therapeutic and toxic effects. Recombinant interferon-$β$, for example, has been shown to induce immunologic effects in the absence of detectable blood levels when given by the subcutaneous route (S. G. Marcus, personal communication). It is also possible that frequent treatment is unnecessary and that a single high dose given weekly or even less frequently may be as effective as lower doses given daily. Protocols used in the treatment of cancer or serious viral infections do not necessarily apply to MS or to other presumably autoimmune diseases. It is important to recognize that if interferons prove to be effective in MS, the level of side effects must be low enough to permit use over several decades, unlike the level of side effects that may be acceptable for short-term use in a fatal disease.

A major problem facing investigators in this field is the multiplicity of interferon preparations now available. Approximately 20 genes code for human α interferons, and at least 14 different subtypes have been prepared by genetic engineering techniques (95,99). Obviously, these cannot all be tested thoroughly in MS. A possible solution is the development of so-called consensus interferon-α, which incorporates amino acid residues on the basis of their frequency of occurrence at each position in the molecule (100). Another solution would be to test mixtures of recombinant α interferons, and yet a third possibility would be to concentrate on interferon-β, of which there is only one molecular species. Recombinant interferon-β appears to incorporate most of the properties of the α interferons, with which it has approximately 30% sequence homology, but is not known to share the immunostimulatory effects of interferon-γ, such as Ia induction and macrophage activation. In addition, natural interferon-β has been tested in MS patients via the intrathecal route with encouraging results (101).

Another important issue in the design of clinical trials is the placebo effect, which is almost certain to occur with any new therapy for MS, particularly one with such extensive advance publicity as interferon. The California natural α trial provides the best documentation of how important the placebo effect can be in assessing the outcome of such a study. It was also apparent in the recombinant α_2 trial in which a possible immunologic correlate, increased NK cell activity in placebo-treated patients, was reported. The original trial of intrathecal interferon-β (101), despite a marked reduction in exacerbations after treatment, suffered from the lack of a placebo-treated control group. Ethical considerations precluded frequent lumbar punctures in the control patients, but without such comparable treatment, the effect of interferon in these patients could not be adequately evaluated. However, a multicenter interferon-β trial with sham lumbar punctures in control patients was recently completed (102) and appears to confirm the earlier results; that is, there was a significant reduction of exacerbations in the interferon-treated group. In the interferon-γ trial, it is obvious that whatever placebo effect may have been present was overcome by the adverse effects of treatment. Because MS is such a variable and unpredictable disease and because interferons are probably most suitable for use in early relapsing-remitting patients who are especially prone to spontaneous improvement, future clinical trials must be carefully controlled and must include appropriate placebo-treated control groups.

VI. CONCLUSIONS

The α and β interferons fulfill several criteria for ideal therapeutic agents in MS. They are well tolerated in moderate doses and are widely available, relatively inexpensive, and easy to administer. Side effects, such as fever, fatigue, myalgias, and arthralgias, which tend to occur after the first few doses, become less prominent with prolonged treatment and are almost immediately reversible upon discontinuation of therapy. In addition, there are no known long-term side effects, such as the irreversible nephrotoxicity that may occur with cyclosporine, the potential for inducing malignant neoplasms that may occur with immunosuppressive agents such as cyclophosphamide or azathioprine, or the protean complications of high-dose corticosteroids.

In MS, a disease that usually begins in young adults, lifelong treatment may be necessary. Thus, ease of administration, low toxicity, and lack of complications with long-term administration are important considerations. In addition, treatment of MS would ideally begin early in the disease before multiple exacerbations occur, leaving the patient with a residual neurologic deficit, and before the disease advances from the relapsing-remitting to the relapsing-progressive or chronic progressive phases. The α and β interferons seem to be most effective in the early relapsing-remitting stage of MS and would be suitable therapeutic agents from this point of view. Because interferon-γ given systemically can induce exacerbations, it may be inferred that modulation of the systemic immune system should also be an effective means of reducing attacks, if the proper agent were administered.

Intrathecal or intraventricular interferon treatment, despite the reports of success by Jacobs et al., is a traumatic procedure that may carry substantial risks of infection and chronic arachnoiditis, especially if performed by inexperienced personnel in large numbers of patients. If a single treatment or series of treatments were curative or resulted in long-term remission, intrathecal or intraventricular treatment might be more feasible. For the present, however, and for purposes of the design of future clinical trials, it probably should be assumed that any effective therapy for MS is likely to require repeated and, perhaps, lifelong treatment. The treatment must be simple to administer and free enough of side effects to be well tolerated by people who are active, ambulatory, employed, and free of disease other than their MS. Only after systemic treatment has been proven ineffective would it be advisable to adopt the intrathecal or intraventricular routes of interferon administration.

REFERENCES

1. McFarlin, D. E., and McFarland, H. F. Multiple sclerosis. *N. Engl. J. Med.* *307*:1183-1188, 1246-1251 (1982).

2. Weiner, H. L., and Hauser, S. L. Neuroimmunology. I. Immunoregulation in neurological disease. *Ann. Neurol. 11*:437-449 (1982).

3. Waksman, B. H., and Reynolds, W. E. Multiple sclerosis as a disease of immune regulation. *Proc. Soc. Exp. Biol. Med. 175*:282-294 (1984).

4. Adams, J. M., and Imagawa, D. T. Measles antibodies in multiple sclerosis. *Proc. Soc. Exp. Biol. Med. 111*:562-566 (1962).

5. Norrby, E. Viral antibodies in multiple sclerosis. *Prog. Med. Virol. 24*: 1-39 (1978).

6. Vandvik, B., Norrby, E., Nordal, H., et al. Oligoclonal measles virus specific IgG antibodies isolated by virus immunoabsorption of cerebrospinal fluids, brain extracts, and sera from patients with subacute sclerosing panencephalitis and multiple sclerosis. *Scand. J. Immunol. 5*:979-992 (1976).

7. Paterson, P.Y., and Whitacre, C. C. The enigma of oligoclonal immunoglobulin G in cerebrospinal fluid from multiple sclerosis patients. *Immunol. Today* 2:111-117 (1981).

8. Utermohlen, V., and Zabriskie, J. B. A suppression of cellular immunity in patients with multiple sclerosis. *J. Exp. Med.* 138:1591-1596 (1973).

9. Greenstein, J. I., McFarland, H. F., Mingioli, E. S., et al. The lymphoproliferative response to measles virus in twins with multiple sclerosis. *Ann. Neurol.* 15:79-87 (1984).

10. Jacobson, S., Flerlage, M. L., and McFarland, H. F. Impaired measles virus-specific cytotoxic T cell responses in multiple sclerosis. *J. Exp. Med.* 162:839-850 (1985).

11. Haase, A. T., Ventura, P., Gibbs, C. J., and Tourtellotte, W. W. Measles virus nucleotide sequences: Detection by hybridization in situ. *Science* 212:672-675 (1981).

12. Kurtzke, J. F., and Hyllested, K. Multiple sclerosis in the Faroe Islands. I. Clinical and epidemiological features. *Ann. Neurol.* 5:6-21 (1979).

13. Kurtzke, J. F., and Hyllested, K. Multiple sclerosis in the Faroe Islands. II. Clinical update, transmission, and the nature of MS. *Neurology* 36: 307-328 (1986).

14. Kurtzke, J. F., Gudmundsson, K. R., and Bergmann, S. Multiple sclerosis in Iceland. I. Evidence of a postwar epidemic. *Neurology* 32:143-150 (1982).

15. Cook, S. C., and Dowling, P. C. Multiple sclerosis and viruses: An overview. *Neurology* 30:80-91 (1980).

16. Johnson, R. T. *Viral Infections of the Nervous System*, Chapter 2. Raven Press, New York, 1982, pp. 263-267.

17. Koprowski, H., DeFreitas, E. C., Harper, M. E. et al. Multiple sclerosis and human T-cell lymphotropic retroviruses. *Nature* 318:154-160 (1985).

18. Rice, G. P. A., Armstrong, H., Paty, D. W., et al. Absence of antibodies to HTLV-III in sera of patients with MS and chronic myelopathy. *Neurology* 36(Suppl. 1):184 (1986).

19. Sibley, W. A., Bamford, C. R., and Clark, K. Clinical viral infections and multiple sclerosis. *Lancet* 1:1313-1315 (1985).

20. Dal Canto, M. C., and Rabinowitz, S. G. Experimental models of virus-

induced demyelination of the central nervous system. *Ann. Neurol. 11*: 109-127 (1982).

21. Panitch, H. S., Gomez-Plascencia, J., Norris, F. H., Cantell, K., and Smith, R. A. Remission of subacute sclerosing panencephalitis in patients treated with intraventricular interferon. *Neurology 36*:562-566 (1986).

22. Smith, R. A., Abramsky, O., Steiner, I., et al. The experimental treatment of subacute sclerosing panencephalitis with interferon. In: *The Biology of the Interferon System 1985* (W. E. Stewart II and H. Schellekens, eds.). Elsevier Science Publishers, Amsterdam, 1986, pp. 505-510).

23. Huttenlocher, P. R., Picchietti, D. L., Roos, R. P., et al. Intrathecal interferon in subacute sclerosing panencephalitis. *Ann. Neruol. 19*:303-305 (1986).

24. Smith, R. A., Norris, F., Palmer, D., Bernhardt, L., and Wills, R. J. Distribution of alpha interferon in serum and cerebrospinal fluid after systemic administration. *Clin. Pharmacol. Ther. 37*:85-88 (1985).

25. Hafler, D. A., and Weiner, H. L. In vivo labeling of blood T-cells: Rapid traffic into cerebrospinal fluid in multiple sclerosis. *Ann. Neurol. 22*: 89-93 (1987).

26. Ebers, G. C., Vinuela, F. V., Feasby, T., et al. Multifocal CT enhancement in MS. *Neurology 34*:341 (1984).

27. Vilcek, J., Gray, P. W., Rinderknecht, E., and Sevastopoulos, C. G. Interferon-gamma: A lymphokine for all seasons. In *Lymphokines*, Vol. 11, (E. Pick, ed.). Academic Press, New York, 1985.

28. DeMaeyer-Guignard, J., and DeMaeyer, E. Immunomodulation by interferons: Recent developments. In: *Interferon 6* (I. Gresser, ed.). Academic Press, New York, 1985, pp. 69-191.

29. Kabat, E. A., Moore, O. H., and Landow, H. An electrophoretic study of the protein components in the cerebrospinal fluid and their relationship to the serum proteins. *J. Clin. Invest. 21*:571-577 (1942).

30. Prineas, J. W., and Wright, R. G. Macrophages, lymphocytes, and plasma cells in the perivascular compartment in chronic multiple sclerosis. *Lab. Invest. 38*:409-421 (1978).

31. Harfast, B., Huddlestone, J. R., Casali, P., et al. Interferon acts directly on human B-lymphocytes to modulate immunoglobulin synthesis. *J. Immunol. 127*:2146-2150 (1981).

32. Neighbour, P. A., and Bloom, B. R. Absence of virus-induced lymphocyte suppression and interferon production in multiple sclerosis. *Proc. Natl. Acad. Sci. USA* 76:476-480 (1979).

33. Salonen, R., Ilonen, J., Reunanen, M., et al. PPD-, and PHA-induced interferon in stable multiple sclerosis: Association with HLA-Dw2 antigen and clinical variables. *Ann. Neurol.* 11:279-284 (1982).

34. Vervliet, G., Claeys, H., Van Haver, H., et al. Interferon production and natural killer cell (NK) activity in leukocyte cultures from multiple sclerosis patients. *J. Neurol. Sci.* 60:137-150 (1983).

35. Santoli, D., Hall, W., Kastrukoff, L., et al. Cytotoxic activity and interferon production by lymphocytes from patients with multiple sclerosis. *J. Immunol.* 126:1274-1278 (1981).

36. Hirsch, R. L., Panitch, H. S., and Johnson, K. P. Lymphocytes from multiple sclerosis patients produce elevated levels of gamma interferon in vitro. *J. Clin. Immunol.* 5:386-389 (1985).

37. Hauser, S. L., Ault, K. A., Levin, M. J., et al. Natural killer cell activity in multiple sclerosis. *J. Immunol.* 127:1114-1117 (1981).

38. Hirsch, R. L., and Johnson, K. P. The effect of recombinant alpha-2 interferon on defective natural killer cell activity in multiple sclerosis. *Neurology* 35:597-600 (1985).

39. Rice, G. P. A., Casali, P., Merigan, T. C. and Oldstone, M. B. A. Natural killer cell activity in patients with multiple sclerosis given alpha interferon. *Ann. Neurol.* 14:333-338 (1983).

40. Merrill, J., Jondal, M., Seeley, J., et al. Decreased NK killing in patients with multiple sclerosis: An analysis on the level of the single effector cell in peripheral blood and cerebrospinal fluid in relation to the activity of the disease. *Clin. Exp. Immunol.* 47:419-430 (1982).

41. Hirsch, R. L., and Johnson, K. P. Natural killer cell activity in multiple sclerosis patients treated with recombinant interferon-alpha$_2$. *Clin. Immunol. Immunopathol.* 37:236-244 (1985).

42. Antel, J. P., Arnason, B. G. W., and Medof, M. E. Suppressor cell function in multiple sclerosis: Correlation with clinical disease activity. *Ann. Neurol.* 5:338-342 (1979).

43. Huddlestone, J. R., and Oldstone, M. B. A. T suppressor (T_G) lymphocytes fluctuate in parallel with changes in the clinical course of patients with multiple sclerosis. *J. Immunol.* 123:1615-1618 (1979).

44. Antel, J. P., Peeples, D. M., Reder, A. T., et al. Analysis of T regulator cell surface markers and functional properties in multiple sclerosis. *J. Neuroimmunol.* 6:93-103 (1984).

45. Reinherz, E. L., Weiner, H. L., Hauser, S. L., et al. Loss of suppressor T cells in active multiple sclerosis: Analysis with monoclonal antibodies. *N. Engl. J. Med.* 303:125-129 (1980).

46. Bach, M.-A., Phan-Dinh-Tuy, F., Tournier, E., et al. Deficit of suppressor T cells in active multiple sclerosis. *Lancet* 2:1221-1223 (1980).

47. Reder, A. T., Antel, J. P., Oger, J., et al. Low T8 antigen density on lymphocytes in active multiple sclerosis. *Ann. Neurol.* 16:242-249 (1984).

48. Mingioli, E. S., and McFarlin, D. E. Leukocyte surface antigens in patients with multiple sclerosis. *J. Neuroimmunol.* 6:131-139 (1984).

49. Hirsch, R. L., Ordonez, J., Panitch, H. S., and Johnson, K. P. T8 antigen density on peripheral blood lymphocytes remains unchanged during exacerbations of multiple sclerosis. *J. Neuroimmunol.* 9:391-398 (1985).

50. Oger, J., Roos, R., and Antel, J. P. Immunology of multiple sclerosis. *Neurol. Clin.* 1:655-679 (1983).

51. Aune, I. M., and Pierce, C. W. Activation of a suppressor T-cell pathway by interferon. *Proc. Natl. Acad. Sci. USA* 79:3808-3812 (1982).

52. Kadish, A. S., Tansey, F. A., Yu, G. S. M., et al. Interferon as a mediator of human lymphocyte suppression. *J. Exp. Med.* 151:637-650 (1980).

53. Abreu, S. L. Suppression of experimental allergic encephalomyelitis by interferon. *Immunol. Commun.* 11:1-7 (1982).

54. Abreu, S. L., Tondreau, J., Levine, S., and Sowinski, R. Inhibition of passive localized experimental allergic encephalomyelitis by interferon. *Int. Arch. Allergy Appl. Immunol.* 72:30-33 (1983).

55. Abreu, S. L. Interferon in experimental autoimmune encephalomyelitis (EAE): Effects of exogenous interferon on the antigen-enhanced adoptive transfer of EAE. *Int. Arch. Allergy Appl. Immunol.* 76:302-307 (1985).

56. Abreu, S. L. Thampoe, I., and Kaplan, P. Interferon in experimental autoimmune encephalomyelitis: Intraventricular administration. *J. Interferon Res.* 6:627-632 (1986).

57. Fog, T. Interferon treatment of multiple sclerosis patients: A pilot study.

In: *Search for the Cause of Multiple Sclerosis and Other Chronic Diseases of the Central Nervous System* (A. Boese, ed.). Verlag Chemie, Weinheim, 1980, pp. 491-493.

58. Ververken, D., Carton, H., and Billiau, A. Intrathecal administration of interferon in MS patients? In: *Humoral Immunity in Neurological Diseases* (D. Karcher, et al., eds.). Plenum Press, New York, 1979, pp. 625-627.

59. Montezuma-de Carvalho, M. J. A treatment for the chronic disabilities of stable multiple sclerosis. *Acta Medicotechnica 31*:155-160 (1983).

60. Johnson, K. P. Systemic interferon therapy for multiple sclerosis: Design of a trial. *Arch. Neurol. 40*:681-682 (1983).

61. Knobler, R. L., Panitch, H. S., Braheny, S. L., et al. controlled clinical trial of systemic alpha interferon in multiple sclerosis. *Neurology 34*: 1273-1279 (1984).

62. Kurtzke, J. F. Further notes on disability evaluation in multiple sclerosis with scale modifications. *Neurology 15*:654-661 (1965).

63. Sipe, J. C., Knobler, R. L., Braheny, S. L., Rice, G. P. A., Panitch, H. S., and Oldstone, M. B. A. A neurological rating scale (NRS) for use in multiple sclerosis. *Neurology 34*:1368-1372 (1984).

64. Rice, G. P. A., Woelfel, E. L., Talbot, P. J., et al. Immunological complications in multiple sclerosis patients receiving interferon. *Ann. Neurol. 18*:439-442 (1985).

65. Panitch, H. S., Francis, G. S., Hooper, C. J., et al. Serial immunological studies in multiple sclerosis patients treated systemically with human alpha interferon. *Ann. Neurol. 18*:434-438 (1985).

66. McFarlin, D. E. Use of interferon in multiple sclerosis. *Ann. Neurol. 18*: 432-433 (1985).

67. Kamin-Lewis, R. M., Panitch, H. S., Merigan, T. C., and Johnson, K. P. Decreased interferon synthesis and responsiveness to interferon by leukocytes from multiple sclerosis patients given natural alpha interferon. *J. Interferon Res. 4*:423-432 (1984).

68. Branca, A. A., and Baglioni, C. Evidence that types I and II interferons have different receptors. *Nature 294*:768-770 (1981).

69. Kamin-Lewis, R. M., Panitch, H. S., and Johnson, K. P. Leukocytes from multiple sclerosis patients respond to alpha and gamma interferons. *J. Neuroimmunol. 9*:221-227 (1985).

70. Kamin-Lewis, R. M., and Johnson, K. P. Has alpha interferon therapy been properly tested. *J. Interferon Res.* in press (1988).

71. Panitch, H. S. Systemic alpha-interferon in multiple sclerosis: Long-term patient follow-up. *Arch. Neurol. 44*:61-63 (1987).

72. Jacobs, L., O'Malley, J. A., Freeman, A., et al. Intrathecal interferon in the treatment of multiple sclerosis. Patient follow-up. *Arch. Neurol. 42*: 841-847 (1985).

73. Camenga, D. L., Johnson, K. P., Alter, M., et al. Systemic recombinant alpha-2 interferon therapy in relapsing multiple sclerosis. *Arch. Neurol. 43*:1239-1246 (1986).

74. Hirsch, R. L., and Johnson, K. P. The effects of long-term administration of recombinant alpha-2 interferon on lymphocyte subsets, proliferation, and suppressor cell function in multiple sclerosis. *J. Interferon Res. 6*: 171-177 (1986).

75. Hirsch, R. L., and Johnson, K. P. Placebo-induced enhancement of natural killer cell activity in a double-blind trial of recombinant alpha-2 interferon in multiple sclerosis patients. In: *Neuroimmunomodulation. Proceedings of the First International Workshop of Neuroimmunomodulation* (N. H. Spector, ed.). IWGN, Bethesda, Maryland, 1985, pp. 219-226.

76. Neighbour, P. A., Miller, A. E., and Bloom, B. R. Interferon responses of leukocytes in multiple sclerosis. *Neurology 31*:561-566 (1981).

77. Vervliet, G., Carton, H., Meulepas, E., and Billiau, A. Interferon production by cultured peripheral leukocytes of MS patients. *Clin. Exp. Immunol. 58*:116-126 (1984).

78. Panitch, H. S., Hirsch, R. L., Haley, A. S., and Johnson, K. P. Exacerbations of multiple sclerosis in patients treated with gamma interferon. *Lancet 1*:893-895 (1987).

79. Poser, C. M., Paty, D. W., Scheinberg, L., et al. New diagnostic criteria for multiple sclerosis: Guidelines for research protocols. *Ann. Neurol. 13*:227-231 (1983).

80. Panitch, H. S., Hirsch, R. L., Schindler, J., and Johnson, K. P. Treatment of multiple sclerosis with gamma interferon: Exacerbations associated with activation of the immune system. *Neurology 37*:1097-1102 (1987).

81. Basham, T. Y., and Merigan, T. C. Recombinant interferon-gamma increases HLA-DR synthesis and expression. *J. Immunol. 130*:1492-1494 (1983).

82. Kelley, V. E., Fiers, W., and Strom, T. B. Cloned human interferon-gamma, but not interferon-beta or -alpha, induces expression of HLA-DR determinants by fetal monocytes and myeloid leukemic cell lines. *J. Immunol.* 132:240-245 (1984).
83. Unanue, E. R., Beller, D. I., Lu,C. Y., and Allen, P. M.Antigen presentation: Comments on its regulation and mechanism. *J. Immunol.* 132:1-5 (1984).
84. Pober, J. S., Gimbone, M. A., and Cotran, R. S. et al. Ia expression by vascular endothelium is inducible by activated T cells and by human interferon. *J. Exp. Med.* 157:1339-1353 (1983).
85. Wong, G. H. W., Bartlett, P. F., Clark-Lewis, I., et al. Interferon-gamma induces the expression of H-2 and Ia antigens on brain cells. *J. Neuroimmunol.* 7:255-278 (1985).
86. Fierz, W., Endler, B., Reske, K., Wekerle, H., and Fontana, A. Astrocytes as antigen-presenting cells. I. Induction of Ia antigen expression in astrocytes by T cells via immune interferon and its effect on antigen presentation. *J. Immunol.* 134:3785-3793 (1985).
87. Steinman, L. S., Rosenbaum, J. T., Sriram, S., and McDevitt, H. O. In vivo effects of antibodies to immune response gene products: Prevention of experimental allergic encephalitis. *Proc. Natl. Acad. Sci. USA* 78: 7111-7114 (1981).
88. Sriram, S., and Steinman, L. Anti I-A antibody suppresses active encephalomyelitis: Treatment model for diseases linked to IR genes. *J. Exp. Med.* 158:1362-1367 (1983).
89. Ling, P. D., Warren, M. K., and Vogel, S. N. Antagonistic effect of interferon-beta on the interferon-gamma-induced expression of Ia antigen in murine macrophages. *J. Immunol.* 135:1857-1863 (1985).
90. Inaba, K., Kitaura, M., Kato, T., et al. Contrasting effect of alpha/beta- and gamma-interferons on expression of macrophage Ia antigens. *J. Exp. Med.* 163:1030-1035 (1986).
91. Bever, C. T., Salazar, A. M., Neely, et al. Preliminary trial of poly ICLC in chronic progressive multiple sclerosis. *Neurology* 36:494-498 (1986).
92. Levine, A. S., Durie, B., Lampkin, B., et al. Poly (ICLC): Interferon induction, toxicity, and clinical efficacy in leukemia, lymphoma, solid tumors, myeloma, and laryngeal papillomatosis. In: *Augmenting Agents in Cancer Therapy* (E. M. Hersch, et al., eds.). Raven Press, New York, 1981, pp. 151-165.

93. O'Gorman, M., and Oger, J. Reduced in vitro IgG secretion following in vivo injection of interferon in multiple sclerosis (MS) patients. *Fed. Proc. 44*:1923 (1985).

94. Basten, A., McLeod, J. G., Pollard, J. D., et al. Transfer factor in treatment of multiple sclerosis. *Lancet 2*:931-934 (1980).

95. Revel, M. Genetic and functional diversity of interferons in man. In: *Interferon 5* (I. Gresser, ed.). Academic Press, London, 1983, pp. 205-239.

96. Rohatiner, A. Z. S., Prior, P. F., Burton, A. C., et al. Central nervous system toxicity of interferon. *Br. J. Cancer 47*:419-422 (1983).

97. Suter, C., Westmoreland, B. F., Sharbrough, F. W., et al. Electroencephalographic abnormalities in interferon encephalopathy: A preliminary report. *Mayo Clin. Proc. 59*:847-850 (1984).

98. Smedley, H., Katrak, M., Sikora, K., et al. Neurological effects of recombinant human interferon. *Br. Med. J. 286*:262-264 (1983).

99. Weissman, C. The cloning of interferon and other mistakes. In: *Interferon 3* (I. Gresser, ed.). Academic Press, London, 1981, pp. 101-134.

100. Alton, K., Stabinsky, Y., Richards, R., et al. Production, characterization and biological effects of recombinant DNA-derived human IFN-alpha and IFN-gamma analogs. In: *The Biology of the Interferon System* (E. DeMaeyer and H. Schellekens, eds.). Elsevier, Amsterdam, 1983.

101. Jacobs, L., O'Malley, J., Freeman, A., and Ekes, R. Intrathecal interferon reduces exacerbations of multiple sclerosis. *Science 214*:1026-1028 (1981).

102. Jacobs, L., Salazar, A., Herndon, R., et al. Multicentre double-blind study of effect of intrathecally administered natural human fibroblast interferon on exacerbations of multiple sclerosis. *Lancet 2*:1411-1413 (1986).

10
Intrathecal Interferon in the Treatment of Multiple Sclerosis

LAWRENCE JACOBS

Baird Multiple Sclerosis Center, Dent Neurologic Institute, Millard Fillmore Hospital, and State University of New York School of Medicine at Buffalo, Buffalo, New York

ANDRES SALAZAR

Walter Reed Army Medical Center and Uniformed Services University of Health Sciences, Bethesda, Maryland

ROBERT M. HERNDON

University of Rochester School of Medicine and Dentristy, Rochester, New York

PETER REESE

Roswell Park Memorial Institute, Buffalo, New York

I. INTRODUCTION

In 1979 we began a preliminary study of the efficacy of intrathecally (IT) administered human fibroblast interferon (IFN-β) as a treatment of multiple sclerosis (MS). The rationale for that trial was the body of evidence suggesting that MS is caused by a previous or ongoing viral infection of the central nervous system (CNS) of a dysimmune host and the known potent antiviral and immunomodulatory effects of the interferons (1–5). We administered the IFN-β intrathecally rather than systemically because previous reserach in animals and humans indicated that systemically administered IFN did not effectively cross the blood-brain barrier (BBB) (5). Moreover, two earlier small clinical studies indicated that systemically administered human leukocyte and fibroblast interferon (IFN-β) were of no benefit in MS (6,7).

Our first reports on this topic, published in late 1981 and early 1982, indicated a beneficial effect of this treatment in terms of the reduction of exacerbation rates in IFN-β recipients, but not controls (8,9). Subsequent to the second publication, the original control patients were crossed over and began receiving IFN-β administered IT (10). This was after they had been observed for approximately 2 years on the study without receiving IFN-β and had shown no change in their exacerbation rates. We also continued to follow up the original recipients. In this report, we present observations on the patients in the preliminary study after more than 5 years (since beginning the study) in the original recipients and 2.9 years (since the crossover) in the original controls. We also describe the design and some preliminary findings of a currently ongoing double-blinded multicenter study of IT IFN-β therapy in MS (11).

II. PATIENTS AND METHODS

A. Preliminary Study

A total of 20 patients with definite MS were included in the preliminary study (Table 1). They were randomly assigned to a group of 10 IFN-β recipients or 10 control patients. Randomization for both groups was performed simultaneously, but because of manpower limitations, the control group was not formally entered into the study until a mean of 0.3 years after the recipients. The disease type was exacerbating-remitting (with residua or progressive) in 7 recipients and 5 controls and stable with residua in 3 recipients and 5 controls. The preliminary study was not blinded because the toxic side effects of IFN-β adminstration that are not reproduced by innocuous placebo would have readily

Table 1 Clinical Features of 20 MS Patinets Included in the Preliminary study[a]

	Recipients (10)	Controls (10)
Age (years)	20-40 (30.2)	12-39 (31.1)
Sex	7F; 3M	8F; 2M
Duration (years)	1-19.4 (8.0)	2.8-20.5 (8.5)
Types	ER-R-4	ER-R-4
	ER-P-3	ER-P-1
	SR-3	SR-5

[a]Means shown in parentheses. Disease types: exacerbating-remitting with residua, ER-R; exacerbating-remitting, progressive, ER-P; stable with residua, SR.

distinguished recipient from control patients. When we initially began the preliminary study we did not know how to alleviate or subdue the toxic side effects of IFN-β administration to the point that adequate blinding could be achieved. The IFN-β was produced by superinduction of human fibroblast cells in the laboratory of J. Horoszewicz at Roswell Park Memorial Institute, Buffalo. The preparation had a specific activity of 1×10^7 interferon reference units (IRU) of IFN-β per milligram of protein. The purified IFN-β was lyophilized, stabilized by the addition of human albumin, and kept in vials containing 2×10^6 or 3×10^6 IRU of the substance (8-10). This IFN-β preparation had undergone testing for toxicity and been approved for the trial by the U.S. Food and Drug Administration. Sterile water (0.2-0.8 ml) and Elliott's B solution (9.2-9.8 ml), were added to the vials of IFN-β prior to injection (8-10).

The IFN-β was administered to the initial recipients by lumbar punctures (LP) performed semiweekly for the first 4 weeks and then once per month for the next 5 months of the study. The dosage administered at the time of each LP was 1×10^6 IRU/m^3. In an attempt to reduce clinical and cerebrospinal fluid (CSF) toxic effects of IFN-β, the dosage and schedule of administration were modified slightly in the controls at crossover. We attempted to administer the IFN-β semiweekly during the first 4 weeks to the controls, but if pleocytosis of 100 ml^{-3} or greater was observed after one of the first eight LP, then the next scheduled LP was delayed by 4-7 days. Thus, it took 5-6 weeks to administer the first eight LP in five controls, whereas the other five underwent the first eight LP in 4 weeks (10). The subsequent five LP when IFN-β was administered to controls occurred at monthly intervals as had been done in the original recipients. Also, the dose of IFN-β administered to the controls was less than that administered to the original recipients. The maximum dosage of IFN-β at the time of each LP in the controls was 1×10^6 IRU, whereas it had been 1×10^6 IRU/m^2 to each of the orignal recipients (10). The initial recipients were hospitalized for at least 1 week and observed for toxic side effects. Experience with the original recipients indicated this period of hospitalization was not necessary, so all of the controls received their IFN-β treatments as outpatients.

The frequencies of exacerbations (standard definition) (12,13) were determined in all of the patients and expressed in terms of exacerbation rates (exacerbations per year) for the duration of the disease prior to and during the study. Before the crossover, the study was controlled internally by comparison of individual patients' prestudy and on-study exacerbation rates and externally by comparison of rates in the recipients and control groups. After crossover, the internal mechanism was used for both groups. The crossover created noncontemporaneous current observation periods (original recipients, 5.3 years; controls after crossover, 2.9 years), but it was thought that testing the efficacy of IFN-β for reducing the control exacerbation rate (as it had in the original recipients) would probably generate more important scientific information than would be gained by observing the controls untreated for another 2 years (10).

Each patient underwent monthly neurologic examinations

during the first 2 years of the study. Thereafter, the original recipients were examined ever 2-4 months and the controls continued on a schedule of monthly evaluations. The severity of patients' symptoms and signs were scored by functional groups and disability status scores (DSS) according to a modified Kurtzke method and in terms of an overall clinical estimate (improved, unchanged, or worsened) compared with their initial status (9,10). When there were discrepancies between Kurtzke's DSS and overall clinical assessments, the latter determinations were used to reflect the patients' clinical conditions. The reasons for making this judgment are given elsewhere (9).

B. Current Ongoing Multicenter Study

In 1983 we began a larger multicenter study of the efficacy of IT administered IFN-β designed to definitively determine whether this treatment is effective in MS as was indicated by the preliminary study (11). The participating centers are the Dent Neurologic Institute (DNI) and Roswell Park Memorial Institute (RPMI), Buffalo, the University of Rochester Medical Center (URMC), Rochester, New York, and the Walter Reed Army Medical Center (WRAMC), Washington, D.C.

The study was designed to include 80 patients with definite MS, each of whom had exacerbating-remitting disease (stable or progressive) of at least 1 year's duration and exacerbation rates of at least 0.6 per year. The only significant finding of the preliminary study was a reduction in exacerbation rate in recipients; therefore, exacerbation rate was to be the major focus of the current study. No patients with chronic progressive disease were included. Although the minimum rate for inclusion was a rate of 0.6 per year, every effort was made to include patients with rates of 1 per year or greater (11). The patients were randomly assigned to a recipient or control group using a stratification based on pretrial exacerbation rates. Ultimately, 76 evaluable patients were included. There are 30 patients at DNI, 21 at URMC, and 25 at WRAMC. The randomization process and all statistical analyses have been performed at RPMI. As in the preliminary study, the patients were assessed in terms of patient exacerbation rates (prestudy versus on-study) and clinical evaluations based on serial neurologic examinations. The treatment and assessment phases have been conducted by two separate clinicians ("treating" and "examining" physicians) at each center. The methods of scoring clinical assessments were the same as in the preliminary study (9, 10). The IFN-β utilized in the current, multicenter trial was produced at at RPMI and underwent the same rigorous testing for purity and toxicity as in the preliminary study.

The treatment phase of the study differed somewhat from that of the preliminary study. Recipients received IFN-β by LP performed once per week for the first 4 weeks of the study and then once per month for the next 5 months (total nine LP with IFN-β administered). In the preliminary study, the IFN-β was administered twice per week for the first 4 weeks and then once per month for the next 5 months (total 13 LP with IFN-β administered). Also, the total dosage of IFN-β administered at each LP was a maximum of 1×10^6 IRU (as in the original controls at crossover) although it had been 1×10^6 IRU/m^2 in the original recipients. We made these changes in treatment schedule and IFN-β dosage in an attempt to reduce clinical and CSF toxicity of IFN-β. A tenth LP was performed at 7 months into the study. This was for CSF analysis only, and no IFN-β was injected at that time.

The controls underwent treatments according to the same schedule as the recipients. However, true LP were performed only at the beginning and end of the study to obtain CSF for analysis. The other eight LP were false LP, in which the routine procedure (skin cleansing and local anesthetic) were followed but the spinal needle advanced only into the subcutaneous tissues, where 5 ml of sterile water was injected. Otherwise the controls underwent all other procedures as the IFN-β recipients.

It was determined in the preliminary study that it was not necessary to routinely hospitalize patients receiving IFN-β. Therefore, in the current study, both recipients and controls received all treatments in a hospital outpatient treatment room. They were observed (with vital signs recorded) for 2 hr after each treatment, and the "treating" physician was available to them thereafter by telephone. They were hospitalized only if severe toxic side effects developed. If hospitalized, they were cared for by the "treating" physician. The "examining physician" did not know which patients were hospitalized, nor did he or she query them in this regard. Cerebrospinal fluid obtained at the time of each LP was analyzed as in the preliminary study (8–10).

As previously stated, we did not attempt to double blind the preliminary study because we did not know how to adequately compensate for the clinical toxic side effects of IFN-β administration that are not reproduced by innocuous placebo. However, while we were designing the current study, we became aware of the work of Mora and associates (14), who administered small oral doses of indomethacin to patients with amyotrophic lateral sclerosis who were undergoing treatment with intrathecal IFN-α. They observed a marked reduction in toxic side effects when indomethacin was administered orally in small doses. Therefore, we administered indomethacin, 25–50 mg orally every 4–6 hr, for 24 hr after each treatment to the recipients. Eleven control patients (at URMC) received indomethacin (same schedule as IFN-β recipients), and 24 control patients (at DNI and WRAMC) did not. Thus, double blinding in the current trial was attempted by the following: (1) use of separate "examining" and "treating" physicians, (2) instructing patients not to discuss toxic side effects or hospitalization with the "examining" physician, and the "examining" physician did not query the patients on those topics, (3) administration of indomethacin in small doses for 24 hr after each treatment, and (4) false LP in the controls.

The primary thrust of the current study was assessment of change in exacerbation rate in recipients and controls. Experience in the preliminary study showed that the change in exacerbation rate is a reliable and clinically meaningful measure of outcome (11). The preliminary study showed a standard deviation (SD) of change in exacerbation rate of 1.15. For the purposes of the current study, the probabilities of type I and II errors were set at 0.05 and 0.20, respectively. The first is the risk of the study results indicating that IT IFN-β is beneficial when in fact it is not; the second, the risk of their indicating that it is not beneficial when in fact it is beneficial. In the current two-arm study, we had an 80% chance of obtaining a significant difference between the control and recipient groups if the true difference in exacerbation rates exceeded 0.65 per year. That difference is considered clinically meaningful. In the preliminary study, an imbalance between the recipients and control arms was introduced by a vagary of randomization. The recipients had a significantly higher pretreatment exacerbation rate than the controls. Although this difference was later adjusted for by a multiple linear regression (10), the occurrence of such an artifact was avoided in the current study. Two strata of patients were identified in the current study: (1) those with less than two exacerbations per year and (2) those with two or more. A biased-coin stratified randomization was employed within each institution to ensure compatability of the treatment arms on the pretreatment exacerbation rate (11). A t statistic will be used to test the effect of treatment on changes in exacerbation rate at the end of the study. Multiple linear regression will also be employed to assess the influence of other potential prognostic variables. Interim analyses have been conducted periodically during the current study to date. A final analysis will be conducted at the end of the study in July 1986, at which time all of the patients will have been followed for at least 2 years since entering the study. The registration and follow-up records of the patients have been sent according to predetermined schedule to the data base at RPMI Biomathematics Department, where all the statistical analysis will be conducted. The key elements of data capture included phone registration, eligibility checking, statistical office randomization of patients, creation and computer entry of data before receipt of all information, and rigorous review and revision of computer-stored data records by the attending physician.

III. RESULTS

A. Preliminary Study

As of June 30, 1982, the recipients had been followed 2.3-2.5 years (mean 2.4 years) and the controls, 2.0-2.2 years (mean 2.1 years) since the beginning of the study. By that time there were a total of 7 exacerbations in 3 recipients and 13 exacerbations in 7 controls. Figure 1 shows the prestudy and on-study exacerbation rates in the two groups as of June 30, 1982. The recipient mean prestudy rate (1.8 per year) was reduced to 0.28 per year during

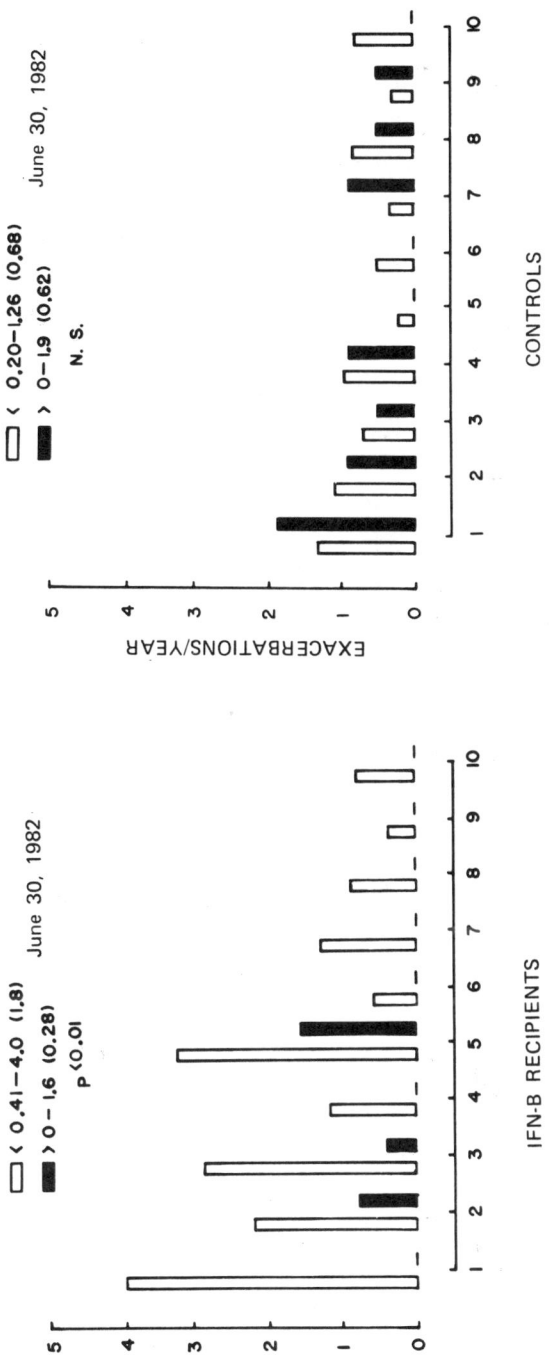

Figure 1 Exacerbation rates of recipients (left) and controls (right) as of June 30, 1982. In this and in Figure 2, open bars indicate prestudy rates; solid bars, on-study rates. Mean duration of study for recipients was 2.4 years; for controls, 2.1 years. There were 7 exacerbations in 3 recipients and 13 exacerbations in 7 controls. Mean prestudy rate of recipients (1.8 per year) was reduced to 9.28 per year during study (P < 0.01). No change in control prestudy and on-study rate (0.68 per year versus 0.62 per year). This was the last assessment in controls before crossover.

the study (P < 0.01, t-test), but there was no change in the rates of the controls before (0.68 per year) or during the study (0.62 per year). The recipient prestudy rate was higher than that of the controls, but by June 30, 1982, this difference changed and the recipient rate was significantly less than that of the controls (P < 0.06, Mann-Whitney U test) (10).

After the June 30, 1982, assessment, a crossover was done and the controls began receiving IT IFN-β according to a schedule that was slightly modified from that of the original recipients (see Sec II). Follow-up assessments were continued on the original recipients. The exacerbation rates of the two groups were not statistically compared with each other after the crossover.

By June 30, 1985, the recipients had been followed for 5.3–5.5 years (mean 5.3 years) since the beginning of the study and the controls had been followed for a mean 2.9 years since the June 30, 1982, crossover. During that period of time there was a total of 11 exacerbations in 3 recipients and 10 exacerbations in 7 controls (i.e., since their crossover). Figure 2 shows the prestudy and on-study rates of recipients and original controls as of June 30, 1985. The recipient prestudy rates are compared with their rates after a mean of 5.3 years since the beginning of the study. The control prestudy rates are compared with their rates after a mean of 2.9 years since the crossover in June 1982. By that time the recipient prestudy rate of 1.8 per year were reduced to 0.2 per year. (P < 0.001, Wilcoxon matched pairs, signed rank). The control mean prestudy rate of 0.68 per year had been reduced to 0.36 per year (P < 0.03, Wilcoxon matched pairs, signed rank).

Table 2 shows the overall clinical assessment of the two groups as of June 30, 1982, and June 30, 1985. The June 30, 1982, assessment shows the patients' condition compared with their condition the start of the study. The June 1985 assessment shows the conditions of the recipients compared with that at the start of the study and the condition of the controls compared with that at the June 1982 crossover. The 1982 assessment revealed that more recipients were improved and fewer recipients were worse than controls, but the difference in clinical conditions between the two groups was not significant. The 1985 assessment (2.9 years after the original controls had been crossed over) revealed no

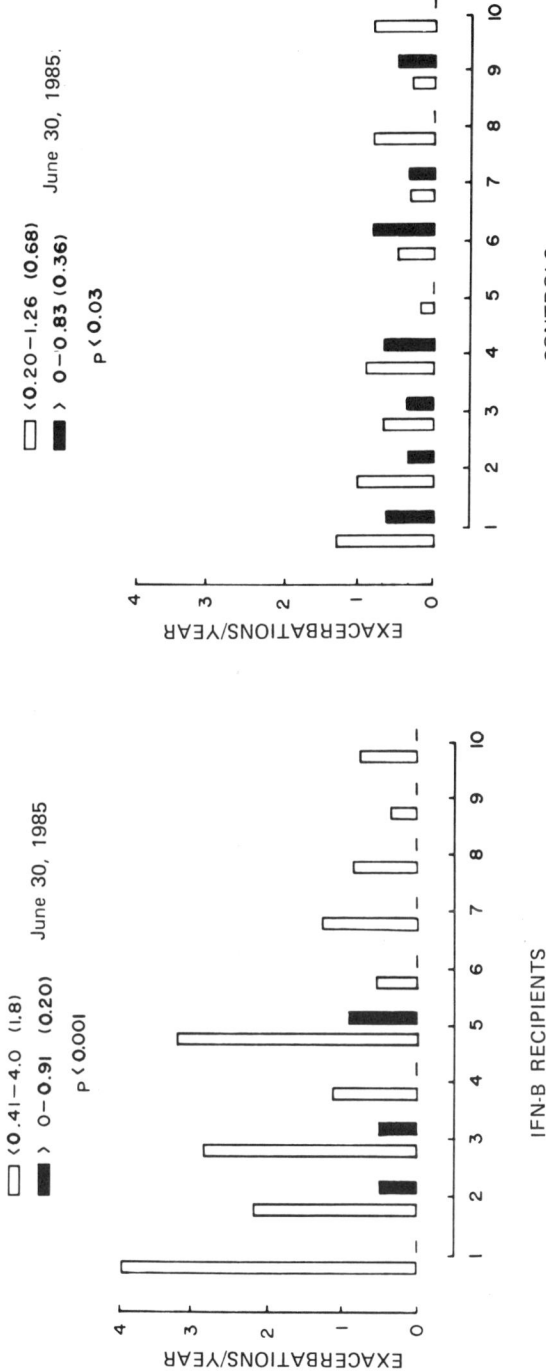

Figure 2 Exacerbation rates of recipients (left) and controls (right) as of June 30, 1985. Mean duration of study for recipients was 5.3 years; for controls, 2.9 years since June 30, 1982, crossover. There were 11 exacerbations in 3 recipients since beginning the study and 10 exacerbations in 7 controls since the crossover. Recipient mean prestudy rate (1.8 per year) was reduced to 0.2 per year ($P < 0.001$). Controls prestudy rate of 0.68 per year was reduced to 0.36 per year ($P < 0.03$).

Table 2 Clinical Conditions of the Patients[a]

	Improved	Unchanged	Worse
June 30, 1982 (precrossover)			
Recipients	5	3	2
Controls	2	4	4
June 30, 1985 (postcrossover)			
Recipients	4	3	3
Controls	4	3	3

[a]The June 1982 assessment compares the conditions of both groups with their conditions at the beginning of the study. The June 1985 assessment compares the recipients' current condition with their condition at the beginning of the study and the controls' current condition with their condition at the time of the June 1982 crossover.

difference between the two groups. There were two more of the original controls in the improved category and one less in each of the unchanged and worsened categories compared with the 1982 assessment (just before crossover). There was one less recipient in the improved and one more in the worsened category compared with the 1982 assessment.

The clinical toxic side effects of treatment were similar in both groups. Headache was most common, experienced by all patients following at least one LP, and two recipients had headache following all LP. Headaches began 6-12 hr following LP and usually lasted 24 hr. Less frequently experienced symptoms were low-grade fevers (38.3°C; six recipients and three controls), weakness (six recipients and four controls), malaise (five recipients and three controls), and myalgia (four recipients and two controls). One to two recipients experienced nausea, vomiting, diarrhea, chills, and rash. Two controls developed sinus and nasal congestion. It must be emphasized that the clinical toxic side effects typically lasted 24-48 hr and then disappeared completely.

Table 3 summarizes the CSF changes observed in these patients during treatment. The data on recipients are from the first 6 months of the study while they were undergoing IT IFN-β treatment; that on the controls was obtained after June 30, 1982, when they began their crossover treatment. The mean maximum pleocytosis observed in individual recipients (510 mm^{-3}) was 3.4 times higher than that observed in individual controls during crossover (148/mm^{-3}). The mean maximum protein level observed in individual recipients (76 mg/dl) was also higher than that observed in individual controls during crossover (61 mg/dl). The maximum elevation of cell counts and protein in the CSF typically occurred between the sixth and ninth LP. The lower levels of pleocytosis and protein in the controls during crossover probably relate to the slightly lower maximum dosage of IFN-β administered at each LP and slight delays in sequential LP depending upon pleocytosis level

Table 3 Cerebrospinal Fluid Changes

	Pleocytosis[a]	Protein[b]
	Preliminary study[c]	
Recipients	38-1750 ml^{-3} (510 ml^{-3})	55-102 mg/dl (76 mg/dl)
Crossed-over controls	70-328 ml^{-3} (148 ml^{-3})	35-91 mg/dl (61 mg/dl)
	Current study	
Recipients	12-566 ml^{-3} (102 ml^{-3})	24-93 mg/dl (55 mg/dl)

[a]Treated recipients during the current study.

[b]The ranges of maximum elevation for individual patients are shown with means of maximum elevation in parentheses.

[c]Recipients and controls after crossover treatment in the preliminary study.

observed in the previous LP (see Sec. II). The CSF cell counts had returned to normal in all the recipients by 1 year following their first IFN-β injections, but the CSF protein remained slightly elevated (mean 46 mg/dl) in seven. A similar decrease in cell counts and CSF protein levels was observed in the controls during successive treatments, but LP were not repeated at 1 year following crossover as had been done in the recipients.

We detected IFN in the CSF (23–52 IRU/ml) of two control patients at the time of their first LP (i.e., before exogenous IFN-β was administered). None of the other patients (recipients or controls) had IFN detected in their CSF prior to treatment. However, 12 patients had detectable levels of IFN in their CSF (3–176 IRU/ml) during the first month of treatment. None of the patients had recordable levels of IFN in the CSF after the first month of treatment. Only one recipient had detectable IFN in the serum concomitant with a recordable level in the CSF. IFN was detected in the CSF of three of eight patients whose conditions improved, all six patients whose conditions were unchanged, and three of six patients whose conditions worsened (9,10).

B. Current Ongoing Study

The final results of this study will not be known until July 1986. However, certain observations have been made to date without endangering its double-blinded status. The randomization process (biased coin and exacerbation rates of less or greater than 2 per year) yielded a recipient and control group that are homogenous (sex, duration of illness, severity of disease, and exacerbation rates). The study was designed to include 80 patients, but only 76 were ultimately randomized into it (difficulty with accession at one center). The double-blinded method has been successful. Administration of small doses of indomethacin has reduced the toxic side effects of IT administered IFN-β to the point that there is no significant difference in the symptoms following treatments in the IFN-β recipients and controls (Table 4). The CSF changes observed in the current study are less severe than in the preliminary study (Table 3). The mean level of maximum

Table 4 Clinical Toxic Side Effects of Treatment in the Current Double-Blinded Study (76 MS Patients)[a]

Toxicity	Recipients		Controls	
	Mean	SD	Mean	SD
Headache	1.65	0.69	1.42	0.78
Nausea and vomiting	0.76	0.74	0.51	0.74
Myalgia	0.88	0.69	0.74	0.78
Lethargy	1.15	0.74	1.00	0.73

[a]Recipients received true LP with IFN-β injected. Controls received false LP with sterile water injected into subcutaneous tissues. Recipients received oral indomethacin for 24 hr after treatments. Controls received placebo indomethacin capsules after treatments. There is no significant difference in the clinical side effects of the two groups.

pleocytosis for individual recipients (102 ml^{-3}) was reduced by 80% compared with that of the preliminary study's original recipients and 31% that of the original controls during crossover treatment. The mean level of maximum elevation of CSF protein for individual recipients (55 mg/dl) is 10–28% less than that observed during treatment in the preliminary study.

IV. DISCUSSION

Continued observation of the patients included in the preliminary study shows a persisting beneficial effect of IT administered IFN-β. The original recipients have experienced a decrease in their exacerbation rate that has become progressively more significant during more than 5 years' follow-up following treatment. The prestudy rate of 1.8 per year that had been reduced to 0.28 per year (p < 0.01) after they had been on the study for a mean of 2.4 years (June 30, 1982) (10) has continued to decrease to 0.2 per year (p < 0.001) as of June 30, 1985, after a mean of 5.3 years of follow-up since the first IFN-β injections. Moreover, the control group also seems to be making a favorable response to the IFN-β treatment. The prestudy rate of 0.68 per year had not changed after they had been followed for a mean of 2.1 years without receiving IFN-β treatment (10). However, the prestudy rate has decreased to 0.36 per year (p < 0.03) during a mean of 2.9 years since the crossover (June 30, 1982) when they began receiving the IT IFN-β treatment.

With but rare exceptions, the treatment phase lasted only 6 months. Two patients were retreated for acute exacerbations 11 and 19 months after they had completed the initial 6 month treatment phase. Both those patients received only single injections of IFN-β in attempts to ameliorate their exacerbations. They have been briefly reported elsewhere (10); their responses to the single injections is the subject of a future report on IT IFN-β treatment of acute exacerbations of MS. In the other patients the beneficial long-term effect of IT IFN-β in reducing exacerbations occurred after a relatively intensive treatment period followed by a relatively long period of time (approximately 4.8 years in original recipients as of June 30, 1985) during which benefit persists without retreatment. However, it is impossible to predict the future courses of these patients, and it may be necessary to subject at least some of them to relatively intensive treatment phases again in the future.

Although the exacerbation rates of MS patients may decrease over time as a natural "burnout" phenomenon, the decreases in rates that we observed (89% in recipients and 47% in controls after crossover) are far in excess of the 15–16% decreases that might be expected to occur as a natural phenomenon (15). How IFN-β administered IT may have exerted a beneficial effect in these patients is unknown. The mechanisms of the actions of IFN are complex and incompletely understood (4,5). It is possible that IFN-β compensated for decreased IFN responsivity of certain immune competent cells of MS patients (5). It may also have normalized impaired suppressor cell activity of MS patients during exacerbation (5). Other possibilities include IFN induction of viral persistence or alteration of abnormal (viral) surface markers on central nervous system target cells to produce its prophylactic effect (2,5). It is known that IFN injected IT does not pool in the lumbar sac but flows upward over the cerebral convexities and presumably comes into direct contact with brain parenchyma (16). Although the mechanisms of its actions are subject to speculation, three studies demonstrate that IFN-β acts in a prophylactic and suppressant fashion on the expression of experimental allergic encephalomyelitis (EAE) in mice (17-19). The IFN-β was more effective and exerted the effects at lower doses when administered intraventricularly than when administered systemically (19).

The toxic side effects experienced by the patients in the preliminary study seemed acceptable for the benefits achieved (8,9). Slight modifications of the administration schedule and total dosage of IFN-β administered at the time of each LP resulted in less pleocytosis and CSF protein elevation experienced by the controls during crossover treatment than by the original recipients during their treatment phase (10). Further reduction of the LP with IFN-β administered from 13 in the preliminary study of 9 in the current study has even further reduced the pleocytosis and CSF protein elevations of patients undergoing IT IFN-β treatment. It should be emphasized that there has been no observable correlation between the CSF changes and clinical toxic side effects observed in any of the patients during IT IFN-β treatment in the preliminary or the currently ongoing study.

That systemically administered IFN does not effectively cross the blood-brain barrier (5,8-10) has prompted several recent studies in which IFN was administered directly into the CSF of patients with CNS diseases (14,20,21). In some of those studies the dosage of IFN administered was higher, the frequency of administration greater, and the duration of treatment longer than in our preliminary or current studies. However, the toxic side effects observed in those studies were similar to our own. The relative consistency with which certain clinical side effects occur when IFN is administered have made adequate double blinding of clinical trials with IFN (systemic or IT) impossible. Benign placebos do not mimick the side effects of IFN (e.g., fever, headache, and myalgia), and most patients soon realize whether they are receiving IFN or placebo simply because of the presence or absence of these side effects. However, it has been discovered that the toxic side effects of IFN (α or β) administered IT may be greatly reduced by the administration of small doses of indomethacin for short periods of time after each IFN treatment (14). This effect may be due, in part, to the inhibition by indomethacin of prostaglandin E_2 synthesis. The incorporation of indomethacin administration (25–50 mg orally every 6 hr for 24 hr) at the time of each treatment into the protocol of our currently ongoing multicenter study has resulted in true double blinding of that study. The indomethacin has so masked the clinical toxicity of IT IFN-β that recipients cannot be differentiated from controls on the basis of toxic side effects experienced. The indomethacin administered may also have played a role in reducing to level of pleocytosis and CSF protein elevation observed in the current study.

The findings of the original preliminary study warranted a larger, more definitive study (11). That study has been designed and conducted to date in such a fashion that it will correct certain shortcomings of the preliminary study and definitively determine whether IFN-β administered IT reduces the exacerbations of MS. The study has the following features: (1) includes approximately four times as many patients as the preliminary study, (2) includes only patients with exacerbating-remitting disease, (3) is conducted at three different clinical centers and a separate statistics center, (4) has separate "treating" and "examining" physicians at each clinical center, and (5) has been successfully double blinded. The results of this study will not be known until July 1986. However, certain interim analyses (that have not endangered the double blinding) have shown that the recipients and controls are homogeneous in all important pretreatment clinical parameters, the posttreatment clinical symptoms and signs have been similar in the two groups, and the CSF changes following treatment have been substantially reduced (compared with the preliminary study) (10) by modifications of treatment schedule and dosage and possibly by administration of indomethacin.

Early studies indicated that systemically administered IFN was of no benefit in MS patients (possibly owing to the failure of IFN to cross the BBB) (6,7). However, a recent study reported a reduction in the exacerbations of MS patients with strictly exacerbation-remitting disease while they were receiving daily intramuscular injections of IFN-α (22). The benefit observed may have resulted from passage of IFN-α from systemic circulation into the CNS through a partial breakdown of the BBB that may occur in MS patients (23) or the systemic immunoenhancing effects of IFN (4,5). It will be extremely important to determine if those patients experience long-term prophylaxis against repeated exacerbations as has been observed in the patients in our preliminary study after IT administration of IFN-β. A subsequent study using lower doses of IFN-α (2×10^6 IRU) administered subcutaneously daily for 12 months showed no benefit of treatment for reducing exacerbation rates, so the effects of systemic treatment may be strongly dose related (24).

The presence of IFN in the CSF but not sera prior to the administration of exogenous IFN-β in 10% of the patients in the preliminary study suggests de novo synthesis of IFN by the CNS in response to the MS disease process (10). In 1968, Sibley and Tourtellotte reported finding IFN activity in 19% of fresh-frozen MS brain specimens (25). It has been suggested that de novo CNS production of IFN may oscillate during the course of MS and play a role in the exacerbation remission cycle (5). Serum and CSF specimens have been obtained for interferon determinations in the current ongoing study, but the results of the assays will not be known until July 1986.

V. ADDENDUM

Subsequent to the original submission of this chapter, the results of the double-blinded, multicenter study have been analyzed and published (26,27). Initially, 76 patients with strictly exacerbating-remitting disease were randomized to the study, but only 69 patients (34 IFN-β recipients and 35 controls) were evaluable at the end of the study (7 either withdrew or were involved in protocol violations). Figure 3 shows the exacerbation rates before and during the study for the IFN-β recipients (interferon) and the

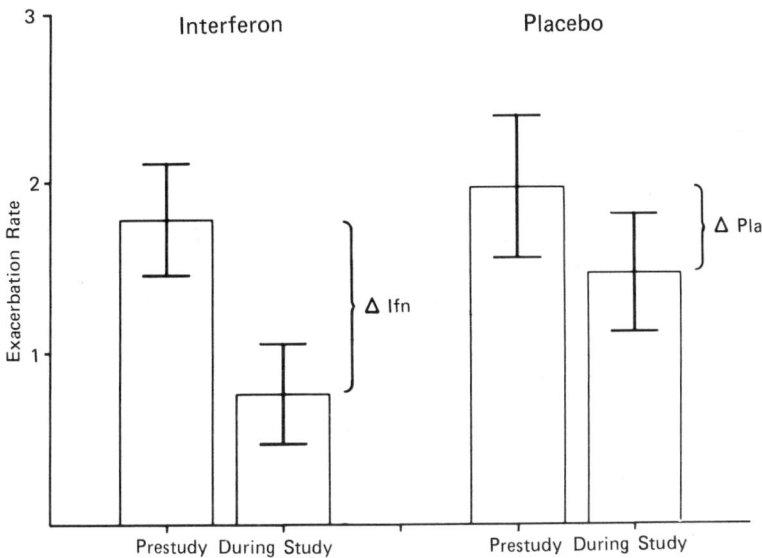

Figure 3 Mean exacerbation rates (exacerbations per year) before and during the study in 34 recipients and 35 controls. Vertical bars: 2 SEM; Δ: change (decreases) in rates observed during study.

controls (placebo). The prestudy exacerbation rates were basically the same in the two groups (means: recipients 1.79, controls 1.98 per year), but the recipient rate during the study (mean 0.76 per year) was significantly lower than that of the controls (mean 1.48 per year) ($p < 0.001$). The rates of both groups decreased during the study, but the change in rate was significantly greater in the recipients than in the controls ($p < 0.04$). The greater reduction in rates in recipients compared with controls was consistently observed at all three of the participating centers.

Clinically, 76.5% of the recipients and 60% of the controls were improved or unchanged and 23.5% of the recipients and 40% of the controls were worse at the end of the study, but this trend for recipients to be improved and controls to be worse did not reach statistical significance ($p = 0.23$). Also, the extent of deterioration was greatest in controls (mean modified Kurtzke score increases:

controls 0.80, recipients 0.32), but this trend was not statistically significant (p = 0.32).

The clinical side effects of treatment (e.g., headache and myalgia) occurred with similar frequency in both groups, except for low-grade fevers, which occurred in more recipients (75%) than controls (31%) (p < 0.001). However, this occurrence did not break the double blinding; questionnaires completed by the patients and examining physicians during the study confirmed that both groups were blinded (examining physician, p = 0.66; patients, p = 0.07). Pleocytosis and CSF protein elevations occurring during treatment in the recipients were temporary, less severe than in the preliminary study (possibly owing to fewer LP with IFN-β injected and the use of indomethacin in the current study) and seemed to generally be unrelated to clinical side effects observed.

Thus, the findings of this study confirmed those of the preliminary study and definitively demonstrated that intrathecally administered IFN-β is effective in exacerbating-remitting MS. It will be important to continue our follow-up of the patients in this study to determine if they obtain a long-term prophylactic effect against exacerbations as did those in the preliminary study. It should also be emphasized that our treatment schedule may not be optimum and that fewer treatments with even lower doses of IFN-β administered intrathecally may provide a similar degree of prophylaxis as observed in this study. It is also possible that systemic interferon therapy may be effective in MS. Recently, Smith et al. (28) identified the interferon-specific C-56 inducible protein in the brains of monkeys following intravenous as well as intrathecal administration of natural IFN-α. This finding demonstrates that interferon administered intravenously (as well as intrathecally) acts directly on brain cells despite low or nonrecordable CSF titers after systemic administration.

ACKNOWLEDGMENTS

Supported by grants from the Baird Foundation, the James H. Cummings Foundation, the Dent Foundation, the Bernard Hoffman Foundation, the Josephine Goodyear Foundation, the Margaret L. Wendt Foundation, the Samuel and Sarah Slepian

Family Foundation, the Losasso Family, the Delaware North Companies, and Grant R01NS19649-01 from the National Institutes of Health.

REFERENCES

1. Cook, D., and Dowling, P. C. Multiple sclerosis and viruses: An overview. *Neurology (N.Y.)* 20:80–91 (1980).

2. Johnson, R. T., Lazzarini, R. A., and Waksman, B. H. Mechanisms of virus persistence. *Ann. Neurol.* 9:616–617 (1981).

3. Hallpike, J. F., Adams, C. W. M., and Tourtellotte, W. W. (eds.). *Multiple Sclerosis.* Williams & Wilkins, Baltimore, 1983, pp. 241–274, 379–412.

4. Stewart, W. E., II. *The Interferon System.* Springer-Verlag, New York, 1979.

5. Salazar, A. M., Gibbs, C. J., Gajudsek, D. C., et al. Clinical use of interferons: Central nervous system disorders. In: *Handbook of Experimental Pharmacology* P. Came and W. A. Carter, Springer-Berlag, Berlin, 1983, Vol. 71, pp. 472–497.

6. Fog, T. Interferon treatment of multiple sclerosis patients: A pilot study. In: *Search for the Cause of Multiple Sclerosis and Other Chronic Diseases of the Nervous System* (A. Boese, ed.). Verlag Chemie, Weinheim, 1980, p. 490.

7. Ververken, H., Carton, H., Billiau, A., et al. Intrathecal administration of interferon in MS patients? In: *Humoral Immunity in Neurological Diseases.* S. Kazrcher, A. Lowenthal, and A. Strosberg, Plenum Press, New York, 1979, p. 625.

8. Jacobs, L., O'Malley, J., Freeman, A., et al. Intrathecal interferon reduces exacerbations of multiple sclerosis. *Science* 214:1026–1028 (1981).

9. Jacobs, L., O'Malley, J., Freeman, A., et al. Intrathecal interferon in multiple sclerosis. *Arch. Neurol.* 39:609–615 (1982).

10. Jacobs, L., O'Malley, J. A., Freeman, A., et al. Intrathecal interferon in the treatment of multiple sclerosis: Patient follow-up. *Arch. Neurol.* 42: 841–847 (1985).

11. Jacobs, L., O'Malley, J. A., and Freeman, A. Intrathecal interferon as

treatment of multiple sclerosis: A planned multicenter study. *Arch. Neurol. 40*:683-686 (1983).

12. Rose, A. S., Kusma, J. W., Kurtzke, J. R., et al. Cooperative study in the evolution of therapy in multiple sclerosis: ACTH vs. placebo in acute exacerbations, preliminary report. *Neurology (N.Y.) 18*:1-10 (1969).

13. Brown, J. R., Beebe, G. W., Kurtzke, J. R., et al. The design of clinical studies to assess therapeutic efficacy in multiple sclerosis. *Neurology (N.Y.) 29*:3-23 (1979).

14. Mora, J. S., Kao, K. P., and Munsat, T. L. Indomethacin reduces the side effects of intrathecal interferon. *N. Engl. J. Med. 310*:126-127 (1984).

15. McAlpine, D., Lumsden, C. E., and Acheson, E. D. *Multiple Sclerosis: A Reappraisal.* Williams & Wilkins, Baltimore, 1972, p. 205.

16. Billiau, A. Interferon therapy: Pharmacokinetic and pharmacological aspects. *Arch. Virol. 67*:121-123 (1981).

17. Abreu, S. L. Suppression of experimental allergic encephalomyelitis by interferon. *Immunol. Commun. 11*:1-7 (1982).

18. Abreu, S. L., Tondreau, J., Levine, S., et al. Inhibition of passive localized allergic encephalomyelitis by interferon. *Int. Arch. Allergy Appl. Immunol. 72*:30-33 (1983).

19. Hertz, F., and Deghenghi, R. Effect of rat and beta human interferon on hyperacute experimental allergic enceophalomyelitis in rats. *Agents Actions 16*:397-403 (1985).

20. Slatkin, N. E., Jaeckle, K. A., Lukes, S. A., et al. Treatment of leptomeningeal gliomatosis with human leukocyte interferon: Results in two patients. *Neurology (N.Y.) 34* (Suppl. 1):151 (1984).

21. Obbens, E. A. M. T., Feum, L. G., Leavens, M. E., et al. Interferon in the treatment of intracranial malignancies: A pilot study. *Neurology (N.Y.) 34* (Suppl. 1):232 (1984).

22. Knobler, R. L., Panitch, H. S., Braheny, S. L., et al. Systemic alpha-interferon therapy of multiple sclerosis. *Neurology (N.Y.) 34*:1273-1279 (1984).

23. Aita, J. F., Bennett, D. R., Anderson, R. E., et al. Cranial CT appearance of acute multiple sclerosis. *Neurology (N.Y.) 28*:251-255 (1978).

24. Kleiner, J. R., Crisp, D. T., Alter, M., et al. Alpha-2 interferon in remitting-relapsing multiple sclerosis. *Am. Coll. Clin. Pharm.* 1986 (In press).

25. Sibley, W. A., and Tourtellotte, W. W. Interferon assay of multiple sclerosis tissue. *Trans. Am. Neurol. Assoc. 93*:124–127 (1968).

26. Jacobs, L., Salazar, A. M., Herndon, R., Reese, P. A., et al. Multicenter double-blind study of effect of intrathecally administered natural human fibroblast interferon on exacerbations of multiple sclerosis. *Lancet, 2*: 1411–1413 (1986).

27. Jacobs, L., Salazar, A. M., Herndon, R., Reese, P. A., et al. Intrathecally administered natural human fibroblast interferon reduces exacerbations of multiple sclerosis: Results of a multicenter, double-blinded study. *Arch. Neurol. 44*:589–595 (1987).

28. Smith, R. A., Landel, C., Cornelius, C. E., et al. Mapping the action of interferon on the primate brain. *J. Interferon Res 6* (Suppl. 1):140 (1986).

11
Treatment of Amyotrophic Lateral Sclerosis with Interferon

RICHARD ALAN SMITH

Center for Neurologic Study, San Diego, California

FORBES H. NORRIS

ALS Research Center, Pacific Presbyterian Medical Center, San Francisco, California

I. INTRODUCTION

The use of interferon for the treatment of amyotrophic lateral sclerosis is predicated on the belief that ALS has a viral etiology (1). This was commented upon by Charcot, who provided the initial clinical description of ALS (2). He noted the clinical similarity between ALS and poliomyelitis and speculated that both diseases might be caused by the same agent. Similarities between the diseases are striking. Asymmetric paralyisis is the hallmark of polio. In the case of ALS a similar distribution of weakness is present early in the course of the disease. The eye musculature, bladder, and bowel are spared in both maladies, as for the most part is the sensory system. In addition to sharing clinical similarities, it has long been noted that patients who have suffered from childhood polio may go on to develop motor neuron disease (3). Poskanzer et al. (4) have reported that the incidence of motor neuron disease in polio survivors is higher than that of the general population, although this has not been observed by others (5).

II. VIRAL STUDIES

The idea that conventional viruses may be the cause of chronic neurologic diseases has been firmly established for both humans and other animals (6). Measles and rubeola virus have been shown to cause chronic encephalitidies. In the case of subacute sclerosing panencephalitis (SSPE), a childhood disease, symptoms typically occur 5-10 years following primary infection. In debilitated patients, JC virus, a member of the papovavirus family, causes progressive multifocal leukoencephalopathy (PML), which shares similarities with multiple sclerosis (MS). In children with combined immune deficiency, polio has been isolated from the brain in patients dying from ill-defined neurologic disorders (7). These cases have not been characterized by affliction of the motor system, as in paralytic polio or ALS.

In sheep a retrovirus is responsible for visna, and in mice a murine picornavirus (Theiler's) is the cause of a demyelinating disorder (8). In the Theiler's model, a naturally occurring viral infection, animals develop a polioencephalitis from which virus can readily be recovered from infected animals. Survivors, however, develop a late-onset neurologic disorder, in which the infected cells contain many copies of the viral genome but little viral protein. It is possible, however, to detect virus using molecular biologic rechniques. Surprisingly, Lansing strain poliovirus can also persist after intracranial injection in mice (9). Virus can be found in asymptomatic animals for months without an apparent immune response.

To pursue a possible viral etiology for ALS, Cremer et al. established tissue cultures from postmorten tissues (10). These were treated in a variety of ways in an effort to establish the presence of virus; none was found. In transmission studies, Gibbs and Gadjusek inoculated subhuman primates intracranially with homogenates of ALS brain and spinal cord (11). No animal became neurologically ill. Some reviewers have concluded these results exclude a viral etilogy for ALS. However, a number of explanations may account for the failure to detect or isolate a virus from infected tissues. A mutant virus may be incapable of replicating outside the CNS, or the virus may be inactivated by antibody or as a result of binding to brain receptor sites. Based on the rationale that viral nucleic acid must be present in viral infection, Kohne and his colleagues screened ALS and control tissues for the presence of polio genome using nucleic acid hybridization (12). The method employs the use of a DNA probe that hybridizes with homologous RNA. Unexpectedly, they found evidence for the presence of polio in the brain of a patient dying from a nonneurologic cause. These observations were extended by Brahic et al., who also found poliolike RNA in the nervous system of a "control case" as well as in a patient dying of amyotrophic lateral sclerosis (see Fig. 1) (13). Using reconstruction experiments, it was found that 30 copies of viral RNA per cell could be detected with this method. As in the earlier study, polio genome was detected in a control case, but in addition 1 of 14 cases of classic ALS were positive for virus.

Although these findings support the notion that picornaviruses may persist in the human nervous system, their significance remains a matter of speculation, in part because recent data suggests that ribosomal RNA may contain sequences that are homologous to viral genomes, including polio (14). The presence of such sequences could result in a false-positive hybridization signal.

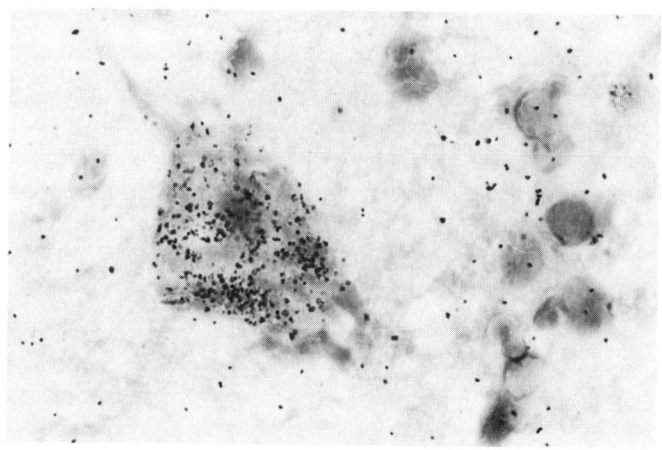

Figure 1 In situ hybridization on frozen sections of spinal cord from a patient with ALS. Sections were hybridized with poliovirus type I [^{3}H]rDNA. Exposure time was 4 weeks. A large neuron in the ventral horn contains RNA sequences that hybridized to the polio cDNA probe.

In no instance, however, has polio been detected in patients with the postpolio syndrome (12,15). However, Dalakas et al. did note signs of viral infection in a group of postpolio patients who exhibited progressive muscular weakness (16). In some patients (7 of 13), oligoclonal IgG bands were noted in the spinal fluid, and some patients had abnormalities of T-cell subsets. One patient had polio antibody in the cerebrospinal fluid (CSF) (normal = 0).

Bartfeldt and colleagues undertook an exhaustive study of the immune status of ALS patients (17). Peripheral blood T- and B-cell counts were normal, as were T-cell suppressor activity, serum immunoglobulins, and immune complexes. Although cellular immunity in ALS patients was normal as judged by skin tests, in vitro immune responses to polio antigens were abnormal. The mean leukocyte migration inhibition factor test (LMIF) response of 38 patients was significantly greater than that of neurologic controls. No difference was noted for adeno-associated virus, measles, or Coxsackie A9. These findings, similar to those reported by Kott et al., suggest ALS patients are sensitized to poliovirus or a related virus, although there was no immunologic evidence for an active polio infection; that is, there was no elevation of humoral antibodies to polio 918).

Looking for indirect evidence of infection, Sibley assayed the spinal cord from two patients dying of ALS for the presence of interferon (19). None was found. Induction of immune interferon in lymphocytes from ALS patients was found to be normal in studies in vitro (17).

Although evidence for a viral etiology for ALS is circumstantial, a number of investigators have treated ALS experimentally with interferon or interferon inducers. Since interferon does not readily cross the blood-brain barrier, the route of administration could have an effect on the outcome.

III. TREATMENT TRIALS

Olsen et al. employed the interferon inducer tilorone (1 g/week) in a double-blind, placebo-controlled trial of 16 ALS patients (20). There was no discernible benefit after 4 months of therapy. Using poly ICLC (another interferon inducer), Engel and Levy treated several patients without success (21). In 1980,

Rissanen et al. reported lack of therapeutic effect with interferon-a after the treatment of two patients with a daily systemic dose of 3×10^6 international units (IU) per day for up to 3 months (22). In a similar study using recombinant interferon-a, Dalakas et al. treated seven patients three times per week with 2×10^6 IU administered subcutaneously (23). Progress was monitored monthly using a modified Norris scale and a scale generated by the clinical examination. At the end of the 4 month treatment period all the patients had worsened. Interferon was not detected in the CSF of any patient 3-24 hr after treatment.

Because systemically administered interferon does not readily cross the blood-brain barrier (24) and interferon inducers are rather unpredictable in their effect (25), a number of workers have employed novel treatment strategies in an effort to ensure the delivery of interferon to the nervous system. Either a high systemic dose has been utilized or the drug has been delivered intrathecally or intraventricularly. In Finland, 10 patients were treated with up to 200×10^6 IU of interferon-a via intravenous infusion for 6 days (26). Hand strength was monitored using a dynamometer. Grip improved in 6 of 10 patients for up to 9 months following treatment. No other measurements were recorded. Treatment was complicated by evidence of neurotoxicity. Some patients became confused or hallucinated or exhibited other worrisome side effects. Fortunately, neurotoxic effects were reversible.

Using the intrathecal route of administration, Mora et al. (27) treated 10 patients weekly for up to 6 months. Of the 10, 6 patients completed the trial. The status of each patient was serially monitored using a sophisticated battery of tests that quantitate neuromuscular function. The slope of deterioration for each function was determined during a treatment and control period. Treatment did not appear to modify the course of the disease. Following intrathecal injections, CSF lymphocytosis was noted (up to 50 cells mm^{-3}) and there was a modest elevation of CSF protein, but no patient developed clinical signs of meningeal irritation.

IV. METHODOLOGY

Because the route of administration was likely to be an important treatment variable, we chose to treat patients with intraventricular administration of interferon in the belief that this may offer the best chance for success. Extrapolating from in vitro studies, there was reason to believe the drug would have to be given at intervals of at least 72 hr to exert a sustained antiviral effect (28). Since animal studies demonstrated that interferons are not notably effective in the case of chronic viral infections, it seemed likely that therapy would have to be continued for a long time (29). Compartmental therapy seemed advantageous, since in the case of intraventricular administration it is certain that the drug has been introduced into the cerebrospinal fluid and that it will then circulate freely throughout the CSF pathway (30). After determining that intraventricular administration of interferon-α was well tolerated in rhesus monkeys, preliminary pharmacokinetic data were obtained in ALS patients bearing Ommaya reservoirs. As reviewed in Chapter 4, it was observed that systemically administered interferon did not readily cross the blood-brain barrier (31). No interferon was seen in the spinal fluid of any of five patients after injections of 18×10^6 IU of IFN-Ra (Roferon) in spite of achieving high serum peaks. After administering 50 million units (mu) of Roferon, the highest CSF titer was 72 pg/ml in one patient. Faced with this result, we turned our attention to study of the pharmacokinetic behavior of intraventricularly administered interferon. Administering as little as 2.5×10^5 IU of partially purified interferon (PIF), we could achieve high CSF titers of interferon (30). As expected, the interferon washed out of the ventricles over 12 hr. It could be detected in the lumbar CSF at 24 hr, demonstrating that intraventricularly injected drug circulated widely throughout the CSF pathway. Since we could not justify intraventricular administration of a placebo or the treatment of a large number of patients, it was decided to conduct an open (uncontrolled) study with a small number of patients. This approach precluded detection of a modest treatment effect, but a change in the course of the disease would probably have been noted since the patients were followed for long periods (up to 36 months). In general, most ALS patients deteriorate in a linear fashion over time. Consequently, it was assumed that we could recognize a "cure" for ALS, but something less than this would be missed. Tyler, commenting on ALS treatment trials, endorsed this treatment strategy: "pick out five patients and treat them for 1½ years; if you had a cure for this disease, you would not need any other trials" (32).

V. RESULTS

At the outset we treated four ALS patients with 2.5×10^5 IU of PIF at weekly intervals for up to 6 months. This was well tolerated after an initial period of adaptation, during which time patients experienced "flulike" symptoms: fever, malaise, and so on. (see Table 1). At periodic intervals, the neuromuscular status of each patient was scored using a modification of the MRC rating system in which individual muscles are graded for strength on a scale of 1-5. No apparent clinical benefit was noted in the initial patients, who continued to deteriorate. Having demonstrated that therapy was well tolerated, the next step was to determine the maximum dose and frequency of administration that could be administered. Accordingly, our protocol was modified so that patients who were subsequently enrolled in the study were treated at once a week intervals for 4 weeks and thereafter at more frequent intervals. Ultimately, it was established that patients could

Table 1 Side Effects Secondary to Intraventricular Injection of 2.5×10^5 IU Leukocyte Interferon

Symptoms	Hours after injection	Range hr/experiment
Headache	4-16	0-12
Fever	3-24	8-16
Chills	3-11	3-5
Fatigue	1-23	2-21
Anorexia	1-6	0-6
Nausea	6-8	0-2
Vomiting	6	0-1
Joint pain	5-6	0-3
Muscle pain	—	0

tolerate 2.5×10^5 IU indefinitely if it was administered at 72 hr intervals. Treatment was administered to three patients for up to 4 months. At this dose, minimal changes were seen in the ventricular CSF (Table 2). A low-grade pleocytosis was common, and CSF protein fluctuated within a narrow range. Patients did well except for noting mild anorexia and fatigue. When one patient was given larger doses, he developed a neurogenic bladder associated with lower extremity numbness. Lumbar CSF protein was mildly elevated (61 mg/dl), whereas ventricular CSF protein was normal (19 mg/dl). On pathologic examination approximately 2 years following treatment, "mild, focal lymphocyte accumulation was seen in the arachnoidea in the lumbar spine along with a single focus of perivascular cuffing by lymphocytes in the cervical cord."

Monitoring the neuromuscular status of each patient, we could demonstrate no convincing effect on the course of the disease (see Fig. 2).

VI. CONCLUSIONS

None of the ALS interferon trials conducted to date would have detected subtle differences in outcomes. A number of understandable factors have prevented researchers from conducting large-scale, double-blind, placebo-controlled trials of ALS with

Table 2 CSF Chemistry During Treatment with Intraventricular Interferon

Patient	Duration of therapy (weeks)	Ventricular	
		WBC (per mm^3)	Protein (mg/ml)
A	13	0–28	10–19
B	14	3–4	4–6
C	17	1–40	10–31

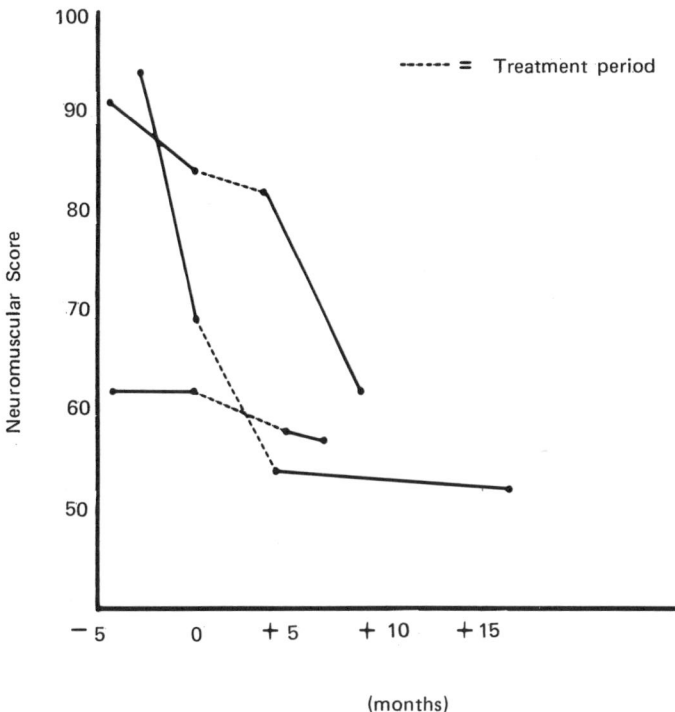

Figure 2 The course of ALS patients treated with intraventricular interferon. The neuromuscular score was determined serially by manual testing of 20 muscles.

interferons. Studies done to date, however, do permit one to conclude that interferon-a does not "cure" ALS. Since all the trials reported to date have employed interferon-a, it is possible that another interferon, alone or in combination, may prove to be an effective therapy for ALS. Considering the lack of any known therapy, it seems reasonable to pursue treatment trials with antiviral drugs, including other interferons.

ACKNOWLEDGMENTS

This work is dedicated to patients Rosalie Mills, Charles Bordner, and Fred Clark, who gave their utmost to participate in these studies. ALS research at the Center for Neurologic Study has been made possible through the generous support of Frances and John Stockton, the James Waldal Fund, and the Thagard Foundation.

REFERENCES

1. Kascsak, R. J., Carp, R. I., Vilcek, J. T., Donnenfeld, H., and Bartfeld, H. Virological studies in amyotrophic lateral sclerosis. *Muscle Nerve* 5:93-101 (1982).

2. Charcot, J. M. Observation communiquée en 1875 à la Société de Biologie par M. Raymond. *Gaz. Méd. Fr.* 225 (1875).

3. Campbell, A. M. G., Williams, E. R., and Pearce, J. Late motor neuron degeneration following poliomyelitis. *Neurology (N.Y.)* 19:1101-1106 (1969).

4. Poskanzer, D., Cantor, H., and Kaplan, G. The frequency of preceding poliomyelitis in amyotrophic lateral sclerosis. In: *Motor Neuron Diseases* (F. Norris and L. Kurland, eds.). Grune and Stratton, New York, 1969, pp. 286-289.

5. Juergens, S. M., Kurland, L. T., Okazaki, P. H. H., and Mulder, D. W. ALS in Rochester, Minnesota, 1925-1977. 30(5):463-470 (1980).

6. Gilden, D. H. Slow virus diseases of the CNS. *Postgrad. Med.* 73(1): 99-106 (1983).

7. Johnson, R. T. Late progression of poliomyelitis paralysis: Discussion of pathogenesis. *Rev. Infect. Dis.* 6:5568-5570 (1984).

8. Lipton, H. L. Theiler's virus infection in mice: An unusal biphasic disease process leading to demyelination. *Infect. Immun.* 11:1147-1155 (1975).

9. Miller, J. R. Prolonged intracerebral infection with poliovirus in asymptomatic mice. *Ann. Neurol.* 9:59-596 (1981).

10. Cremer, N. E., Oshiro, L. S., Norris, H., and Lennette, E. H. Cultures of tissues from patients with amyotrophic lateral sclerosis. *Neurology (N.Y.)* 29:331-333 (1973).

11. Gibbs, Jr., C. J., and Gajdusek, D. C. Amyotrophic lateral sclerosis, Parkinson's disease, and the amyotrophic lateral sclerosis-parkinsonism-dementia complex on Guam: A review and summary of attempts to demonstrate infection as the etiology. *Br. Med. Assoc.* 132-140, 1971.

12. Kohne, D. E., Gibbs, C. J., White, L., Tracy, S. M., Meinke, W., and Smith, R. A. Virus detection by nucleic acid hybridization: Examination of normal and ALS tissues for the presence of poliovirus. *J. Gen. Virol.* 56:223-233 (1981).

13. Brahic, M. D., Smith, R. A., Gibbs, Jr., C. J., Garruto, R. M., Tourtellotte, W. W., and Cash, E. Detection of picornavirus sequences in nervous tissue of amyotrophic lateral sclerosis and control patients. *Ann. Neurol.* 18(3):337-343 (1985).

14. McClure, M. A., and Perrault, J. Poliovirus genome RNA hybridizes specifically to higher eukaryotic rRNAs. *Nucleic Acids Res.* 13(19): 6797-6897 (1985).

15. Viola, M. V., Myers, J. C., Gann, K. L., Gibbs, Jr., J. C., and Roos, R. P. Failure to detect poliovirus genetic information in amyotrophic lateral sclerosis. *Ann. Neurol.* 5(4):402-403 (1979).

16. Dalakas, M. C., Sever, J. L., Madden, D. L., Papadopoulos, N. M., Shekarchi, I. C., Albrecht, P., and Krezlewicz, A. Late postpoliomyelitis muscular atrophy: Clinical, virologic, and immunologic studies. *Rev. Infect. Dis.* 6(2):S562-S567 (1984).

17. Bartfeld, H., Dham, C., Donnenfeld, H., Jashnani, L., Carp, R., Kascsak, R., Vilcek, J., Rapport, M., and Wallenstein, S. Immunological profile of amyotrophic lateral sclerosis patients and their cell-mediated immune responses to viral and CNS antigens. *Clin. Exp. Immunol.* 48:137-147 (1982).

18. Kott, E., Livni, E., and Zamir, R. Cell-mediated immunity to polio and HLA antigens in amyotrophic lateral sclerosis. *Neurology (N.Y.)* 29:1040 (1979).

19. Johnson, R. T. Virologic studies and summary of Soviet experiments on the transmission of ALS to monkeys in motor neuron diseases. In: (F. H. Norris and L. T. Kurland, eds.). Grune and Stratton, New York, 1969.

20. Olson, W. H., Simons, J. A., and Halaass, G. W. Therapeutic trial of tilorone in ALS: Lack of benefit in a double-blind, placebo-controlled study. *Neurology (N.Y.)* 18:1293-1295 (1978).

21. Salazar, A. M., Gibbs, Jr., C. J., Gajdusek, D. C., and Smith, R. A. Clinical use of interferons: Central nervous system disorders. In: *The Handbook of Experimental Pharmacology* Vol. 71. 1984, pp. 472-497.

22. Rissanen, A., Palo, J., Myllyla, G., and Cantell, K. Interferon therapy for ALS. *Ann. Neurol.* 7(4):392 (1980).

23. Dalakas, M. C., Aksamit, A. J., Madden, D. L., and Sever, J. L. Administration of recombinant human leukocyte $_2$-interferon in patients with amyotrophic lateral sclerosis. *Arch. Neurol. 43*:933-935 (1986).

24. Habif, D. V., Lipton, R., and Cantell, K. Interferon crosses the blood-cerebrospinal fluid barrier in monkeys. *Proc. Soc. Exp. Biol. Med. 149*: 287-289 (1975).

25. Guggenheim, M. A., and Baron, S. Clinical studies of an interferon inducer, polyriboinosinic-polyribocytidylic acid [poly (I)·poly (C)], in children. *J. Infect. Dis. 136*:50-58 (1977).

26. Farkkila, M. A., Iivanaien, M. V., Roine, R. O., and Cantell, K. Effect of interferon on the course of amyotrophic lateral sclerosis. *ALS Rev. 5*(2): 38 (1986).

27. Mora, J. S., Munsat, T. L., Kao, K.-P., Finison, L. J., Hedlund, W., Bradley, G. A., Scheife, R., and Georgiades, J. A. Intrathecal administration of natural human interferon alpha in amyotrophic lateral sclerosis. *Neurology (N.Y.) 36*:1137-1140 (1986).

28. Lab, M., and Koehren, F. Maintenance and recovery of the interferon-induced antiviral state. *Proc. Soc. Exp. Biol. Med. 153*:112-118 (1976).

29. Hilfenhaus, J., Weinmann, E., Majer, Barth, R., and Jaeger, O. Administration of human interferon to rabies virus-infected monkeys after exposure *J. Infect. Dis. 135*:846 (1977).

30. Smith, R. A., Kingsbury, D., Alksne, A., James, H., and Cantell, K. Distribution of interferon in cerebrospinal fluid after systemic, intrathecal and intraventricular administration. *Ann. Neurol. 12*:81 (1982).

31. Smith, R. A., Norris, F., Palmer, D., Bernhardt, L., and Wills, R. J. Distribution of alpha interferon in serum and cerebrospinal fluid after systemic administration. *Clin. Pharmacol. Ther. 37*(1):85-88 (1985).

32. Shafer, S. Q., and Olarte, M. R. Methodological considerations for clinical trials in motor neuron disease (discussion). In: *Human Motor Neuron Diseases* Rowland, ed.). Raven Press, New York, 1982, pp. 559-568.

12
Effects of Interferons on Malignant Brain Tumors

KINTOMO TAKAKURA and OSAMU NAKAMURA*

University of Tokyo Hospital, Tokyo, Japan

ALLAN J. YATES

College of Medicine, The Ohio State University, Columbus, Ohio

I. INTRODUCTION

The antiproliferative properties of interferons have stimulated considerable interest in these compounds as anticancer agents. Their potential value in treating human gliomas has also been widely recognized and has formed the basis for studies both in vitro and in vivo to determine their usefulness against these tumors. Although the results to date are somewhat promising, it is becoming apparent that the mechanisms through which interferons affect the biology of gliomas in situ are quite complex. The type of glioma, mode, site and schedule of delivery, type of interferon, and concurrent therapeutic agents, as well as the effects on the immune system, have all been identified as playing a role in the therapeutic outcome. Undoubtedly, many other factors will be found that also participate in determining the clinical response of a patient with a brain tumor to interferon therapy.

---

* *Present affiliation*: Tokyo Metropolitan Komagome Hospital, Tokyo Japan.

This chapter presents information derived from basic studies conducted both in vitro and using experimental animals and clinical investigations on patients with malignant gliomas and medulloblastomas. Although it is evident that interferons can have a therapeutically beneficial effect on the biology of these neoplasms, it is also obvious that considerably more research is required to define more specifically the interactive determinants responsible for the variable responses of malignant brain tumors to this form of therapy. Only with the availability of such information will it be possible to choose the specific interferon, or combination of interferons, and deliver it in such a manner that will optimize the therapeutic response for each patient with a brain tumor.

II. IN VIVO STUDIES

The recent development of cell culture and recombinant genetic techniques has made it possible to synthesize a large quantity of various interferons (IFN). The suppressive effect of human fibroblast IFN-β on malignant gliomas was first reported by Nagai et al. in 1980 (1,2).

Study groups to evaluate the clinical efficacy of IFN on various malignant neoplasms and other viral diseases have been separately organized for each type of IFN under the supervision of the General Committee for Evaluation of Interferons, organized by the Japanese Ministry of Health and Welfare. Since 1979, the effect of various IFN on malignant brain tumors, mainly malignant gliomas, have been evaluated in phase I and II studies by our Brain Tumor Study Subcommittee.

The results obtained from the study group on the effects of two human fibroblast IFN-β, two recombinant IFN-α, and a human lymphoblast IFN-α on malignant gliomas and our clinical experience with the long-term administration of human fibroblast IFN-β are summarized in the first part of this report on in vivo studies.

Since it is difficult to evaluate the effects of human IFN in an in vivo situation, from an experimental point of view the tumor model transplanted to nude mice is useful to determine the therapeutic effects of IFN. In the second part the results obtained from our studies on the antitumor effects of IFN in nude mice are summarized. The effects of IFN-β administration alone and the possible enhancement of its antitumor action by combined use with radiation and chemotherapy in nude mice bearing human glioma transplants are reported with a view to determining more effective usage of IFN in the suppression of malignant brain tumors.

A. Clinical Effects of Interferons on Malignant Brain Tumors

1. Patients, Materials, and Methods

Patients. Patients with primary malignant brain tumors, mainly glioblastoma multiforme, malignant astrocytoma (grade III), and medulloblastoma, were selected for the studies regardless of whether they were primary or recurrent cases. Few cases of other kinds of malignant gliomas or tumors other than metastatic were included. The following criteria were adopted for the selection of patients:

1. Established histologic diagnosis
2. The presence of measurable tumor on computed tomographic (CT) scans
3. The absence of double cancers
4. Preferably grade 0-3 performance status (PS); a few patients with grade 4 status were, however, included
5. The absence of serious accompanying complications
6. The absence of effects of previous treatment: at least 1 month's lapse of time from any previous radiotherapy or at least 2 weeks' washout period following any chemotherapy
7. Age under 75 years

Pregnant patients and those with allergic diathesis were excluded. Informed consent for the use of IFN treatment was obtained from the patient or the patient's family prior to the study. The numbers of evaluable cases for each type of IFN are shown in Table 1.

Table 1 Effect of Interferons on Malignant Brain Tumors[a]

Interferon	Total number of cases	CR	PR	NC (MR)	PD	Effectiveness rate (%)	Reference
β (fibroblast HuIFN-β)[b]	54	4	8	26 (4)	16	22.2	Nagai (1983)(3)
β (fibroblast, MR-21)[c]	37	0	5	7 (1)	15	13.5	Takakura (1985)(4)
α (recombinant, r-IFN-αA. Ro22-8181)[d]	39	0	4	25 (2)	10	10.3	Takakura (1985)(4)
α (recombinant, r-IFN-α$_2$, Sch30500)[e]	35	0	7	17 (1)	11	20.0	Kitamura (1985)(5)
α (lymphoblast, Interferol-α)[f]	38	1	1	24 (5)	12	5.3	Furue (1985)(6)

[a]Abbreviations: CR, complete response; PR, partial response; NC, no change; MR, minor response; PD, progressive disease. effectiveness rate, number of CR+PR cases per total number of cases.
[b]Human fibroblast interferon, Toray.
[c]Human fibroblast interferon, Mochida.
[d]Recombinant interferon-αA, Takeda & Roche.
[e]Recombinant interferon-α$_2$, Yamanouchi and Essex, Japan.
[f]Human lymphoblast interferon-α, Midori, Jyuji.

Interferons and Methods of Application. Five different types of IFN were used:

1. IFN-β (human fibroblast IFN-β), Feron, Toray) (3), 3–9 × 10^6 IU, IV daily

2. IFN-β (human fibroblast IFN-β, MR-21, Mochida) (4), 5 × 10^6 IU, IV daily; 10 × 10^6 IU, IV three times a week; or 50 × 10^6 IU IV, twice a week

3. IFN-α (recombinant IFN-βA, Ro22-8181, Takeda-Roche Japan and USA) (7), 3–50 × 10^6 IU, IM, daily or every other day

4. IFN-α (recombinant IFN-$α_2$, Sch 30500, Yamanouchi-Essex Japan) (5), 3 × 10^6 IU, IM, daily or every other day

5. IFN-α [lymphoblast (Namelva strain) IFN-α, Interferol α, Mirodi Jyuju) (6), 3–9 × 10^6 IU, IM, daily or every other day

Each dose was increased appropriately after confirmation of its safety until an optimum dose permitting successive administration of IFN could be continued for at least 4 weeks in order to evaluate the effects. Intrathecal or local administration of IFN was followed whenever possible, but the dose of administration was reduced by one-tenth of the above-mentioned initial doses and increased gradually after checking for side effects.

Evaluation of Effectiveness and Side Effects. Evaluation of the clinical response was based primarily upon findings of the CT scans and conformed with the criteria approved by the Japanese Society for Cancer Therapy: complete response (CR), disappearance of tumor on CT scan; partial response (PR), more than 50% decrease in two-dimensional size of the tumor; minor response (MR), more than 25% and less than 50% decrease in the tumor size; no change (NC), less than 25% decrease or increase in the tumor size; progressive disease (PD), more than 25% increase in the tumor size.

Effectiveness rate was calculated by the number of CR and PR cases divided by the total number of cases. Exclusion from the evaluable cases in this study was based on the following criteria:

(1) combined chemotherapy was performed during the period of the study; (2) the duration of IFN administration was less than 4 weeks; (3) IFN treatment was started without the above-mentioned lapse of time after previous radiotherapy or chemotherapy; and (4) the final histologic diagnosis was not primary malignant brain tumor. The side effects of each type of interferon were accumulated from all cases, regardless of whether they were evaluable or nonevaluable.

2. Results

Of 203 evaluable cases accumulated for studies on the effects of five different interferons, 168 cases were glioblastoma multiforme or malignant astrocytoma (grade III). The other 35 cases included 11 medulloblastomas, 6 astrocytomas (grade II), 4 oliogdendrogliomas, 2 ependymomas, 2 immature teratomas, and 10 other tumors. The numbers of evaluable cases for each type of IFN are summarized in Tables 1 and 2. The effectiveness of IFN on malignant brain tumors is shown in Table 1. The effectiveness rates were 22.2% for human fibroblast IFN-β (HuIFN-β), 13.5% for human fibroblast IFN-β (MR-21), 10.3% for recombinant IFN-α (r-IFN-α A), 20.0% for recombinant IFN-α (r-IFNα2), and 5.3% for lymphoblast IFN-α (Interferol-α).

The effectiveness of IFN on malignant glioma (glioblastoma multiforme and malignant astrocytoma grade III) is summarized in Table 2. The effectiveness rates were 16.7% for human fibroblast IFN-β (HuIFN-β), 13.8% for human fibroblast IFN-β (MR-21), 17.1% for recombinant IFN-α (r-IFNα A), 16.7% for recombinant IFN-α (r-IFN-α 2), and 5.6% for lymphoblast IFN-α (Interferol-α). There were five cases of complete response: one glioblastoma multiforme, two medulloblastomas and one other glioma by human fibroblast IFN-β, and one malignant astrocytoma by lymphoblast IFN-α.

Effects of Human Fibroblast IFN-β (HuIFN-β) (3). The effectiveness of human fibroblast IFN-β was studied in detail. Human fibroblast IFN-β (HuIFN-β) was administered to 31 primary and 23 recurrent cases. The effectiveness rates were 32.3% for primary cases and 5.7% for recurrent cases. In malignant glioma cases, no difference in effectiveness rates was observed between intravenous

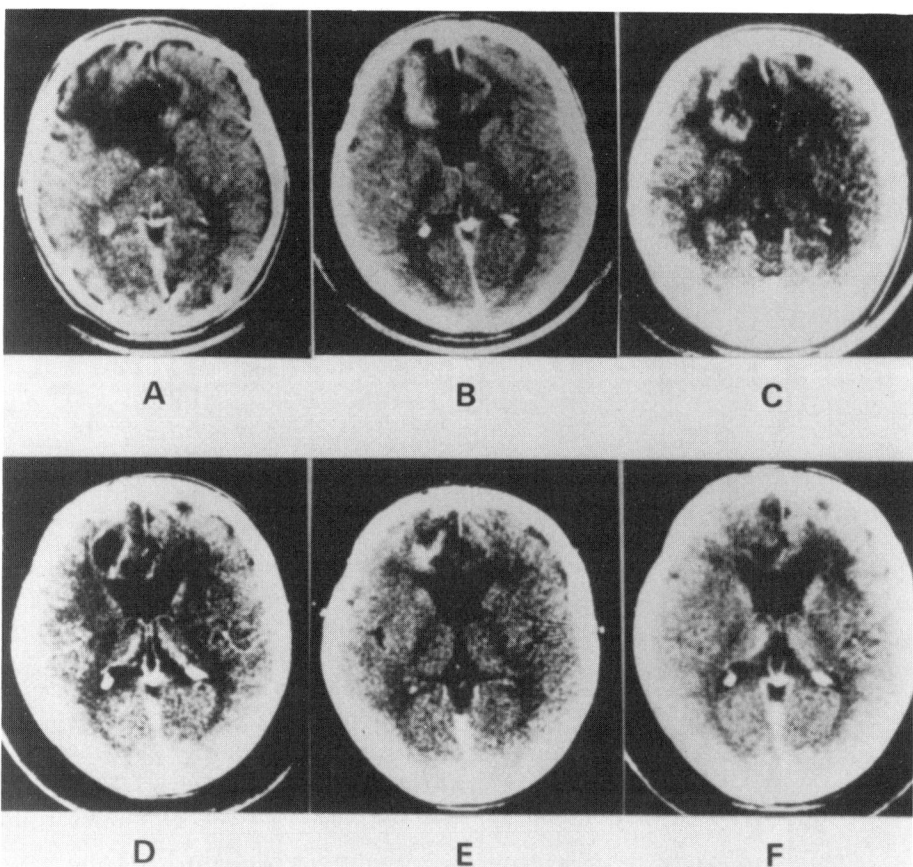

Figure 1 CT scans of case 1, 30-year-old female, malignant astrocytoma. (A) Before treatment. (B) After surgical removal and chemoradiotherapy. (C) Before IFN-β treatment. (D) At 5 months of IFN-β treatment (1.7×10^8 U). (F) At 24 months of IFN-β treatment (3.8×10^8 U). At 46 months after the start of IFN-β treatment, no recurrence of the tumor has been noted.

This patient was treated with HuIFN-β alone for almost 4 years after the initial radiotherapy and chemotherapy. It is therefore attributed to the effect of HuIFN-β that the tumor has remarkably regressed on CT scan.

Case 2. An 11-year-old girl with glioblastoma multiforme in the pineal region complained of headache and nausea at the end of January 1985, at the age of 11 years, and left hemiparesis appeared 1 week later. CT scan revealed a large tumor in the pineal region with extension into the right parietal lobe accompanying hydrocephalus. Ventricular-peritoneal shunting and radiotherapy were performed at another hospital under the diagnosis of pineal germ cell tumor. Since the tumor size on CT scan did not show regression after local radiotherapy of 20 Gy, she was referred to our clinic for diagnosis and further treatment. She was operated on March 26, 1985, and the tumor was diagnosed as glioblastoma multiforme. After the partial removal of the tumor, radiotherapy (28 Gy to the whole brain and 12 Gy to the local tumor site) with chemotherapy consisting of ACNU and vincristine were administered. From June 14, 1985, she was treated with intravenous administration of interleukin-2 for 4 weeks. On August 26, treatment with HuIFN-β (3×10^6 IU/day, twice a week) was started. On December 6, 1985, combined treatment with IFN and vincristine (1 mg/day, IV, once a week for 2 months) was started. During 6 months' treatment with IFN, the residual tumor on CT scan disappeared almost completely, and she has returned to school.

This case suggested that combined treatment with HuIFN-β and vincristine was effective in suppressing growth of glioblastoma multiforme.

B. Effects of Interferon on Experimental Brain Tumors

1. Materials and Methods

Mice. Specific pathogen-free nude mice of both sexes with a genetic background of BALB/cA were used. They were at least 5 weeks old when used and were assigned to experimental groups of three to eight each.

MALIGNANT BRAIN TUMORS

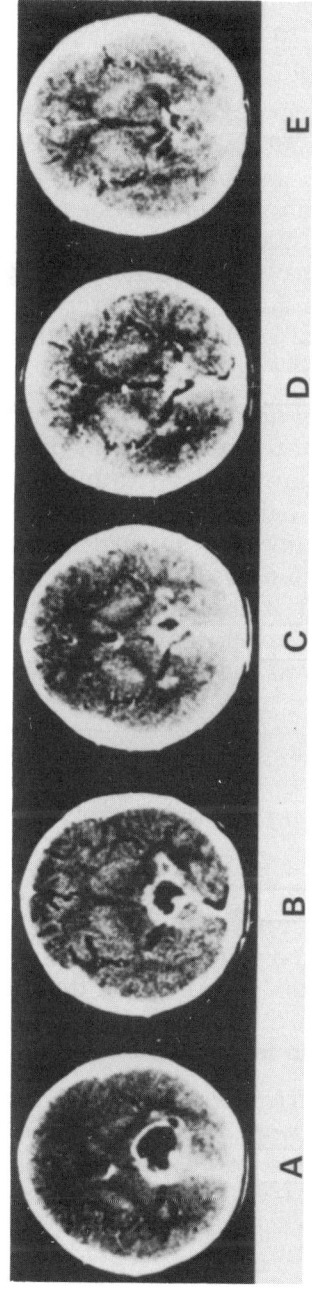

Figure 2 CT scans of case 2, 11-year-old girl, glioblastoma multiforme. (A) Before treatment. (B) After surgical removal. (C) After chemoradiotherapy (May 31, 1985). (D) Before IFN-β treatment. (E) At 4 months after the start of IFN-β treatment (total dose 1.4×10^8 U).

Tumor. Human glioma cell lines (six strains) that had been maintained at the Central Institute for Experimental Animals, Kawasaki, for more than 20 serial transplantations in mice after excision of the tumors from patients were studied (8).

Transplantation of Tumors. Each animal received a subcutaneous transplant (3 mm^3 cube of tumor tissue) injected into the right axillary region by means of a trocar. Treatment was begun when the transplanted tumor volume, defined as ½(longer diameter) × (shorter diameter)^2, reached approximately 100–300 mm^3. In the experiments that involved radiation therapy, subcutaneous tumor transplantation was made by injection into the right thigh in both treated and control groups in order to limit irradiation to the neoplastic lesion.

Evaluation of Therapeutic Response. Tumor response was assessed by measurement of the tumor volume twice weekly over a period of 3 weeks after the start of treatment. A tumor growth curve was drawn on the basis of these measurements and the therapy-control (T/C) ratio was calculated according to the method of the Battelle Columbus Laboratories (9). The treatment was rated as effective (+) if the animal showed a T/C ratio of ≤42% and was considered positively effective (++) in cases in which the tumor volume was reduced to less than at the initiation of treatment.

HuIFN-β Preparation. The HuIFN-β (Toray) used was produced by superinduction with poly IC, cycloheximide, and actinomycin D in mass cultures of human preputial fibroblast cells in multitrays (10).

Antitumor Effect of HuIFN-β: Study with Six Glioma Cell Lines. Mice were given an intraperitoneal injection of IFN-β (5 × 10^6 IU/kg) daily for 21 days. The tumor volume was measured twice weekly over a period of 3 weeks after the start of treatment, and the therapeutic response was evaluated by the method of the Battelle Columbus Laboratories (9).

Changes in Antitumor Effect with Route of Administration and Dose of HuIFN-β: Study with Glioma Cell Line GL-5-JCK. The effect of HuIFN-β was investigated for three different routes of administration: intravenous via the tail vein, subcutaneous into the perilesional area, or intratumoral. The IFN was injected at high and low dose levels of 25×10^6 IU/kg, and 5×10^6 IU/kg, respectively, by IV or SC routes, whereas intratumoral injections were made at the low dose level alone. Animals received IFN daily for a period of 7 days, and T/C ratio data calculated from biweekly measurements of the tumor volume during the 3 week period were statistically analyzed by the U test (one-sided, 1%) for significance of intergroup differences.

Effect of HuIFN-β Therapy in Combination with Other Treatments: Study with Glioma Cell Line GL-2-JCK. HuIFN-β Therapy Combined with Other Anticancer Drug. Mice in group 1 were given an intraperitoneal injection of adriamycin at a dose of 8 mg/kg (maximal tolerated dose, 12 mg/kg) on day 1, alone or in combination with HuIFN-β injected IP in doses of 500×10^4 IU/kg daily for 21 days beginning on day 1. The antitumor responses of animals receiving adriamycin alone and those receiving adriamycin plus IFN were compared with the response of animals given IFN alone, the T/C ratio being 63%, as previously reported.

Mice in group 2 received a single IP dose of 20 mg/kg (maximal tolerated dose, 60 mg/kg) of ACNU on day 1, alone or in combination with HuIFN-β injected IP in doses of 500×10^4 IU/kg daily from day 1 through day 21. Antitumor responses were compared among the groups of mice receiving IFN alone, ACNU alone, or ACNU plus IFN.

HuIFN-β Therapy Combined with Radiotherapy. Responses were compared between a group of mice given irradiation (dose, 390 rads) on day 1 and HuIFN-β injected IP in doses of 500×10^4 IU/kg daily from day 1 through day 21, a group receiving the same dose of irradiation alone, and a group of mice given irradiation (dose, 650 rads) on day 1 and daily IP injections of HuIFN-β in doses of 500×10^4 IU/kg for 21 days beginning on day 1, a group given the same dose of irradiation alone, and a group receiving HuIFN-β alone.

For irradiation, mice were restrained under Nembutal anesthesia. The right hindleg with tumor transplant was irradiated exclusively with a Toshiba telecobalt unit (source-skin distance, 11 cm). The dose rate was 130 rad/min.

2. Results

Antitumor Effect on HuIFN-β. In two of six glioma strains, the tumor reduction rate (treated-control values) treated with HuIFN-β was evaluated as effective by the method of the Battelle Columbus Laboratories (Table 4).

Changes in Antitumor Effect with Route of Administration and Dose of HuIFN-β. Tumor regression was progressively enhanced over the period from day 4 to day 10 in all groups receiving HuIFN-β injections by any of the three different routes studied. Maximal effect was observed on day 10, at which point the T/C ratio was 33% by IV route (high dose) and 35% by SC route (low dose); hence there was little or no difference in antitumor effect between the routes. The regressions were statistically significant in all groups except a low-dose group, as assessed by U test (one-sided, 1%).

The inhibition of tumor growth was dose dependent during the period from day 4 to day 10 by the IV route as well as by the SC route (Table 5).

Table 4 Evaluation of Therapeutic Response[a]

Drugs	Tumors					
	Epe-1	Epe-2	GL-2	GL-3	GL-4	GL-5
HuIFN-β 5×10^6 IU/kg	77(−)	94(−)	63(−)	35(+)	71(−)	39(+)

[a]The tumor response was assessed by measurement of the tumor volume twice weekly over a period of 3 weeks after the start of treatment. A tumor growth curve was drawn from the data, and the therapy-control (T/C) ratio was calculated according to the method of the Battelle Columbus Laboratories (9). The treatment was rated as effective (+) if the animal showed a T/C ratio of ≤42%, and it was considered positively effective (++) in cases in which the tumor volume became reduced to less than that at initiation of treatment. (GL, glioblastoma; Epe, ependymoma).

Table 5 Comparison of the Effect of HuIFN-β by the Route of Administration[a]

Route	Dose	T/C value (%)					
		Day 4	7	10	14	18	21
IV	High	<u>59</u>	<u>41</u>	<u>33</u>	<u>35</u>	<u>43</u>	<u>49</u>
	Low	<u>76</u>	<u>52</u>	<u>43</u>	<u>47</u>	<u>52</u>	<u>57</u>
SC	High	<u>65</u>	<u>51</u>	<u>35</u>	<u>36</u>	<u>38</u>	<u>50</u>
	Low	70	<u>64</u>	<u>56</u>	<u>61</u>	<u>61</u>	<u>65</u>
IT	High	—	—	—	—	—	—
	Low	<u>64</u>	<u>51</u>	<u>41</u>	<u>46</u>	<u>52</u>	<u>64</u>

[a]High, 25×10^6 IU/kg. Low, 5×10^6 IU/kg. Underscored values are significant (U test).

Effect of HuIFN-β' Therapy Combined with Other Treatment. HuIFN-β' Therapy Combined with Adriamycin. The antitumor effect was inconspicuous with HuIFN-β alone (T/C ratio, 63%) and was similarly poor with adriamycin alone (T/C ratio, 48%). Treatment with combined regimens, however, produced a tumor regression (+) with a T/C ratio of 36% (Fig. 3).

HuIFN-β' Therapy Combined with ACNU. Animals given HuIFN-β alone showed a T/C ratio of 63%. The T/C ratio was no better than 44% in the group receiving ACNU alone because the dose (20 mg/kg) was one-third of the maximal tolerated dose. With a combination of the two drugs, an apparently greater degree of regression occurred (Fig. 4).

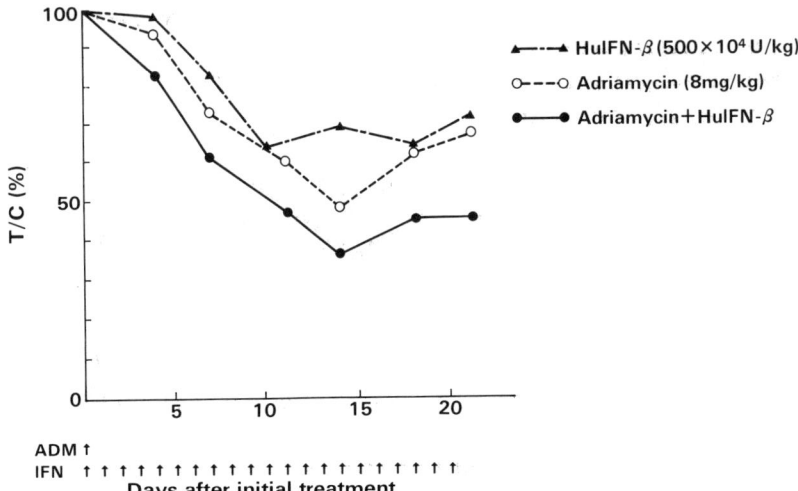

Figure 3 HuIFN-β therapy combined with adriamycin. The antitumor effect was inconspicuous with HuIFN-β alone (T/C ratio, 63%) and was similarly poor with adriamycin alone (T/C ratio, 48%). Treatment with combined regimens, however, produced a (+) tumor regression with a T/C ratio of 36%.

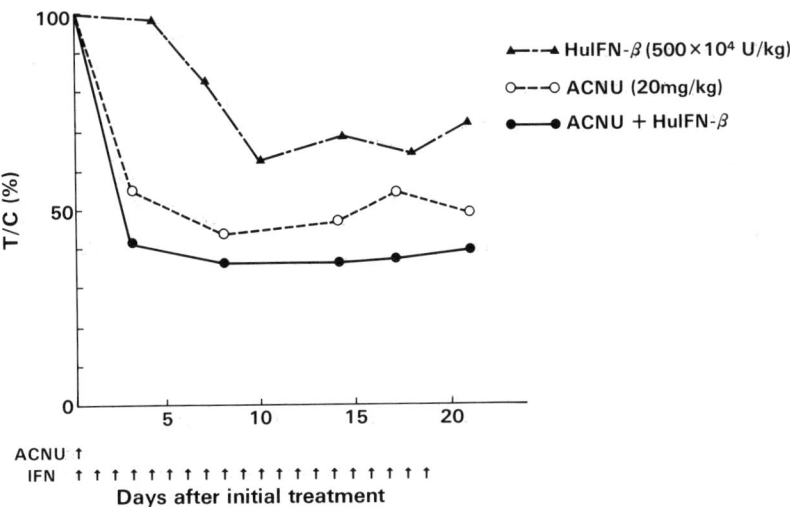

Figure 4 HuIFN-β therapy combined with ACNU. Animals given HuIFN-β alone showed a T/C ratio of 63%. The T/C ratio was no better than 44% in the group receiving ACNU alone because the dose (20 mg/kg) was one-third of the maximal tolerated dose. With a combination of the two drugs, an apparently greater degree of regression occurred.

HuIFN-β' Therapy Combined with Radiation. The T/C ratio was 63% in the group given HuIFN-β alone and 61% in the group receiving radiation therapy alone (390 rad). The antitumor effect was enhanced in the group receiving combined IFN and radiation therapy (T/C ratio, 35%). This trend was even more conspicuous with an increased radiation dose of 650 rad, that is, a T/C ratio of 26% in the combined treatment group compared with 63% with HuIFN-β alone and 51% with radiotherapy alone (Fig. 5).

3. Discussion

Various attempts have been made to adapt the use of IFN to the treatment of human malignant neoplasms (10-14). Several investigators have recently reported the clinical effectiveness of IFN on malignant gliomas (15-22). Although the suppressive effects on gliomas were different in each type of IFN, the data were analyzed based on a very limited number of cases and different methods of administration; therefore it is difficult to evaluate properly the efficacy of each type of IFN. It is now generally thought that the antitumor effect of IFN is not as great as previously expected when administered alone in spite of the rarity of serious adverse reactions. It should be stressed that the studies on the effect of long-term IFN administration as described in this report are necessary to evaluate definitely the effect of IFN.

In our laboratory studies on human gliomas transplanted into nude mice, IFN produced a significant antitumor effect against only two of the six glioma cell lines tested and was not noticeably more potent than commonly used anticancer drugs, such as ACNU and vincristine, in suppressing malignant neoplastic growth (8). Based on the results of basic research that demonstrated an enhanced tumor-suppressive effect of IFN in combination with radiotherapy and chemotherapy, studies on combined treatment should be conducted in the coming years.

With regard to the antitumor effects of IFN administered in combination with other anticancer drugs, a noteworthy amount of laboratory work has been reported (23-31). From these reports, the antitumor effects of the combined use of IFN are evident with a wide variety of anticancer drugs, such as ACNU, BCNU, bleomycin, mitomycin C, adriamycin, aclacinomycin,

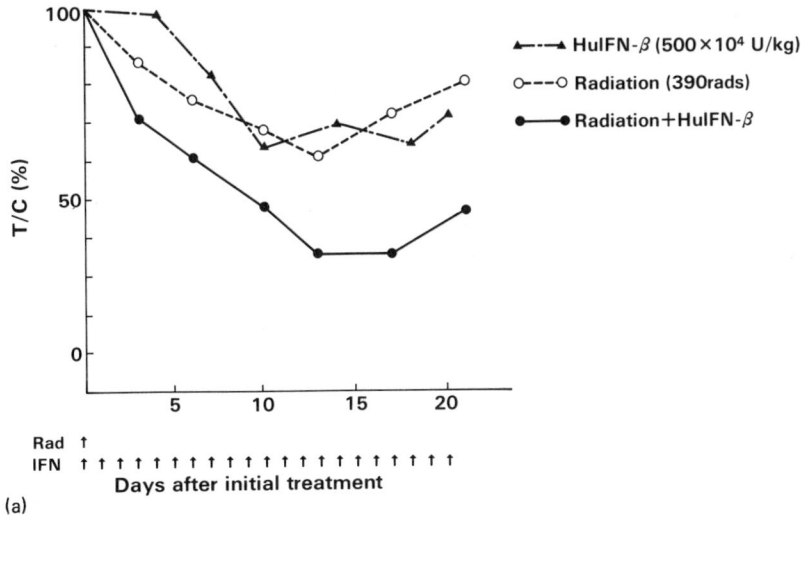

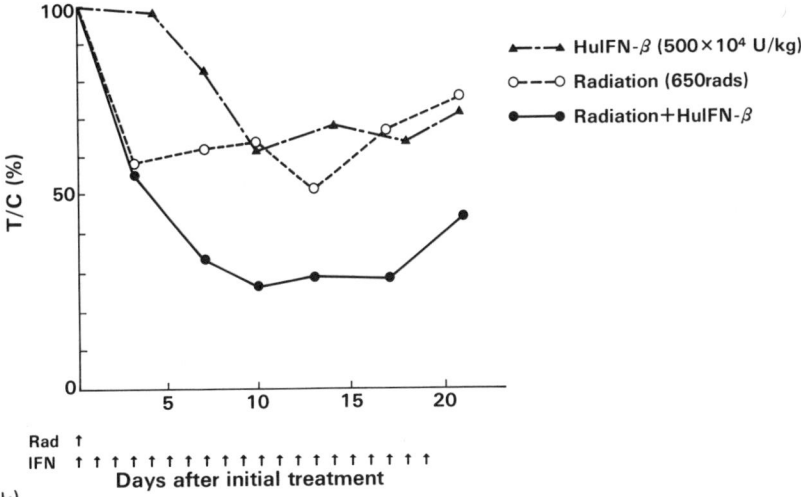

Figure 5 HuIFN-β therapy combined with radiation. (a) The T/C ratio was 63% in the group given HuIFN-β alone and 61% in the group receiving radiation therapy (390 rad). The antitumor effect was enhanced in the group receiving combined IFN-radiation therapy (T/C ratio, 35%). (b) This trend was more conspicuous with an increased radiation dose of 650 rad, that is, a T/C ratio of 26% in the combined treatment group compared with 63% with HuIFN alone and 51% with radiotherapy alone.

actinomycin D, pepleomycin, Cytosine arabinoside, 5-fluorouracil, cyclophosphamide, vincristine, vindesin, and vinblastine. Most effects were nevertheless in the category of additive rather than potentiating, and tumor responses have not necessarily been consistent, varying with the tumor cell line and type of IFN preparation. Much remains to be clarified with respect to the underlying mechanisms in the majority of these drugs.

Talas et al. first reported in 1978 a protective effect of IFN against radiation hazards (32). Reports of the antitumor effects of the combined use of IFN with radiotherapy as yet are few. It was observed by Miyoshi et al. (33) in their study on Sarcoma 180 cells in vitro that a 24 hr exposure of tumor cells to IFN after irradiation resulted in a synergistic antitumor effect, whereas when the cells were treated in reverse sequence the overall beneficial effect tended to be reduced because cells pretreated with IFN were protected from damage by radiation. Itoh (34) observed essentially the same tendency in their experiments on a cultured cell line derived from human carcinoma of the base of the oral cavity: a synergistic effect of IFN and radiation was noted in cultures given IFN after irradiation, whereas no such effect could be seen in cultures irradiated after treatment with IFN. They noted that the synergistic effect of IFN with radiation may be ascribed to the inhibition of cellular recovery from radiation-induced injury, in that analysis of the radiation dose-response curve revealed a significant difference in D_q between a control group and combined treatment groups but no significant intergroup difference in D_0.

In addition to these studies in vitro, Ortaldo and McCoy (35) noted significant prolongation of mean survival time of mice receiving 3×10^4 IU of IFN following "lethal irradiation." The investigators inferred that the protective effect of IFN may be due at least in part to improvement of depressed immune function by IFN, on the grounds that the animals given IFN after irradiation showed elevated natural killer (NK) activity. IFN has been described to have the properties of cytotoxic T-cell killing (36), activation of monocyte function (37), and stimulation of production of the leukocyte migration inhibitory factor, in addition to augmentation of NK and ADCC activities (38). As discussed below it is very likely that some of these activities are involved in the protective effect of IFN.

Reports of clinical studies on the antitumor effect of IFN given in combination with other drugs, particularly those encompassing the evaluation of the effect of combined regimens, have been few. Winkler et al. (39) investigated the therapeutic response to treatment with methotrexate and adriamycin, alone or in combination with IFN, in 151 cases of osteosarcoma and found that the presence or absence of IFN in therapy regimens had no significant relation to therapeutic response. The use of IFN in combination with radiotherapy in patients with carcinoma has also been reported (40,41). According to Arai et al. (40), there was a significantly greater percentage of long-term survivors in a group receiving radiotherapy before treatment with IFN. The two satisfactory responders in our series of cancer patients received IFN therapy instituted 2-4 months after the completion of radiotherapy; this as well as the present data in mice are of profound interest when viewed with reference to the findings discussed earlier. Further study will be necessary to explore the effect of IFN as maintenance therapy after antitumor radio- and/or chemotherapy as a potentially effective method of IFN dosing.

III. IN VITRO STUDIES

A major goal of studying the effects of interferons on cultured glioma cells is to gain an understanding of their effects on gliomas in human patients. However, there are several reasons for caution in directly applying the results of such studies to the clinical situation. The major obvious difference is that cells in culture are in a much less complex environment than in vivo, where a host of factors could be oeprating that are absent in vitro. Owing to the selective pressures of the culture conditions, only a minority of human gliomas placed in culture develop into permanent cell lines (approximately 15%) (42-44), and the cells that grow in vitro may not be representative of the heterogeneous population of cells in the tumor from which they were derived. Culture conditions may allow the growth of some populations of cells that are of little clinical significance while suppressing other major cell populations. Because of drift in the biologic characteristics of cells from passage to passage and their genetic instability, phenotypic characteristics of glioma clones can also vary with time in culture, and it is possible that responses to interferons may also vary on such bases. Primary explants and three-dimensional colonies eliminate some of this variation, but the number of cells available from such cultures is quite limited, and it is difficult to perform many quantitative studies on these populations of cells.

Nevertheless, in vitro systems also have several advantages. The interferons can be added directly to the growth medium, and samples of the medium are readily obtained at different times (45). This provides the investigator with the ability to control and monitor the concentration of interferons in the immediate environment of the glioma cells. The availability of well-characterized lines and clones of glioma cells (both human and animal) facilitates the reproducibility of experimental conditions and allows comparisons of results from studies on different types of cultured glioma cells. Growth conditions can be easily varied using different growth media, culture substrata, such additives as growth factors, antibodies, and drugs to study their interactive effects with interferons on biologic characteristics of glioma cells. Morphologic changes in glioma cells in response to interferon can be examined directly at the light microscopic level, and electron microscopic studies of cultured cells can easily be done. The effects of interferons on interactions between glioma and nonneural (e.g., immune) cells can also be studied, In short, several interactive mechanisms that could influence the final clinical result of interferon therapy can be isolated and examined separately. Four such mechanisms have been studied using cultured glioma cells: (1) growth inhibitory effects of interferon; (2) effects of interferons on the activity of natural killer cells against glioma cells; (3) effects of interferon on the resistance of glioma cells to NK cytolysis; and (4) biochemical responses of glioma cells to interferons. These are discussed below.

A. Effect of Human Interferons on Growth of Cultured Human Glioma Cells

It is now well established that all three major types of interferon (IFN-α, IFN-β, and IFN-γ) have growth inhibitory effects on several different types of tumor cells. Thus it is of interest that cultures of both human glioma and fetal brain cells will produce IFN in response to Sendai virus and polyribosinic-polycytidilic acid (46). Some of these cell lines produced 4000–8000 U/ml medium in response to Sendai virus, 60,000 U/ml in response to superinduction, and up to 80,000 U/ml if the cells were first primed with a low dose of IFN. Characterization of the IFN produced using heat treatment, determinations of antiviral activity in heterologous cells, and antisera neutralization indicates that it is of the β type. It has been determined from clinical studies that IFN has some deleterious, usually reversible effects on the nervous system (47), raising the possibility that some of the generalized neurologic manifestations seen with infectious and neoplastic involvement of the brain may be due to local production of IFN. The effects of exogenous or endogenously produced interferon on the developing nervous system is an important question that has yet to be thoroughly addressed.

Lundblad and Lundgren (48) first demonstrated that the growth of cultured human glioma cells is inhibited by IFN. Using the cell line U-251 MG, they found that as little as 10 units (U) IFN-β per milliliter culture medium had a growth inhibitory effect and that growth was virtually completely inhibited by 500 U/ml. The cells were also inhibited by IFN-α but not to the same degree, a finding corroborated by Slimmer et al. (4) for a clone derived from a glioblastoma multiforme. Analyses of cell cycle parameters using thymidine incorporation and flow cytometric analyses indicated that both IFN-α and IFN-β allow the cells to enter S phase, but they stop synthesizing DNA prematurely. Korosue et al. (50) synchronized the growth of a human glioma cell line (KNS-42) with a double-excess thymidine method and studied the rate of thymidine incorporation after block reversal. Labeling of cells exposed to HuIFN-β was considerably less with both pulse- and continuous-labeling methods. Thymidine labeling of cells following release from growth arrest by HuIFN-β began to increase

2 hr and peaked 3 hr after removal of HuIFN-β. Mitotic figures appeared later, and their peak number was reached at 12 hr after changing to medium without HuIFN-β. These findings were interpreted to mean that HuIFN-β prevented the cells from entering S phase. The discrepancy in the conclusions of these two studies may be due either to the different techniques and sources of HuIFN-β used or to biologic differences in the cell lines studied.

A growth inhibitory effect of a HuIFN-β preparation on cell lines cultured from human glioblastoma multiforme, astrocytoma, and neuroblastoma (not specified whether central or peripheral in origin) tumors was also demonstrated (45). the astrocytoma and glioblastoma cells were all quite sensitive, their growth being inhibited by 50% with only 30 U HuIFN-β per milliliter culture medium or less. The neuroblastoma cells were less sensitive, requiring 30–300 U/ml to be inhibited to the same degree. This differential sensitivity to the growth inhibitory effects of IFN among different human glioma lines has also been noted by other investigators. Growth of KNS-42 cells is only slightly inhibited by 500 U HuIFN-β/ml, and 1×10^4 U/ml is cytocidal. The HuIFN-β preparation used by Cook et al. (45) caused morphologic changes in the cells (pyknosis and cytoplasmic changes described as cytolysis) at 3×10^3 U/ml. However, parallel studies with mock IFN were not described for either of these investigations, so the specificities of these effects are not beyond question. Although data were not shown, Cook et al. (45) state that similar results had been obtained using explants of brain tumors.

We also have found that cells cultured from different neural sources have different sensitivities to the growth inhibitory effects of HuIFN-β (51). The three most sensitive cell lines, of eight studied, were from glioblastoma multiformes that were inhibited 36–84%. An anaplastic astrocytoma and a schwannoma cell line were each inhibited approximately 15%, and cells derived from human fetal brain and an oligodendroglioma were virtually uninhibited by 1000 U/ml (Table 6). Thus it seems that the degree of sensitivity to the growth inhibitory effects of HuIFN-β generally correlates with the degree of anaplasia of the tissues from which the cells were derived. Regardless of the degree of sensitivity, growth inhibition was dose dependent, and even less sensitive cells

Table 6 Effect of IFN-β on Cell Growth of Cultured Neural Cells[a]

Cell line	Passage	Original tissue	Cell density[b]		% Inhibition[b]
			Mock	IFN	
CHI	10	Fetal brain	25.8 ± 1.5[c]	23.6 ± 1.3	8.6
CHII	13	Fetal brain	76.6 ± 1.5	82.1 ± 3.9	-7.2
12-10	8	Oligodendroglioma	25.9 ± 0	26.4 ± 1.4	-1.9
8-25	3	Schwannoma	26.6 ± 2.7	22.0 ± 1.18	17.3
7-1	7	Anaplastic astrocytoma	26.2 ± 1.9	22.5 ± 0.9	14.1
1-29A	4	Glioblastoma	43.3 ± 11.2	27.7 ± 2.4	36.1
12-18	32	Glioblastoma	89.1 ± 0.4	24.0 ± 1.0	73.1
U251-MG	20[d]	Glioblastoma	112.2 ± 5.3	19.3 ± 1.2	83.7

[a]During early log phase, cultures were exposed to 1000 IU IFN-β per milliliter culture medium for 3 days. Cells were harvested when control cultures were confluent.
[b]Percentage inhibition = 100(1-IFN/mock).
[c]Mean ± SE of the results (cells/cm^2).
[d]The passage level for U251-MG refers to the number of passages it underwent in our laboratory.
Source: From Reference 51.

grown from fetal brain were inhibited with higher concentrations (Table 7). However, there was no correlation between the degree of growth inhibition and the antiviral effect of HuIFN-β on these cell lines, all of which were quite sensitive to the latter. This was noted previously in studies on a clone derived from a human glioblastoma multiforme (49).

The effects on growth of different exposure times to HuIFN-β were studied using a glioblastoma cell line (12-18). Cells were grown in medium lacking IFN to mid-log phase, at which time medium was changed to that containing 1000 U HuIFN-β per milliliter. After time intervals between 1 and 96 hr, IFN-containing medium was removed, the cells were washed, and fresh medium without IFN added. Cells were harvested and counted when control cultures unexposed to IFN were confluent. Cell densities of cultures exposed to IFN were expressed as percentages of densities for cultures exposed in the same way to mock IFN. No growth inhibitory effect was seen in cultures exposed to IFN for up to 12 hr, but cell densities of cultures exposed for 24 hr were only 60%, and those exposed for 48 hr only 30% of those for mock IFN controls (Fig. 6). This suggests that prolonged exposure to IFN may b necessary to achieve the maximum clinically useful growth inhibitory effect that might be achieved by direct local infusions of tumor beds.

Prolonged exposure from the time of plating of two glioma cell lines (U-251 MG and U-118 MG) to 100 U HuIFN-α per milliliter inhibited their growth rates for 2-3 weeks, but subsequently growth returned to normal even in the presence of HuIFN-α (52). The mechanism of this was not determined but could be due either to the later proliferation of IFN-insensitive cells or to the development of IFN resistance. Combined exposure of these cells to HuIFN-α and irradiation did not have a synergistic growth inhibitory effect greater than that of either modality separately. This is different from the results of experiments described below in which nude mice bearing transplanted human gliomas were treated with IFN-β and radiation.

The point along the growth curve at which IFN is added also has an effect on the final density to which neural cultures grow (51). The only time when human fetal brain cells were inhibited

Table 7 Dose-Response Effect of IFN-β on Cell Growth[a]

Cell line	Control	Dose of IFN-β or equivalent of mock IFN (IU)							
		10		100		1000		5000	
		Mock	IFN	Mock	IFN	Mock	IFN	Mock	IFN
CHII	90.1 ± 5.5[b]	74.3 ± 2.5	84.5 ± 0.7	79.7 ± 6.5	97.3 ± 2.2	76.6 ± 1.5	82.1 ± 3.0	66.1 ± 1.7	52.3 ± 3.5
12-18	99.3 ± 3.5	82.3 ± 6.9	89.0 ± 7.1	97.2 ± 5.0	66.1 ± 0.8	89.1 ± 0.4	24.0 ± 1.0	100.4 ± 2.8	3.0 ± 0.2
U251-MG	134.2 ± 1.2	91.3 ± 2.1	107.6 ± 5.5	124.6 ± 12.2	70.3 ± 6.1	112.2 ± 5.3	18.3 ± 1.2	—[c]	—

[a]Cultures were exposed to IFN-β or mock IFN for 3 days during early log phase of growth. cultures were harvested, and cells were counted when control cultures were confluent (after more than four population doublings).
[b]Mean ± SE of the results (cells/cm^2) from at least three separate cultures.
[c]Not done.
Source: From Reference 51.

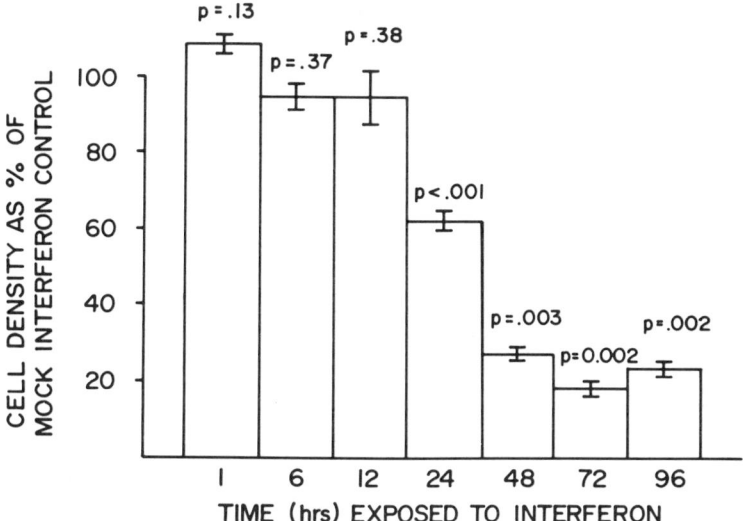

Figure 6 Effects of different exposure times to IFN (1000 IU/ml medium) on growth of 12-18. Cells were harvested when control cultures (unexposed to either IFN or mock IFN) had reached confluency (approximately four population doublings). Results are for cell densities of IFN-exposed cells as the percentage of mock IFN-exposed cells. Columns, mean of at least three cultures; bars, SE. The p values were obtained using Student's t-test in paired comparisons with values for samples treated with mock IFN over the same time period. (From Ref. 51.)

by HuIFN-β was when it was added during the log phase of growth, and the degree of inhibition was slight. However, the earlier that HuIFN-β was added to cultures of glioblastoma multiforme cells, the lower were the final cell densities (Fig. 7). An obvious interpretation is that the IFN is inhibiting the cultures soon after it is added, so they are harvested with cell densities close to what they were at the time the IFN was added. However, inhibition of cell growth at the concentration of IFN used was not due to a cytocidal effect because there were no differences in cell densities between control and treated cultures when it was added at confluency of either fetal brain or glioma cell cultures.

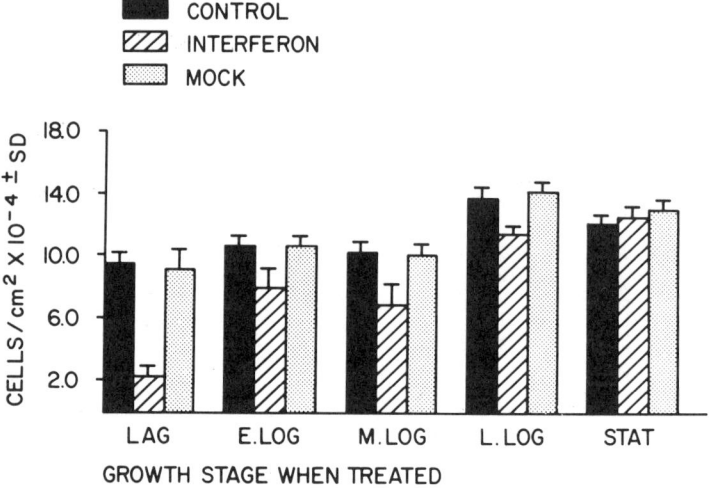

Figure 7 Effect on growth of glioblastoma (12-18) cells exposed to IFN (1000 IU/ml medium) for 3 days during different stages of growth curve. Columns, mean of at least three cultures; bars, SE. The ordinate values were obtained by multiplying cell density by 10^{-4}. Lag, first 3 days after plating; E, early; M, middle; L, late (referring to logarithmic phase by growth curve); STAT, stationary growth phase at confluency. (From Ref. 51.)

For interferon to have a biologic effect, it must first bind to a receptor at the surface of the cell. Some gangliosides (especially GM_2) bind to and neutralize the biologic effects of interferon, so it was suggested that ganglioside may be at least part of the interferon receptor (53-56). If it were, then it may be possible to augment the responsiveness of a cell to interferon by increasing the amount of ganglioside at its surface. An increase in the sensitivity to cholera toxin of cells following their incubation with GM_1 ganglioside, which is the receptor for this toxin, was previously demonstrated (57). The growth of cultured human fetal brain cells is inhibited by some gangliosides but not by 1000 U HuIFN-β per milliliter growth medium. The 12-18 line of human glioblastoma cells is inhibited by HuIFN-β but not gangliosides. Therefore, this is an excellent model to test whether preincubation of either human glioma or fetal brain cells with gangliosides makes the cells more responsive to interferon. We conducted an extensive series of experiments to test this possibility (51). The results of one of these experiments is shown in Figure 8. This demonstrates that the human fetal brain cells (CHII) were slightly inhibited by a mixture of gangliosides isolated from human brain but were insensitive to HuIFN-β either with or without preincubation with gangliosides. Growth of the 12-18 glioblastoma cells was inhibited by the interferon, but this effect was not augmented by preincubating the cells with gangliosides isolated from normal human brain. It was thought that perhaps the dose of HuIFN-β used was causing the maximum possible amount of growth inhibition of 12-18 cells, so the experiment was repeated with one-tenth the concentration of HuIFN-β, but similar results were obtained. GM_2 had been shown to be the ganglioside with the most potent effect of neutralizing interferon. Therefore, these experiments were performed once more but using purified GM_2 isolated from the brain of a patient with Tay-Sachs disease. Again, there were negative results. From this we concluded that the growth inhibitory effects of HuIFN-β cannot be augmented by preincubating the cells with gangliosides. Furthermore, it seems unlikely that the receptor for HuIFN-β consists solely of ganglioside, but these experiments do not prove that ganglioside is not part of the receptor complex.

B. Effects of Interferon on Natural Killer Cytolysis of Human Glioma Cells

Natural killer cells are described morphologically as large granular lymphocytes that attack and lyse a variety of cultured tumor cells without prior exposure to them. Using an in vitro chromium release assay (58,59), we tested the ability of human NK cells to lyse cultured human glioma, fetal brain, and schwannoma cells and found these targets to be relatively insensitive to NK attack (60). The process leading to NK cytolysis involves two steps: (1) binding the NK cells to the target; and (2) lysis of the target cells. Using single cell assays we found that the resistance of some glioma cells is mainly due to a low frequency with which the NK cells bind to the glioma targets. Binding of NK cells to some other

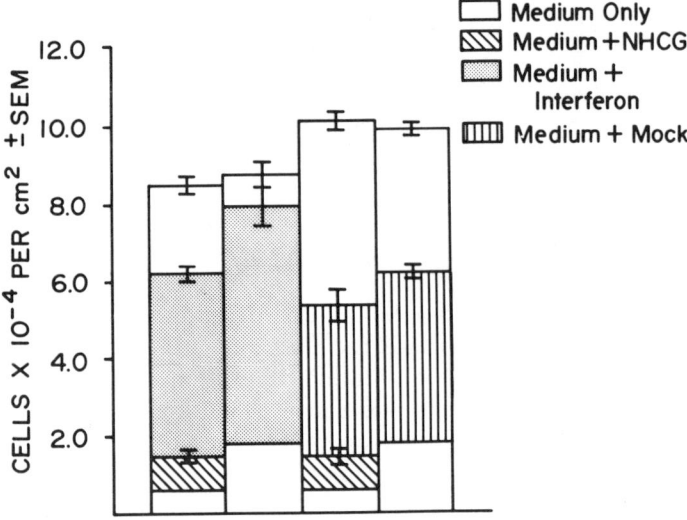

Figure 8 Cell densities of cultures of human fetal brain cells (CHII) of IFN (1000 IU/ml medium), mock IFN, and 50 μm NHCG. Several flasks were seeded in medium at 5000 cells/cm². After 1 day of growth, cell counts were performed on at least three flasks. All remaining cultures were washed; one-half received medium with NHCG and the other half, medium only. Cells from several flasks were counted 2 days later, and the medium changed in the remaining, half of which received IFN and half mock IFN. Cell counts were made 3 days later, and medium in all remaining flasks was changed to standard medium. All remaining cultures were harvested when a series of parallel cultures grown only in standard medium had reached confluency. Each column represents one series of treatment combinations. Each segment of the column is coded to represent the medium in which the cells were grown for that part of the experiment. The time sequence of treatment progresses from the bottom to the top of each column. The cell density at the termination of each stage of this progression is represented by the horizontal lines in each column. Each value is the mean of at least three cultures; bars, SE. The ordinate values were obtained by multiplying cell density by 10^{-4}. (From Ref. 51.)

glioma cells is reasonably high, but the glioma cells that bind to NK are resistant to subsequent cytolytic events. Still other glioma cells have both low frequencies of binding and are resistant to cytolysis (60).

Exposure of NK cells to IFN prior to mixing them with the target cells in assays for NK activity increases the cytolytic activity of the NK cells toward many types of nonneural cells. We found a similar phenomenon using human glioma and fetal brain cells as targets. Preincubation of the NK cells with either HuIFN-α or HuIFN-β increased the percentage specific lysis of these target cells. The magnitude of this increase varied among the cell lines tested, and although the increase for some cell lines was several-fold, the percentage specific lysis never exceeded 40% with an effector-target ratio of 50:1. By comparison, the NK-sensitive control lymphoblastoid cell line Molt-4 and the control resistant Raji line have specific lyses of approximately 80 and 40%, respectively. Therefore, even with the interferon activation of the NK cells these neural targets remain fairly resistant to NK cytolysis.

Several types of nonneural cells become more resistant to NK attack following their exposure to IFN (61,62). We examined this phenomenon for fetal brain and glioma cells by adding 1000 U HuIFN-β per milliliter growth medium when the cells were in the late log phase of growth. They were harvested 3 days later and used as targets in a chromium release assay to determine their sensitivities to cytolysis by IFN-activated NK cells. The results of these studies are seen in Figure 9. One fetal brain (CH-I) and one glioma (U-251MG) cell line were extremely resistant to NK attack, and pre-exposure to HuIFN-β had no measurable effect on this resistance. The other fetal brain cell line was slightly more sensitive, but HuIFN-β had no effect on it, either. Exposure of the other three glioma cell lines to HuIFN-β made them more resistant to NK cytolysis, but this was most pronounced for I29-A and 7-24 cells. From this it is concluded that HuIFN-β can increase the resistance of human glioma cells to NK cytolysis.

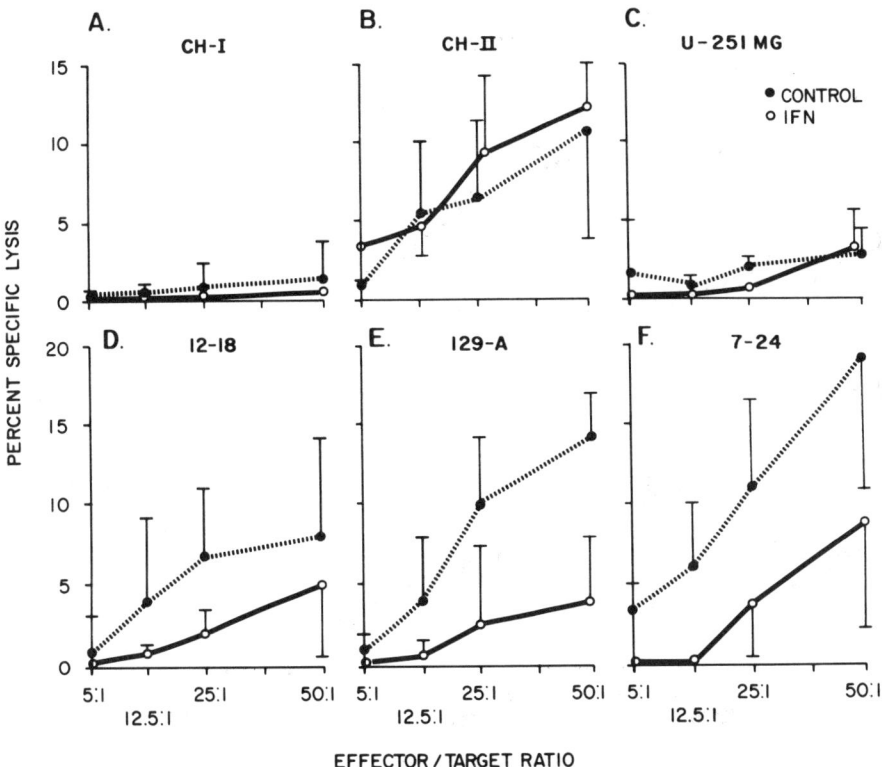

Figure 9 The indicated cell lines were cultured 3 days in medium alone (control ●▥▥●) or medium supplemented with 1000 U/ml human IFN (○—○) and tested for their sensitivity to NK cytolysis in a standard 4 hr ^{51}Cr release assay. The results represent the means of three separate experiments. The vertical bars show standard deviations. (From Ref. 63.)

C. Biochemical Effects of Interferon on Human Glioma Cells

Concurrent with the growth inhibitory effect of 5000 U HuIFN-β per milliliter medium on the human glioma cell line KNS-42, there are changes in the morphology and chemical composition of these cells (50). The volume of treated cells increases, and they have larger and more cytoplasmic processes. These changes correlate with greater amounts of total cellular protein and glial fibrillary acidic protein. We also found a larger amount of total protein in IFN-treated neural cells but not as large as that found by the previous authors (63). This effect may vary considerably among cell lines.

Studies on lymphoid cells have shown that IFN can alter the cellular composition of glycolipids, and it has been suggested that such changes may be responsible for alterations in the NK susceptibility of IFN-treated cells (64,65). We found a consistent increase in the amount of total neutral glycolipid in both fetal brain and glioma cells exposed to HuIFN-β (63). Separation and quantitation of specific neutral glycolipids using high-performance liquid chromatography showed that in all cell lines studied the major ones were cerebroside with nonhydroxy fatty acids, ceramide dihexoside, ceramide trihexoside, and globoside. Lesser amounts of hydroxy fatty acid containing cerebroside, asialo GM_1, and asialo GM_2 were present. There were differences in the molar percentage distributions of these compounds among the cell lines, and IFN treatment caused a major change in the distribution of these glycolipids in two glioma cell lines (I29-A and 7-24). In both of these there was a greater proportion of glycolipids with longer oligosaccharide chains. As mentioned earlier, these are the same two glioma lines that had the largest decrease in sensitivity to NK cytolysis. From this we conclude that the total amount of glycolipid (and perhaps total glycoconjugate) may be one of the factors responsible for the resistance of a cell to NK attack. The oligosaccharides of these compounds can interact with each other through hydrogen bonds, and they contribute to the rigidity of the cell surface (66–68). Therefore, it is possible that collectively they could be acting like a scaffolding over the cell surface, and when present in high enough quantities provide sufficient structural stability to the membrane for it to resist the cytolytic effects of NK attack long enough for counterlytic mechanisms to repair the damaged membrane (69,70). Although this remains speculative, it is possible to test this hypothesis experimentally.

The mechanisms through which IFN is causing changes in the glycolipid composition are obscure. The oligosaccharide portion of the molecules are synthesized in the Golgi apparatus by means of specific glycosyltransferases, and the intact molecules are transported to the plasmalemma into which they are inserted. Degradation occurs mainly in the lysosome as a consequence of glycosidases. Either accelerated synthesis or retarded breakdown could lead to the observed changes. A model of glycosyltransferase regulation involves intracellular levels of cyclic AMP, which in some cells increases in response to IFN (71,72). Such a mechanism may be involved in glioma cells, but this has yet to be shown. Glycosyltransferase activities may also be increased as a result of induced synthesis of new enzyme, but this has not been studied, either.

IV. SUMMARY

The effects of different interferons on human malignant brain tumors in patients, nude mice, and cell culture have been studied. Of 203 evaluable patients with primary brain tumors treated with interferons, the best overall effectiveness rate (22%) was with human fibroblast IFN-β. The clinical effectiveness rates for three different types of IFN-a varied between 5 and 20.0%. There were five cases considered to be complete responses. In primary cases the effectiveness rate of human fibroblast IFN-β was 32%; for recurrent cases it was only 6%. The effects of IFN in vivo were also assessed using nude mice into which human glioma cells were transplanted. Treatment with HuIFN-β was considered to be effective in two of six glioma strains studied. The route of administration (intravenous, subcutaneous, or intratuumor) had no effect on outcome. Combinations of HuIFN-β with adriamycin, ACNU, or radiotherapy were more effective than each modality alone.

Interferons added to growth media inhibit the growth of cultured human glioma cells in a dose-dependent fashion. This effect is greater when it is added soon after plating, and IFN must be present for at least several hours to be growth inhibitory. Preincubation of the cells with gangliosides did not augment the growth inhibitory effect of HuIFN-β. Human glioma cells are generally resistant to the cytotoxic effects of human natural killer cells, but this activity is increased by preincubating NK cells with either IFN-α or IFN-β. Exposure of the glioma targets to IFN-β makes some of them more resistant to NK cells and this is associated with an increased amount of neutral glycolipid, suggesting that this group of biochemicals may play a role in the resistance of glioma cells to NK.

It is concluded that interferon therapy could have a role in treating some human gliomas, but further studies are required to define this more precisely. The mechanisms through which IFN affects glioma biology are complex and probably involve: (1) growth inhibition of the tumor cells; (2) augmentation of natural killer cell activity; and (3) effects on the sensitivity of glioma cells to NK cytolysis.

ACKNOWLEDGMENTS

This work was supported in part by the Cancer Research Fund from the Ministry of Health and Welfare, the Scientific Research Grant from the Ministry of Education, Science and Culture, and the Japan Brain Foundation. It was also supported by PHS grant CA-31564 and P30-CA16058 awarded by The National Cancer Institute, DHHS, the Department of Pathology, College of Medicine, The Ohio State University.

REFERENCES

1. Nagai, M., Arai, T., and Kohno, S. Clinical application of fibroblast interferon for malignant brain tumors. *J. Jpn. Soc. Cancer Ther. 15*:758 (1980).

2. Nagai, M., Arai, T., Kohno, S., and Kohase, M. Interferon therapy for malignant brain tumors. In *The Clinical Potential of Interferons* (R. Kono and J. Vilcek, eds.). University of Tokyo Press, Tokyo, 1982, pp. 257-272.

3. Nagai, M. Clinical trials of human fibroblast interferon (HuIFN-β) on malignant brain tumors. *J. Jpn. Soc. Cancer Ther. 18*:60-68 (1983).

4. Takakura, K. Clinical trials of interferon-β (Mr-21) on malignant brain

tumors. Report on interferon research. Mochida Pharma. Co., Tokyo, 1985, pp. 1-18.

5. Kitamura, K. Phase II study of interferon-α 2 (Sch 30500) for brain tumors. *Rinsho Iyaku (J. Clin. Ther.-Med.)* 1:43-58 (1985).

6. Furue, H. Phase II clinical study on interferon-α, produced from human lymphoblast (interferon-α for malignant tumor). *Rinsho Iyaku (J. Clin. Ther.-Med.)* 1:1103-1121 (1985).

7. Takakura, K., and Cooperative Study Group of Ro 22-8181 in Japan. Phase II study of recombinant human interferon α A(Ro 22-8181) in malignant brain tumors. In: *Recent Advances in Chemotherapy* (J. Ishigami, ed.). University of Tokyo Press, Tokyo, 1985, pp. 983-984.

8. Nakamura, O., Maruo, K., Ueyama, Y., Nomura, K., and Takakura, K. Antineoplastic effects of Hu-IFN-β and other anticancer drugs on malignant brain tumors in athymic nude mice. *Neurol. Surg.* 13:503-508 (1985).

9. Ovejera, A. A., and Houchens, D. P. Selection of potential anticancer agents using human tumor xenografts athymic nude mice. Contract 1-CM-67099, NCI.

10. Nakamura, O., Takakura, K., and Kobayaski, S. Effect of human interferon in the treatment of malignant brain tumors. *UCLA Symp. Mol. Cell. Biol.* 24:465-477 (1982).

11. Blomgren, H., Cantell, K., Johansson, B., Lagergren, C., Fingborg, W., and Strander, H. Interferon therapy in Hodgkin's diseases. *Acta Med. Scand.* 199:527-532 (1976).

12. Ikic, D., Padovan, I., Broadarec, I., Knezcviv, M., and Soos, E. Application of human leukocyte interferon in patients with tumor of the head and neck. *Lancet* (8228):1025-1027 (1982).

13. Merigan, T. C., Sikora, K., Breeden, J. H., and Rosenberg, S. A. Preliminary observations on the effect of human leukocyte interferon on non-Hodgkin's lymphoma. *N. Engl. J. Med.* 299:1449-1453 (1978).

14. Strander, H., Cantell, K., Jakobsen, P. A., Nilsonne, U., and Soderberg, G. Exogenous interferon therapy of osteogenic sarcoma. *Acta Orthop. Scand.* 45:958-959 (1974).

15. Boethius, J., Blomgren, H., Collins, V. P., et al. The effect of systemic human interferon-alpha administration to patients with glioblastoma multiforme. *Acta Neurochir. (Wien)* 68:239-251 (1983).

16. Duff, T. A., Borden, E., Bay, J., et al. Phase II trial of interferon-β for treatment of recurrent glioblastoma multiforme. *J. Neurosurg.* 64:408-413 (1986).
17. Hirakawa, K., Ueda, S., Nakagawa, Y., et al. Effects of human leukocyte interferon on malignant brain tumors. *Cancer* 51:1976-1981 (1983).
18. Mahaley, M. S., Jr., Urso, M. B., Whaley, R. A., et al. Immunobiology of primary intracranial tumors. IX. Phase I study of human lymphoblastoid interferon. *J. Biol. Response Mod.* 3:19-25 (1984).
19. Mahaley, M. S., Jr., Urso, M. B., Whaley, R. A., et al. Interferon as adjuvant therapy with initial radiotherapy of patients with anaplastic gliomas. *J. Neurosurg.* 61:1069-1071 (1984).
20. Nagai, M., and Arai, T. Clinical effect of interferon in malignant brain tumours. *Neurosurg. Rev.* 7:55-64 (1984).
21. Obbens, E. A. M. T., Feun, L. G., Leavens, M. E., et al. Phase I clinical trial of intralesional or intraventricular leukocyte interferon for intracranial malignancies. *J. Neuro-oncol.* 3:61-67 (1985).
22. Salford, L. G., Stromblad, L. G., Nordstrom, C. M., et al. Intratumoral administration of interferon in malignant gliomas. *Acta Neurochir. (Wien)* 56:130-131 (1981).
23. Aapro, M. S., Alberts, D. S., and Salmon, S. E. Interactions of human leukocytes interferon with vinca alkaloids and other chemotherapeutic agents against human tumors in clonogenic assay. *Cancer Chemother. Pharmacol.* 10:161-166 (1983).
24. Brostram, L. A. The combined effect of interferon and methotrexate on human osteosarcoma and lymphoma cell lines. *Cancer Let.* 10:83-90 (1980).
25. Chirigos, M. A., and Pearson, J. W. Cure of murine leukemia with drug and interferon treatment. *JNCI* 51:1367-1368 (1973).
26. Gresser, I., Maury, C., and Tovey, M. Efficacy of combined interferon, cyclophosphamide therapy after diagnosis of lymphoma in AKR mice. *Eur. J. Cancer* 15:97-99 (1978).
27. Inoue, M., and Tan, Y. H. Enhancement of actinomycin D and *cis*-diamminedichloroplatinum induced killing of human fibroblast by α-interferon. *Cancer Res.* 43:5484-5488 (1983).
28. Kuwata, T., Fuse, A., and Morinaga, N. Combined effects of interferon

and antitumor drugs on the growth of human transformed cells in vitro. Int. Soc. Chemotherapy Proc. 10th Int. Congr. of Chemotherapy. 1978, pp. 1103-1106.

29. Namba, M., Miyoshi, T., Kanamori, T., Nobuhara, M., Kimoto, T., and Ogawa, S. Combined effects of 5-fluorouracil and interferon on proliferation of human neoplastic cells in culture. *Gann (Jpn. J. Cancer Res.) 73*: 819-824 (1982).

30. Oku, T., Imanishi, J., and Kishida, T. Assessment of antitumor cell effect of human leukocyte interferon in combination with anticancer agents by a convenient assay system in monolayer cell culture. *Gann (Jpn. J. Cancer Res.) 73*:667-674 (1982).

31. Slater, L. M., Wetzel, M. W., and Cesario, T. Combined interferon-antimetabolite therapy of murine L1210 leukemia. *Cancer 48*:5-9 (1981).

32. Talas, M., nd Szolgay, E. Radioprotective activity of interferon inducers. *Arch. Virol. 56*:309-315 (1978).

33. Miyoshi, T., et al. Effects of interferon on the growth of irradiated sarcoma 180 cells in vitro. *Igaku no Ayumi (Tokyo) 112*:526-528 (1980).

34. Ito, H. Antitumor and radiation sensitizing effect of human leukocyte interferon in vitro. *Nippon Acta Radiol. 41*:551-558 (1981).

35. Ortaldo, J. R., and McCoy, J. L. Protective effects of interferon in mice previously exposed to lethal irradiation. *Radiat. Res. 81*:262-266 (1980).

36. Lindahl, P., Leary, P., and Gresser, I. Effects of interferon on cells. In: *Viruses and the Immune System* (A. Geraldes, ed.). Academic Press, London, 1975, pp. 471-482.

37. Schultz, R. M., Popmatheakis, J. D., and Chirigos, M. A. Interferon; an inducer of macrophage activation by polyanions. *Science 197*:674-676 (1977).

38. Herberman, R. B., Ortaldo, J. R., and Bonnord, G. D. Augmentation by interferon of human natural and antibody-dependent cell-mediated cytotoxicity. *Nature 177*:221-223 (1979).

39. Winkler, K., et al. Adjuvant chemotherapy in osteosarcoma: Effects of cisplatinum, BCD and fibroblast interferon in sequential.

40. Arai, T., Nagai, M., and Watari, T. Combination therapy of interferon and radiation to malignant brain tumors. *J. Jpn. Soc. Cancer Ther. 19*: 139 (1984).

41. Miyoshi, T., et al. Preliminary study of children's brain tumors treated by interferon (IFN-a) and radiation. *J. Jpn. Soc. Cancer Ther. 19*:140 (1984).

42. Ponten, J., and Macintyre, E. H. Long term culture of normal and neoplastic human glia. *Acta Pathol. Scand. 74*:465 (1968).

43. Shapiro, J. R., Yung, W. A., and Shapiro, W. R. Isolation, karyotype, and clonal growth of heterogeneous subpopulations of human malignant gliomas. *Cancer Res. 41*:2349 (1981).

44. Westermark, B., Ponten, J., and Hugosson, R. Determinants for the establishment of permanent tissue culture lines from human gliomas. *Acta Pathol. Microbiol. Scand.* [A] *81*:791 (1973).

45. Cook, A. W., Carter, W. A., and Nidzgorski, F. Human brain tumor-derived cell lines: Growth rate reduced by human fibroblast interferon. *Science 219*:881–883 (1983).

46. Larsson, I., Lanstrom, L.-E., Larner, E., Lundgren, E., Miorner, H., and Strannegard, O. Interferon production in glia and glioma cell lines. *Infect. Immun. 22*:786–789 (1978).

47. Iivanainen, M., Laaksonen, R., Niemi, M.-L., Farkkila, M., Bergstrom, L., Mattson, K., Niiranen, A., and Cantell, K. Memory and psychomotor impairment following high-dose interferon treatment in amyotrophic lateral sclerosis. *Acta Neurol. Scand. 72*:475–480 (1985).

48. Lundblad, D., and Lundgren, E. Block of a glioma cell line in S by interferon. *Int. J. Cancer 27*:749–754 (1981).

49. Slimmer, S., Masui, H., and Kaplan, N. O. Antiproliferative assay for human interferons. *Methods Enzymol. 79*:419–422 (1981).

50. Korosue, K., Takeshita, I., Mannoji, H., and Fukui, M. Interferon effects on multiplication, cytoplasmic protein and GFAP content and morphology in human glioma cells. *J. Neuro-Oncol. 1*:69–76 (1983).

51. Yates, A. J., Stephens, R. E., Elder, P. J., Markowitz, D. L., and Rice, J. M. Effects of interferon and gangliosides on growth of cultured human glioma and fetal brain cells. *Cancer Res. 45*:1033–1039 (1985).

52. Nederman, T., and Benediktsson, G. Effects of interferon on growth

rate and radiation sensitivity of cultured, human glioma cells. *Acta Radiol. Oncol.* 21:231-234 (1982).

53. Ankel, H., Besancon, F., and Krishnamurti, C. Intrerferon-carbohydrate interaction. *ACS (Am. Chem. Soc.) Symp. Ser.* 128:391-405 (1980).

54. Besancon, F., and Ankel, H. Binding of interferon to gangliosides. *Nature* 252:478-480 (1974).

55. Besancon, F., Ankel, H., and Basu, S. Specificity and reversibility of interferon ganglioside interaction. *Nature* 259:576-578 (1976).

56. Krishnamurti, C., Besancon, F., Justesen, J., Poulsen, K., and Ankel, H. Inhibition of mouse fibroblast interferon by gangliosides. Differential effects on biological activity and on induction of (2'-5') oligoadenylate synthetase. *Eur. J. Biochem.* 124:1-6 (1982).

57. Fishman, P. H., Moss, J., and Vaughan, M. Uptake and metabolism of gangliosides in transformed mouse fibroblasts. *J. Biol. Chem.* 251:4490-4494 (1976).

58. Opremcak, E. M., Bankenhaster, K., and Whisler, R. L. NK and K cell characteristics of human lymphocytes enriched for subpopulations isolated from NK tumor cell conjugates. *Cell. Immunol.* 58:415-425 (1981).

59. Timonen, T., and Saksela, E. Isolation of human NK cells by density gradient centrifugation. *J. Immunol. Methods* 36:285-291 (1980).

60. Yates, A. J., Icard-Lipekalns, C., Sirinek, L. P., Stephens, R. E., Elder, P. J., Liepkalns, V. A., and Whisler, R. L. Natural killer activity against cultured human neural tumor, and fetal brain cells. *Cell. Immunol.* 90: 485-492 (1985).

61. Hansson, M., Kiessling, R., Andersson, B., and Welsh, R. M. Effect of interferon and interferon inducers on the NK sensitivity of normal mouse thymocytes. *J. Immunol.* 125:2225-2231 (1980).

62. Welsh, R. M., Karre, K., Hansson, M., Kunkel, L. A., and Kiessling, R. W. Interferon-mediated protection of normal and tumor target cells against lysis by mouse natural killer cells. *J. Immunol.* 126:219-225 (1981).

63. Yates, A. J., Stephens, R. E., Markowitz, D. L., Elder, P. J., Sirinek, L. P., and Whisler, R. L. Resistance to natural killer cytolysis and neutral glycolipid composition of cultured human glioma and fetal brain cells. *J. Neuropathol. Exp. Neurol.* 44:371-383 (1985).

64. Yogeeswaran, G., Gronberg, A., Hansson, M., Delianis, T., Kiessling, R.,

and Welsh, R. M. Correlation of glycosphingolipids and sialic acid in YAC-1 lymphoma variants with their sensitivity to natural killer-cell-mediated lysis. *Int. J. Cancer 28*:517-526 (1981).

65. Young, W. W., Jr., Durdik, J. M., Urdal, D., Hakomori, S., and Henney, C. S. Glycolipid expression in lymphoma cell variants: Chemical quantity, immunologic reactivity, and correlations with susceptibility to NK cells. *J. Immunol. 126*:1-6 (1981).

66. Bach, D., and Sela, B. A. A differential scanning calorimetry study of the interaction of gangliosides with peanut lectin, serotonin and daunomycin. *Biochim. Biophys. Acta 596*:186-191 (1980).

67. Bertoli, E., Maserini, M., Sonnino, S., Ghidoni, R., Cestaro, B., and Tettamanti, G. Electron paramagnetic resonance studies on the fluidity and surface dynamics of egg phosphatidylcholine vesicles containing gangliosides. *Biochim. Biphys. Acta 647*:196-202 (1981).

68. Holmgren, J., and Lindholm, L. Cholera toxin, ganglioside receptors, and the immune response. *Immunol. Commun. 5*:737-756 (1976).

69. Collins, J. L., Patek, P. Q., and Cohn, M. Tumorigenicity and lysis by natural killer cells. *J. Exp. Med. 153*:89-106 (1981).

70. Hudig, D., Djobadze, M., Redelman, D., and Mendelsohn, J. Active tumor cell resistance to human natural killer lymphocyte attack. *Cancer Res. 41*:2803-2808 (1981).

71. Dawson, G., McLawhon, R., and Miller, R. J. Opiates and enkephalins inhibit synthesis of gangliosides and membrane glycoproteins in mouse neuroblastoma cell line N4TG1. *Proc. Natl. Acad. Sci. USA 76*:605-609 (1979).

72. Dawson, G., McLawhon, R., and Miller, R. J. Inhibition of sialoglycosphingolipid (ganglioside) biosynthesis in mouse clonal lines N4TG1 and NG108-15 by beta-endorphin, enkephalins, and opiates. *J. Biol. Chem. 255*:129-137 (1980).

13
Interferons and Neurologic Disease: Epilogue

DAVID GOLDSTEIN and ERNEST C. BORDEN

University of Wisconsin Clinical Cancer Center, Madison, Wisconsin

The future role of interferons (IFN) in the treatment of neurologic disorders can be viewed based upon its roles as an antiviral agent, an immune modulator, and an antiproliferative agent.

IFN are usually synthesized early in response to viral disease. Viruses that cause delayed or chronic illness, however, may also be influenced. The use of IFN is supported by the responses in rabies (Hovanessian et al.) and in subacute sclerosing panencephalitis (Panitch et al.), both discussed in this volume, in addition to responses in progressive multifocal leukoencephalopathy and herpesvirus (1), in chronic hepatitis B (2), and in the virally induced papillomas and condylomas (3). In these diseases, persistent viral expression somehow overcomes normal immune responses and causes ongoing damage either by direct effects or indirectly by a continuing ineffective endogenous inflammatory response. Although the mechanism by which IFN act in these diseases is unclear, correction of subtle immune defects or reduction in viral antigen load may allow for effective viral clearance. The induction of endonucleases such as that induced by $2',5'$-oligoadenylate synthetase may be important in these antiviral effects (4,5).

In multiple sclerosis (MS), an immune modulatory rather than an antiviral effect may be important. Unlike the clinical experience with hepatitis B virus, there appears to be a prolonged effect after cessation of IFN. The rather complex interactions of IFN with the immune system and their effects on exacerbations of MS were recently reviewed (1). Salazar has suggested that fluctuating levels of IFN may correlate with initiation and subsequent termination of the attacks; that is, higher levels lead to remission, possibly by increased suppressor activity or change in neural cell antigen expression. The work reviewed in this volume suggests that IFN holds its greatest promise as long-term prophylaxis against exacerbations in early relapsing-remitting disease.

Chapter 9 by Panitch and Johnson and Jacobs et al. in Chapter 10 reviewed the favorable results in MS of both leukocyte and fibroblast IFN. Panitch et al. (5), however, have data to suggest that IFN-γ is likely to exacerbate the disease. The explanation is likely to be more complex than just the potentially harmful effect of HLA-DR induction and possible increased antigenicity (5). Since class II antigen expression can be induced by crude leukocyte preparations (6) and by IFN-β (7), both of which show promise in this condition, other effects of IFN-γ need to be considered. Alternative possibilities include enhancement of interleukin-1 (IL-1) release by IFN-γ (8). IL-1 has been produced in vitro by stimulation of microglial cells (9) and has also been shown to induce glial cell proliferation (10); thus an increase in its production could be implicated in the IFN-γ-induced exacerbations.

The variability in effects of IFN on immunologic parameters in patients (3) probably better reflects the insensitivity of our current tests than a lack of real modulation. The therapeutic response in multiple sclerosis supports this thesis. Alternative ways of looking at immune activation, such as IL-2 receptor number and functional macrophage assays, are being investigated by several groups, including ours, to provide more sensitive measures of immune modulation. Nevertheless, it already seems clear that there is a dose threshold above which there is no further increment and possibly a decrease in natural killer (NK) cell activity enhancement and $2',5'$-oligoadenylate synthetase induction (11-13). Thus, despite the poor response to recombinant 2×10^6 MU IFN-α reported Chapter 9 by Panitch and Johnson, exploration of low-dose regimens in multiple sclerosis should continue.

Identifying the optimal IFN presents a major challenge. As Panitch et al. point out, the diversity of functions of the different subtypes of IFN-α are only beginning to be explored. A recent paper showed marked differences in increases in antigen expression with different α subtypes in vitro (14); clinical differences of two IFN-α subtypes have also been defined (15). The use of the lymphoblastoid IFN-α with its combination of subtypes represents one approach.

Introduction of a stable recombinant IFN-β molecule into the clinic (16) has led to initiation of studies in MS patients. The responses reported by Jacobs et al. with natural IFN-β are grounds for optimism (17). The development of IFN-β is a model for recombinant production of molecules designed for a specific biologic effect. Recombinant production of IFN-β in *Escherichia coli* resulted in a molecule with impaired potency. Subsequent substitution of cysteine by serine has overcome earlier problems of abnormal disulfide bonds and produced a compound equipotent with natural fibroblast β in much more available quantities.

An alternative approach in developing IFN has been the production of compounds combining different subtypes of IFN-α (18). One approach is to create *hybrids*, compounds that combine complementary segments of different IFN. Another is the synthesis of *consensus* molecules that contain the amino acid sequences found to be the most common among several different subtypes (18). Such consensus molecules already exist and are undergoing clinical trials. Future development of potent IFN with minimal side effects, however, requires a greater understanding of how the immune modulating and systemic side effects are mediated. Ultimately such consensus molecules may combine complementary aspects of all three IFN subtypes.

The question of route of administration is also of considerable importance. In the case of proteins like IFN, which are rapidly cleared from circulation, the most appropriate route for maximal immunomodulation may be intradermal, that is, intralymphatic

(19). An even more complicating factor is the issue of the blood-brain barrier, as discussed by Smith et al. In Chapter 11, they have evidence suggesting that systemic IFN therapy can also result in induction of IFN-induced proteins in the central nervous system (CNS) (20), although the intraventricular route is to be preferred. The clinical data for multiple sclerosis and glioma (see below) also support further investigation of local, that is intraventricular or intrathecal application.

As in malignant disease, single agents may have limited effectiveness, with rapid return of symptoms after cessation of treatment. Thus combination therapy with other antiviral agents, such as acyclovir, will be explored, as in vitro data show significant synergism (21). The in vitro data from antiproliferative studies have shown synergism between types I and II IFN (22) and other lymphokines, most notably TNF (23), combinations that are being actively explored in cancer trials. Similar interactions may prove to be therapeutic in neurologic disorders. Despite the negative effects of IFN-γ as a single agent, the availability of a murine animal model of MS—experimental allergic encephalitis (24,25)—lends itself to the exploration of possible cooperation of IFN either in sequence or jointly.

Neurologic malignancy remains an uncertain area. Early studies using human fibroblast IFN have been encouraging, as Takakura has documented. As with MS, it may be that local therapy will give much higher response rates (26) than the median response rate reported in the literature (3). Since the antiproliferative response of IFN appears to be a linear dose response, the use of indomethacin to reduce side effects, shown by Jacobs, is encouraging as it may increase the therapeutic index.

The data from our program at the University of Wisconsin (27, 28) and other laboratories (as cited in Chapter 12 by Takakura et al.) regarding synergism of IFN with both chemotherapy and radiotherapy suggest the future direction for gliomas and indeed probably all solid tumors. In this regard, work with the lipid-soluble drugs, such as BCNU, VP-16, and *Vinca* alkaloids, should be explored further in vitro and in phase I trials. Similarly, Takakura et al. have shown interesting data regarding the in vitro use of IFN as an adjuvant to radiation. Other studies in several malignant cell lines support the synergistic effect of IFN after, rather than preceding, radiotherapy (29). As with other tumor studies, it is reasonable to suspect that IFN is far more likely to be effective in the adjuvant setting with a small tumor burden, particularly from an immune modulating perspective.

A totally different area of investigation with regard to the impact of IFN on the central nervous system appears in the work of Blalock (30) and others in the expanding field of neuroimmunology (31). Several groups have shown that stimulated lymphocytes can produce neuropeptides, such as ACTH and γ-endorphin, by activation of the propiomelanocortin gene concurrently with production of IFN (32–34). Blalock's group has also demonstrated that mice injected intracerebrally with crude human IFN-a showed analgesia and catatonia similar to that induced by β-endorphin and morphine, which could be reversed by naloxone (35). They further demonstrated competition in vitro with [^{3}H]dihydromorphine for binding to the opiate receptor with IFN-a, but not with IFN-β or IFN-γ (35). Subsequent experiments with recombinant IFN-a in vivo using microiontopheretic technqiues of direct application to rat cerebra have shown that the actions of IFN on the brain cannot be blocked by naloxone and indeed have an excitatory effect on neurons (in contrast to the depressive effect of morphine) (36).

Taken together, such data imply that activation of lymphocytes may be associated with release of other peptides in association with IFN, which could thus be the source of some of the neurologic toxicity, particularly of IFN-a. We are currently using different lymphokines to explore the effect of endorphin blockade in animal models to decide whether it will improve tolerance to IFN without compromising efficacy. Since both β-endorphin and ACTH modulate the immune system (37,38), their blockage could have a negative impact and thus negate any reduction in side effects.

Other effects of IFN-γ on the nervous system have recently been reported. Decreases in cerebrospinal fluid 5-hydroxyindoleacetic acid in response to treatment have been shown (39). This may be related to effects of IFN-γ showing increases in

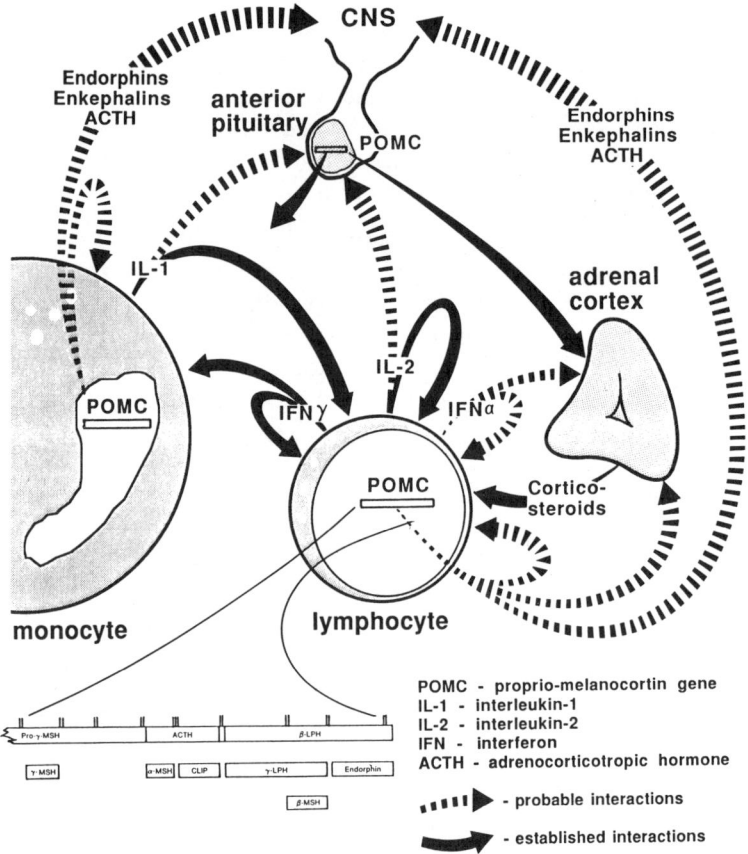

Figure 1 Interactions among the immune, nervous, and endocrine systems.

tryptophan metabolism (40). Since serotonin has been shown to suppress class II Ag expression (41), increased serotonin degradation may be one of the mechanisms allowing for the increases in antigen expression seen in response to IFN-γ. The exacerbation with IFN-γ of such diseases as MS mentioned earlier may be related to an alteration in tryptophan metabolism. It is relevant to note that the decreases in serotonin seen during IFN-γ therapy were not associated with the types of neurotoxicities reported with IFN-α (3,39). It is thus possible that we can expect a spectrum of neurologic side effects according to the type of IFN used and the resulting associations of either neuropeptide release or tryptophan degradation.

The increases in corticosteroids after IFN-γ (42), IFN-β (43), and IFN-α (44) suggest another mechanism by which CNS effects could occur. In this case, although the increases are only moderately elevated above the upper limit of normal, significant elevations in free cortisol, which could have profound effects, may occur.

These coupled interactions among the IFN, the CNS, and the endocrine systems serve to underscore potential links between the immune and nervous systems via neuropeptides, IFN, and other cytokines. As Blalock has suggested, the immune system appears to be linked in a direct way with the CNS, resulting in the opportunity for profound reciprocal interactions (Fig. 1).

Future developments in this area will undoubtedly result in unexpected therapeutic options in a variety of neurologic disorders. As reviewed in this volume, the need exists to probe these horizons further. IFN will likely prove a prototype for dissecting the role of other cytokines in the therapy of neurologic disease.

REFERENCES

1. Salazar, A. M., Gibbs, C. J., Gajdusek, D. C., and Smith, R. A. Clinical use of interferons: Central nervous system disorders. In: *Handbook of Experimental Pharmacology*, Vol. 71, 1984, pp. 472–497.
2. Dooley, J. S., Davis, G. L., Peters, M., Waggoner, J. G., Goodman, Z., and

Hoofnagle, J. H. Pilot study of recombinant human α-interferon for chronic type B hepatitis. *Gastroenterology 90*:150-157 (1986).

3. Goldstein, D., and Laszlo, J. Interferon therapy in cancer: From imaginon to interferon. *Cancer Res. 46*:4315-4329 (1986).

4. Revel, M., Kimchi, A., Shulman, L., Fradin, A. Shuster, R., Yakobson, E., Chernajovsky, Y., Schmidt, A., Shure, A., and Bendori, R. Role of interferon-induced enzymes in the antiviral and antimitogenic effects of interferon. *Ann. N.Y. Acad. Sci. 350*:459-472 (1980).

5. Panitch, H. S., Hirsch, R. L., Haley, A. S., and Johnson, K. P. Exacerbations of multiple sclerosis in patients treated with gamma interferon. *Lancet 1*:893-895 (1987).

6. Revel, M. The interferon system in man. In: *Antiviral Drugs and Interferon: The Molecular Basis of Their Activity* Becker, (ed.). Martinus Nijhoff, Boston, 1984, pp. 358-433.

7. Spear, G. T., Paulnock, D. M., Jordan, R. L., Meltzer, D. M., Merritt, J. A., and Borden, E. C. Enhancement of monocyte class I and II histocompatibility antigen expression in many by in vivo interferon-β. *Clin. Exp. Immunol.* in press, (1987).

8. Arenzana-Seisdedos, F., Virelizier, J. L., and Fiers, W. Interferons as macrophage-activating factors. III. Preferential effects of interferon-γ on the interleukin 1 secretory potential of fresh or aged human monocytes. *J. Immunol. 134*:2444-2448 (1985).

9. Giulian, D., and Lachman, L. B. Interleukin-1 stimulation of astroglial proliferation after brain injury. *Science 228*:497-499 (1985).

10. Giulian, D., Baker, T. J., Shi, L. N., and Lachman, L. B. Interleukin 1 of the central nervous system is produced by ameboid microglia. *J. Exp. Med. 164*:594-604 (1986).

11. Edwards, B. S., Merritt, J. A., Fuhlbrigge, R. L., and Borden, E. C. Low doses of interferon α result in more effective clinical natural killer cell activation. *J. Clin. Invest. 75*:1908-1913 (1985).

12. Laszlo, J., Huang, A. T., Brenckman, W. D., Jeffs, C., Koren, H. S., Cianciolo, G., Metzgar, R., Cashdollar, R., Cox, E., Buckley, C. E., Tso, C. Y., and Lucas, V. S. Phase I study of pharmacological and immunological effects of human lymphoblastoid interferon given to patients with cancer. *Cancer Res. 43*:4458-4466 (1983).

13. Merritt, J. A., Ball, L. A., Sielaff, K. M., Meltzer, D., and Borden, E. C.

Modulation of 2,′5′-oligoadenylate synthetase in patients treated with alpha-interferon: Effects of dose, schedule, and route of administration. *J. Interferon Res.* 6:189 (1986).

14. Greiner, J., Fisher, P., Pestka, S., and Schlom, J. Differential effects of recombinant human leukocyte interferons on cell surface antigen expression. *Cancer Res.* 46:4984-4990 (1986).

15. Hawkins, M. J., Borden, E. C., Merritt, J. A., Edwards, B. S., Ball, L. A., Grossbard, E., and Simon, K. J. Comparison of the biologic effects of two recombinant human interferons alpha (rA and rD) in humans. *J. Clin. Oncol.* 2:221-226 (1984).

16. Hawkins, M. J., Horning, S., Konrad, W., Anderson, S., Sielaff, K. M., Rosno, S., Schiesel, J., Davis, T. E., DeMets, D., Merigan, T., and Borden, E. C. Phase I evaluation of a synthetic mutant of β-interferon. *Cancer Res.* 45:5914-5920 (1985).

17. Jacobs, L., Salazar, A. M., Herndon, R., Reese, P., Freeman, A., Josefowicz, R., Cuetter, A., Husain, F., Smith, W. A., Ekes, R., and O'Malley, J. A. Multicentre double-blind study of effect of intrathecally administered natural human fibroblast interferon on exacerbations of multiple sclerosis. *Lancet* 2:1411-1413 (1986).

18. Altrock, B. W., Fagin, K. D., Hockman, H. R., Fish, E. N., Goldstein, L., Chang, D., Duker, K., and Stebbing, N. Antiviral and antitumor effects of a human interferon analog, IFN-αCon 1, assessed in hamsters. *J. Interferon Res.* 6:405-415, (1986).

19. Bocci, V. Immunomodulators as local hormones: New insights regarding their clinical utilization. *J. Biol. Respir. Mod.* 4:340-352 (1985).

20. Smith, R. A., Landel, C., Cornelius, C. E., and Revel, M. Mapping the action of interferon on primate brain. *J. Interferon Res.* 6(Suppl.):140 (1986).

21. Eppstein, D. A., and Marsh, Y. V. Potent synergistic inhibition of herpes simplex virus-2 by 9-[1,3-dihydroxy-2-propoxy)methyl] guanine in combination with recombinant interferons. *Biochem. Biophys. Res. Commun.* 120:66-73 (1984).

22. Schiller, J. H., Groveman, D. S., Schmid, S. M., Willson, J. K. V., Cummings, K. B., and Borden, E. C. Synergistic antiproliferative effects of human recombinant α54- or β-ser interferon with γ-interferon on human cell lines of various histogenesis. *Cancer Res.* 46:483-487 (1986).

23. Lee, S. H., Aggarwal, B. B., Rinderknecht, E., Assisi, F., and Chiu, H.

The synergistic anti-proliferative effect of γ interferon and human lymphotoxin. *J. Immunol. 133*:1083-1086 (1984).

24. Abreu, S., Tondreau, J., Levine, S., and Sowinski, R. Inhibition of passive localized experimental allergic encephalomyelitis by interferon. *Int. Arch. Allergy Appl. Immunol. 72*:30-33 (1983).

25. Hertz, F., and Deghengi, R. Effect of rat and β-human interferons on hyperacute experimental allergic encephalomyelitis in rats. *Agents Actions 16*:397-402 (1985).

26. Nagai, M., and Arai, T. Clinical effect of interferon in malignant brain tumors. *Neurosurg. Rev. 7*:55-64 (1984).

27. Borden, E. C., Sidky, Y., Groveman, D. S., and Bryan, G. T. Antitumor effects of polyribonucleotides for mouse transitional cell carcinoma enhanced by cyclophosphamide. *Cancer Res. 45*:45-50 (1985).

28. Cummings, K. B., Schmid, S. M., Bryan, G. T., and Borden, E. C. Antiproliferative activity of recombinant interferons α and β for human renal carcinoma cells. Supra-additive activity with elevated temperature or vinblastine. *World J. Urol. 3*:230-233 (1986).

29. Gould, M. N., Kakria, C. K., Olson, S., and Borden, E. C. Radiosensitization of human bronchogenic carcinoma cells by interferon beta. *J. Interferon Res. 4*:123-128 (1984).

30. Blalock, J. E. The immune system as a sensory organ. *J. Immunol. 312*:1067-1069 (1984).

31. Goetzel, J. (ed.). Proceedings of a conference on neuromodulation of immunity and hypersensitivity. *J. Immunol. 135*(Suppl.):739s-862s (1985).

32. Harbour-McMenamin, D., Smith, E. M., and Blalock, J. E. Bacterial lipopolysaccharide induction of leukocyte-derived corticotropin and endorphins. *Infect. Immun. 48*:813-817 (1985).

33. Westly, H. J., Kleiss, A. J., Kelley, K. W., Wong, P. K. Y., and Yuen, P.-H. Newcastle disease virus-infected splenocytes express the proopiomelanocortin gene. *J. Exp. Med. 163*:1589-1594 (1986).

34. Zurawski, G., Benedik, M., Kamb, B. J., Abrams, J. S., Zurawski, S. M., and Lee, F. D. Activation of mouse T-helper cells induces abundant preproenkephalin mRNA synthesis. *Science 232*:772-775 (1986).

35. Smith, E. M., Dion, D. L., and Blalock, J. E. Opiate receptor mediated effects of IFN-alpha and lymphocyte derived endorphin-like peptides. *Prog. Clin. Biol. Res. 192*:259-264 (1985).

36. Reyes-Vazquez, C., Weisbrodt, N., and Dafny, N. Does interferon exert its actions through opiate receptors. *Life Sci.* 35:1015-1021 (1984).
37. Fischer, E. G., and Falke, N. E. B-endorphin modulates immune functions. A review. *Psychother. Psychosom.* 42:195-204 (1984).
38. Johnson, H. M., Torres, B. A., Smith, E. M., Dion, L. D., and Blalock, J. E. Regulation of lymphokine (γ-interferon) production by corticotropin. *J. Immunol.* 132:246-250 (1984).
39. Farkkila, M., Iivanainen, M., Harkonen, M., Laakso, J., Mattson, K., and Cantell, K. Neurotransmitter changes induced by recombinant γ-interferon in patients with lung cancer. *J. Interferon Res.* 6(Suppl. 1) (1986).
40. Byrne, G., Lehmann, L. K., Kirshbaum, J. G., Borden, E. C., Lee, C. M., and Brown, R. R. Induction of tryptophan degradation in vitro and in vivo: A gamma-interferon-stimulated activity. *J. Interferon Res.* 6:389-396 (1986).
41. Sternberg, E. M., Trial, J., Parker, C. W. Effect of serotonin on murine macrophages: Suppression of Ia expression by serotonin and its reversal by 5-ht$_2$ serotonergic receptor antagonists. *J. Immunol.* 137:276-282 (1986).
42. Nolten, W. E., Schiller, J. H., Borden, E. C., Dixon, R. M., and Ehrlich, E. N. Interferon stimulates cortisol production in cancer patients. *Clin. Res.* 34:932A (1986).
43. Laszlo, J., Ellinwood, E., Gockerman, J., et al. Elevation in corticosteroids after gamma interferon therapy. *Proc. Am. Soc. Clin. Oncol.* 5: 895 (1986).
44. Roosth, J., Pollard, R. B., Brown, S. L., and Meyer, III, W. J. Cortisol stimulation by recombinant interferon-α_2. *J. Neuroimmunol.* 12:311-316 (1986).

Index

2-5A dependent RNase, 50-52
2-5A synthetase, 13, 43, 45-46, 50, 52-54, 67, 73, 161-163, 165-171, 177, 318-319
  cDNA, 52
Absolute bioavailability F(abs), 104, 110
Absorption, 109-110, 122
Acid phosphatase, 73
ACTH, 322
Actinomycin D, 67
Activated Killer cells, 75
Acyclovir, 149, 154
Adams, F., 137, 139
Administration: 169, 210, 224
  adaptation, 136
  brain tumor therapy, 310
  intracerebral, 139, 169
  intradermal, 320
  intrathecal, 115, 123, 136, 192-196, 210, 229-231, 240-241, 253, 256, 268, 279, 321

[Administration]
  intraventricular, 115, 123, 136, 192-196, 198-199, 210, 213, 231, 256, 268-271, 321-322
  routes, 119-121, 158-159, 228, 280, 282, 288, 290, 310, 320-321
  side effects, 135, 231
  systemic, 115, 123, 210, 217, 268-269
  tolerance, 119
  toxicity, 136
AIDS-related complex, 54
Alkaline phosphatase, 72
Amyotrophic Lateral Sclerosis:
  endogenous IFN, 268-271
  etiology, 264-267
  immunity, 267
  polio genome, 266
  treatment trials, 268-271
  viral studies, 265-266
Animal models, 109, 158, 160,

[Animal models]
163, 166, 170, 210, 212, 276, 286-289, 293, 301, 310
Antagonistic effect, 73
Antibody: 19, 74, 82
  antirabies, 177
  Ia determinants, 225
  measles, 188
  mouse brain, 173
  neutralization, 160, 162-163
  production, 19, 74
  protein, 189
  rabies virus, 173
  Sendai virus, 217, 219
  SSPE, 188
Antibody-dependent cell-mediated lysis (ADCC), 72, 75, 78, 81, 295
Anticellular effects, 67, 82
Antigen:
  antibody production, 74
  expression, 320
Antiparasitic activity, 21
Antiproliferative effects, 18-19, 56, 66, 71, 74
Antitumor activity, 17, 19, 26, 66
Antiviral effect, 3, 15-16, 54, 66, 70, 82, 169, 177
Antiviral proteins, 67
Apparent volume distribution, 107
Arai, T., 296
Arvin, A., 152
Assay Techniques: 77
  chromium release, 81
  enzyme linked immunosorbent (ELISA), 11
  macrophage, 319
  pharmacokinetic, 108
  plaque reduction, 9
  radioimmunoassays (RIA), 11
  single-cell, 81
  T-cell suppressor, 212
Athymic mice, 174-176, 179

ATP, 55
Autoimmune disorders, 22, 81
Azacytidine, 57

Baer, G. M., 160
Baron, S., 146
Bartman, C. R., 194
B cell helper factor, 73
B cells, 71, 74
Behan, P. O., 194
Behavioral change, 137
Beta-2 microglobulin, 46, 73
Bever, C. T., 225
Bhayani, H., 70
Billiau, A., 115
Bioavailability, 104-105
  intramuscular site, 110
Biochemical effects, 308-310
Biologic properties, 7, 67
Biopterin, 74
Blalock, J. E., 322
Blood-brain barrier, 103, 115, 122-123, 168, 170, 177, 188, 192-193, 210-211, 224-225, 241, 246, 253, 256-258, 260, 268, 321
Bocci, V., 109, 119
Bohoslawec, O., 114
Bone marrow suppression, 25-26, 70
Brain:
  measles, 189
  SSPE, 189
Brain tumors: 275-311, 321
  animal model, 276-277, 286, 288-290, 293, 310
  combination therapy, 289, 291, 293, 295-296, 310
  in-vitro studies, 296-298, 301, 303-305, 307-308, 310-311

INDEX

[Brain tumors]
  treatment with interferon, 276, 279-280, 282, 290
Bye, A., 194

Calcium pulse techniques, 77
cAMP, 12, 310
Cantell, K., 6, 110, 146
Catabolism, 109, 117, 119, 122
Catalano, L. W., 146
cDNA, 46
Cell:
  cycle, 67, 70
  growth, 70
  lines, 72-73
  proliferation, 70-72
  regulation, 43
  types, 82
Cellular:
  differentiation, 67, 71-72
  immunity, 20 (see also Immunity)
  origin, 5, 7
Central nervous system (CNS), 136, 187, 298
Cerebrospinal fluid (CSF), 71, 80-81, 188, 192, 209, 217, 222, 224, 243, 246, 252-254, 256-258, 260, 271, 322
  IgG, 217
  titers, 253
c-fos proto oncogene, 46
Cholera toxins, 304
Chromium-release, 77
Chromosomal localization, 53
Chromosome 7, 55
Chromosome 9, 7, 8, 65
Chromosome 11, 53
Chromosome 12, 8, 53, 55
Chromosome 21, 12, 21

Class II antigens, 73
Clearance, drug, 106
Clearance, renal, 107
c-myc:
  gene, 56
  inhibition, 46
  PDGF, 56
  RNA, 56
Colony stimulating factor, 26
Combination therapy, 26, 289, 291, 293, 295-296, 301, 310, 321-322
Concanavalin A, 66, 80, 82, 212
Concentration, 110
Condyloma, 23, 318
Consensus molecules, 320
Cook, A., 299
Corticosteroids, 323
CSF (see Cerebrospinal fluid)
Cyclic AMP, 12, 310
Cyclic GMP, 12
Cytochrome P_{450}, 48, 119
Cytokines, 323
Cytoplasmic enzymes, 72, 83
Cytoprotection, 78
Cytotoxicity, 75-77, 79, 82, 211

Daudi cells, 44, 56
Dawson, J. R., 187
Definition, 7
Disease:
  amyotrophic lateral sclerosis, 25, 193, 246, 264, 266
  aplastic anemia, 70
  brain tumor, 321
  carcinoma cell line, 295-296
  cerebrovascular accident, 80
  chickenpox, 152, 154
  condyloma acuminatum, 23, 318
  Down's syndrome, 21

[Disease]
  encephalitis, 145, 265
  experimental allergic encephalitis (EAE), 212-213, 225, 227-228, 256, 321
  Grave's, 22
  Guillain-Barre syndrome, 5, 24
  hairy cell leukemia, 23, 136
  hepatitis, 22
  herpes:
    orolabial, 123, 146-149, 154
    genital, 149-151, 154
    keratitis, 22
    zoster, 24
  influenza, 22
  juvenile laryngeal papillomatosis, 23, 318
  leukemia, 72
  measles, 187
  meningeal carcinomatosis, 193
  meningoencephalitis, 80
  multiple leukoencephalopathy, 318
  multiple sclerosis, 5, 24, 79, 80-82, 123, 136, 193, 208, 210-211, 213-217, 219, 222, 240, 265, 319, 321
  Newcastle, 79
  osteosarcoma, 6, 296
  poliomyelitis, 264, 266-267
  postherpetic neuralgia, 24
  postpolio syndrome, 267
  progressive multifocal leukoencephalopathy (PML), 265, 318
  psoriasis, 123
  rabies, 157-179, 318
  Reye's syndrome, 5, 24
  rheumatoid arthritis, 22, 123
  rhinovirus, 22
  sarcoma, 295
  shingles, 152-153

[Disease]
  subacute sclerosing panencephalitis (SSPE), 187-194, 265, 318
  tumors, 22
  upper respiratory infection, 209-210
  viral (*see* Virus)
  visna, 265
  warts, 23
Distribution, 114-116, 122
Divergent evolution, 8
DNA methylation, 57
Dopamine, 139
Down-regulation, 71, 219
Drug:
  hepatic, 106
  metabolism, 119
  protein bound, 108
  tissue bound, 108
  volume distribution, 107
Durant, R. H., 190-191
Dyken, P. R., 191

Effects, 1
Effector cells, 75
eIF-2 initiation factor: 50, 54-55, 161
  phosphorylation, 14, 161
  protein synthesis, 14
  reticulocytes, 14
Einhorn, S., 71
Electroencephalogram (EEG), 136, 138-139, 179, 188, 193, 196, 198
Elimination half-life, drug, 105
Encephalopathy, 137
Endocrine system, 323
Endogenous IFN, 123 (*see* Interferon)

INDEX

Endonuclease, 13, 318
Endoribonuclease, 167
Endorphin, 139, 322
Endotoxin, 75
Epithelial cells, 65
Erythroid cells, 70
Excretion, 109
Experimental use, 3

Falcoff, R., 70
Färkkilä, M. 136
Farrar, W. L., 68
Fc receptor, 20, 70, 72, 75
Febrile response, 48
Feedback inhibition, 83
Feedback suppression, 70
Fenje, P., 158
Fetal brain cells, 303-305
Fever, 25, 66, 148
Fibroblasts, 65
Fog, T., 213

Gangliosides, 304-305, 310
Gene regulation, 46
Genes, interferon, 65-66
Glial fibrillary acidic protein, 309
Glial proliferation, 319
Glioma cells, 293, 297-298, 304, 309, 311
Glucocorticoid, 13, (see 2-5 A Synthetase)
Glycolipids, 309-310
Glycosylated proteins, 119

Glycosyltransferase, 310
Growth factors, 83
Growth inhibition, 67, 70, 72, 297-298, 310-311
Haase, A. T., 189
Haddad, F. S., 190
Haverkos, H. W., 147
Hemagglutinin, 189
Hematopoiesis, 70
Heparin, 55
Hepatic clearance, 106
Hepatic extraction ratio, 106
Heremans, H., 114
Herpes Zoster (see Disease)
Hirsch, R. L., 222
Histocompatibility antigens, 46, 48
Histones, 54, 55
History, 1, 5
HIV, 54
HL60, 72
HLA: 73
   antibody production, 82
   cytotoxicity, 82
   DR antigen, 68, 70, 72, 80, 82, 224, 319
   expression, 224, 319, 323
   interferon-gamma, 82
   interferon production, 80
Homology, 8
   viral, 266
Host immune response, 168
HTLV-1, 209
HTLV-3, 209
Huddlestone, J., 82
Humes, J. L., 68
Huttenlocher, P. R., 196
Hybrid molecules, 320
Hydrogen peroxide, 73
5-Hydroxylindoleacetic acid, 322

Ia determinants, 224-225
IgG:
  B cells, 74
  receptors, 72
  secretion, 71
IgM, 74
IL-1, 82
IL-1-IL-2 circuit, 82
IL-2 receptor: 68
  production, 70
  sequestration by T cells, 69
Immune:
  activation, 319
  complex, 79
  parameters, 267
  response, 69, 177, 210, 241
  suppression, 21, 68, 152-153, 171, 173, 176-177, 179
Immunoglobulin:
  secretion, 71
  synthesis, 211, 226
Immunologic effects, 219, 241
Immunologic markers, MS, 217
Immunoregulatory defects, 210, 222
Immunoregulatory effects, 19, 66-67, 241
Immunoregulatory molecules, 73
Immunosuppressive therapy, 230
Inflammatory cells, 210
Inclusion bodies, SSPE, 188-189
Indomethacin:
  side effects, 253, 257, 321
  toxicity of interferon, 246
Inducers, 7, 159, 161, 176, 194, 225, 267-268
Induction: 3, 7, 15, 67-68, 162, 169, 170-171, 177, 260
  double stranded RNA, 65
  HLA-DR antigen, 224
  leukotriene, 68
  lipopolysaccharides, 65
  phorbol myristate acetate (PMA), 66

[Induction]
  polymers, 65
  rabies vaccine, 160-161
  suppression, 68
  transcriptional, 45
  viruses, 15, 65, 68
Infection:
  athymic mice, 175
  bacterial, 21
  central nervous system, 81
  experimental, 179
  genital, 149
  herpes, 24
  malnourished children, 190
  natural history, 154
  protozoan, 21
  rabies virus, 161-163, 173
  varicella, 152-154
  viral, 15, 162, 164, 318
    response, 82
  zoster, 153-154
Inflammation, 73
Interferon:
  absorption, 122
  activity, 81
  administration, 115
  animal models, 109
  athymic mice, 175
  biochemical effects, 308-309
  bone marrow, 70
  brain, 116, 165
  brain maturation, 298
  brain tumor, 275-311
  catabolism, 122
  cell volume, 73
  class comparison, 66
  classes, 65
  CNS, effect, 298
  combinations, 229
  concentration profiles, 110
  consensus, 229, 320
  correlation between effects, 301
  corticosteroids, 323
  CSF, 80-81, 192, 258

INDEX

[Interferon]
- diffusion in brain, 165
- distribution, 114, 116, 122
- dosage, 228
- EAE, 212, 256
- endogenous, 123, 223, 258
- exogenous, 158
- families, 7
- gangliosides, 305
- genital herpes, 149-150, 154
- glial fibrillary acidic protein, 309
- glioma studies, 279, 291, 297-299, 301, 308-309, 311
- glycolipids, 309
- growth inhibition, 297, 311
- herpes, 145-154
- HLA expression, 80, 319
- Ia determinants, 225
- inducers, 145-154, 159, 161, 176, 194, 225, 268
- induction of, 15, 65, 67, 74, 80, 160-162, 319
- induction of mRNA, 15
- induction of proteins, 15, 74, 162, 171, 177, 319-320
- interferon-gamma, 80
- interleukin, 75
- in pathogenesis, 21
- lymphoblastoid, 213
- lymphotoxin, 74
- macrophages, 211
- mapping, 260
- morphologic effects, 308
- mouse, 171
- myeloid cells, 72
- neuroblastoma line, 166-169, 177
- neutralization, 162-163
- opiate receptors, 322
- pharmacokinetics, 108, 193
- physiologic, 157
- production, 79-80, 82

[Interferon]
- rabies: 171, 173, 176-177
  - prophylaxis, 158-159
- radiation, 295, 322
- recombinant, 320
- relapse in MS, 319
- resistance, 19
- responsiveness in MS, 82
- selection of, 320
- SSPE, 194, 196, 198-199
- systemic, 213
- T cells, 211-212
- titers: 192, 224-225, 258
  - in blood, 81
  - in csf, 192, 224, 243, 252-254, 258, 267
  - in rat brain, 166
- titers & viral infectivity, 164-165
- toxicity (see side effects)
- tumor necrosis factor, (74
- viral strain, 179
- varicella, 152-153

Interferon-α: 70, 73, 83
- administration, 121
- absorption, 110, 122
- antagonism to alpha interferon, 73
- antibody production, 74
- bioavailability, 110
- catabolism, 117, 122
- Fc receptors, 72
- HLA antigens, 73
- induction, 72, 225
- inhibition, 83
- mixtures, 229
- multiple sclerosis, 220-221, 223
- phagocytosis, 73
- prostaglandins, 70
- purity, 110
- retinoic acid, 70
- species, 66
- subcutaneous infusion, 121

Interferon-β:
  animal model, 276
  antagonism to gamma interferon, 73
  antibody production, 74
  absorption, 110, 122
  bioavailability, 110
  biochemical effects, 309
  biologic effect, 67
  brain tumor, 276-277, 280-282, 290-291
  catabolism, 117, 122
  combination therapy, 291
  cell volume, 73
  concentration, 110
  EAE, rat model, 212
  fetal brain cell line, 301, 303-305
  gene regulation, 53
  glioma cell line, 298-299, 301, 304-305, 308
  glycolipids, 309
  induction, 68, 225
  inhibition, 83, 301, 303
  intrathecal administration, 253
  longterm administration, 282
  multiple sclerosis, 227, 229, 241, 245, 320
  production, 242, 298
  prostaglandins, 70
  retinoic acid, 70
  side effects, 241, 253
  titers, 253
  toxicity, 241, 246, 252
Interferon-γ: 68-69, 70, 72, 83
  absorption, 110, 122
  ADCC, 72
  catabolism, 117, 122
  cell maturation, 83
  cell proliferation, 70
  cell volume, 73
  concentration, 110
  corticosteroids, 323
  CSF, 224, 322

[Interferon-γ]
  cytotoxicity, 79
  erythroid cells, 70
  Fc receptors, 72
  feedback inhibition, 83
  growth factors, 83
  growth inhibition, 72
  5-hydroxyindolacetic acid, 322
  HLA-DR, 68, 82
  induction, 66, 76
  induction-augmentation, 68
  interleukins, 68-69, 82, 319
  macrophage, 68, 70, 82-83
  monoclonal antibody, 70
  multiple sclerosis, 82, 224-225, 230, 319
    HLA antigens, 224, 319
    Ia determinants, 224-225
    NK cell, 224
  myeloid cells, 70
  N-acetylglucouronidase, 72
  neopterin, 74
  NK cells, 70
  phase I studies, 121
  production, 69-70, 82, 224
  prostaglandin, 70, 82
  serotonin, 70
  side effects, 224
  synergy with alfa interferon, 70, 83
  T cells, 68-70, 82-83
  tryptophan metabolism, 322-323
Interleukins, cytotoxicity, 79
Interleukin-1, 68, 75, 82, 319
Interleukin-2, 66, 68-70, 319
Intracerebral administration (see Administration)
Intrathecal administration (see Administration)
Intraventricular administration (see Administration)
in-vitro, 71, 79-80, 82, 219, 222, 224, 226, 228, 296-297, 299, 301, 303-307, 310

in-vivo, 71
Isoprinosine (Inosiplex), 191-192, 196, 198-199
Issacs, A., 1, 5
Issacs and Lindemann, 1, 5, 65
Itoh, H., 295

Jacobs, L., 220, 231, 319, 320-321
Johnson, K. P., 319, 329
Joncas, J. H., 192
Jones, C. E., 191

Kaplan, N. M., 158
Kuhls, T. L., 151

Landel, C. P., 116
Leucine aminopeptidase, 73
Leukemia cells, 72
Leukocytes, 75, 194, 196, 214, 219
Leukocyte migration inhibitory factor (LMIF), 267, 295
Leukotriene B4, 68
Lindemann, J., 1, 5
Lipoxygenase, 68
Lipopolysaccharides, 65
Lundblad, D., 298
Lundgren, E., 298
Lymphoblastoid cells, 13, 65, 194, 213, 226
Lymphocytes, 53, 70
Lymphotoxin, 74
Lysosomal enzymes, 72
Lytic effects, 19, 78

Macrophage, 20, 65, 67-68, 70, 74-75, 211, 319
Macrophage activating factor (MAF), 73
Macrophage inhibitory factor (MIF), 73
Magnetic resonance imaging, 226
Matrix protein, 189
Mattson, K., 137
McCoy, J. L., 295
Mechanism of action, 5, 76, 192, 255-256, 311
Memory impairment, 137
Mendelson, J., 151
Metabolism, tryptophan, 322-323
Metallothionein-II, 46
Microfilaments, 67
Microglobulin, 46
Micronuclear cells, 189
Mitogens, 46, 74
Mixed lymphocyte reaction (MLR), 72, 75
Miyoshi, T., 295
Monoclonal antibody, 55, 66, 68, 70, 109
Monocytes, 72, 75
Mono-oxygenases, 48
Montezuma-de Carvalho, M. J., 213
Morphologic effects, 308-309
mRNA: 3, 5, 209
  activation, 7
  induction, 12, 67
  micronuclear cells, 189
  synthesis, 5
  transcription, 46
Multiple sclerosis, 265, 321 (see Disease)
  animal models, 210
  blood-brain barrier, 210-211
  CSF, 211, 217, 253, 258
  epidemiology, 209
  HLA antigen, 80, 224, 319
  IgG, 217, 226

[Multiple sclerosis]
  immunologic markers, 79, 217, 221-222, 319
  immunoregulatory defects, 210
  inflammatory cells, 210-211
  interferon 81, 208-231, 240-260, 319-320
    gamma, 22, 79, 224-225, 230, 319
    production, 79-80, 211, 219, 222, 228, 246, 258
    responsiveness, 82
  interleukin, 79, 319
  measles, 209
  MRI scan, 226
  NK cells, (see listing)
  oligoclonal antibody, 209
  pathogenesis, 209-210
  poly ICLC, 225-226
  placebo effect, 214, 221-222, 319
  prostaglandins, 79, 81
  relapses, 224-225, 319
  respiratory infection, 209
  T cells, 212, 219, 255
  treatment, 81-82, 213-214, 217, 219-221, 224-234, 240-260, 319-320
  trial design, 227-228, 246, 257
Mx Protein, 14, 46, 48, 50
Mycoplasma, 68
Myeloid cells, 70, 72

N-Acetylglucouronidase, 72
Namalva cells, 56
Naphthyl acetate esterase, 72
Natural killer cells: 18, 20, 65-66, 68, 70, 75-77, 211, 229, 295, 297, 307, 309, 311, 319

[Natural killer cells]
  activation, 75, 80-81, 192
  activity, 82, 192, 211-212, 219, 221, 228, 307
  assay, 81
  augmentation, 295, 307
  CSF studies, 81
  cytolysis, 76-77, 192, 211, 305, 307
  glioma cell, 305, 307, 310-311
  glycolipids, 309, 311
  growth inhibition, 70
  HLA, 80
  interferon, 80-81
  lysis, 76-78, 305, 307, 311
  multiple sclerosis, 79, 80-82, 221, 224, 228
  placebo effect, 221, 229
  production of interferon, 68
  resistance to, 307, 311
  response, 221, 224
  responsiveness, 221
  target cell binding, 78
  twin studies, 80
Neopterin, 74
Nephectomy, 117
Nervous system disorders, 24
Nervous system, rabies, 179
Neuroblastoma cell line, 168-169, 177
Neuronal excitability, 193
Neurons, rabies, 166
Neuropeptides, 322-323
Neurophysiology, neurons, 322
Neurotoxicity, 123, 193, 228, 268 (*see* Side effects and Toxicity)
Neurotransmitters, 74, 139
NP protein, 190
Nor-dihydroguaiaretic acid, 68
N-ras RNA, 56

Obrecht, R., 139
OKT3, 70
OKT4+ cells, 66, 70, 72
OKT8+ cells, 66, 70, 72
OK10, 72, 82
2′,5′-Oligoadenylate synthetase (see 2-5A synthetase)
Oligoclonal IgG, 209
Oligonucleotides, 167–168, 177
Olsen, G. A., 146
Oncogene, ras, 56–57
Opiate receptors, 322
Organic polymers, 65
Ortaldo, J.R., 295
Ouabain, 67
Oxygen intermediates, 72

Panitch, H. S., 196, 319, 320
Pan-T monoclonal antibody, 70
Papilloma, 318
Patients, immunocompromised, 153–154
Pathogenesis, 21, 162–163, 174–175, 177, 179
Paty, D., 226
Pazin, G. J., 147, 149
Peripheral blood leukocyte (PBL), 74, 80–81
Peripheral nervous system, 136
Phagocytosis, 73
Pharmacokinetics, 103–109, 193, 269
2′-phosphodiesterase, 50
Phorbol Myristate Acetate, 66
Phospholipase A2, 78
Physiology, neurons, 322
Phytohemmaglutinin, (PHA), 66, 68–69, 71 80
Placebo effect, 214, 221, 229

Plasma cells, 74, 211
Plasma concentration, 110
Plasma concentration time curve, 104
Pokeweed mitogen, 74
Poly ICLC, 75, 159–161, 167, 194, 225–226, 267
Polymorphonuclear leukocytes, 73, 75
Postic, B., 158
Precursor cells, 82
Predictive factors, MS, 220
Priming, 53
Production: 6, 8, 157, 162, 211, 298
  cell types, 65, 68
  efficiency of, 21
  fetal brain cell, 298
  glioma cell line, 298
Properties, 6
Prostaglandins: 51, 70–71, 75, 257
  induction, 48, 79, 81–82
  inhibition of interferon, 82
  MS, 81
Protein complex, 70
Protein kinase: 14, 43, 50, 54, 162, 165, 169–170, 177
  adenovirus, 54
  heparin, 55
  p21, 56
  p65, 54
  p67, 139
  p68, 54–55
Proteins:
  antiviral, 3
  C56, 260, 321
  effector, 3
  eIF initiation, 14
  IFN action, 6–7
  induction of, 13–14
  inhibition, 54

[Proteins]
P68, 55
synthesis, 6-7, 14, 54, 78
Proteolytic degradation, 117
Proto-oncogene, 43, 46, 55
Psychomotor behavior, 137

Rabies:
  animal models, 158-164, 166-168, 170-171, 173
  2-5A synthetase, 168, 177
  cell culture, 166
  clinical features, 157-158
  EEG abnormalities, 179
  host immunity, 168, 171, 173, 176
  neutralization antibody, 160
  poly ICLC, 160-161
  replication, 162, 166
  sleep alterations, 179
  strain differences, 160, 175
  treatment, 158, 161
  vaccine, 158, 161
Radiation protection, 295
Raefsky, E. L., 70
Raji cells, 56
Receptor: 219, 304, 322
  degradation, 67
  gene dosage, 12
  IFN-beta, 305
  interactions, 12, 44
  regulation, 45, 219
  types, 44
Recombinant DNA technique, 6, 8
Recombinant interferons, 24, 76, 220, 222, 227, 320
Recycling, 75, 77
Regulation by PGE2, 75
Renal transplant, 149

Reticular activating system, 140
Reticulocytes, eLF-2 initiation factor, 14
Retinoic acid, 70
Retrovirus, 209
Reuanen, M., 194
Rhesus monkey, 269
Rice, G., 82
Risk, W. S., 190
RNA:
  double-stranded, 13-14, 50, 65
  message, 3, 5, 46, 209 (see mRNA)
  ribosomal, 266
RNase L (*see* Proteins, induction of)

Salazar, A., 319
Secondary structure, 8
Second messengers, 45
Sendai virus, 6, 66, 217
Sensory ganglia, latency, 154
Serotonin, 323
Serum concentration, 110, 122
Serum IgG, 217
Sibley, W.A., 209
Side effects: 24, 198, 225, 230, 253, 322
  bone marrow suppression, 26
  clinical trials, 193, 282
  effect on blinding, 242
  hypersomnia, 139
  immunosuppressive therapy, 230
  indomethacin, 321
  intrathecal administration, 231, 241
  intraventricular administration, 198, 231, 270-271, 322
  laboratory, 282
  mechanism, 139

INDEX

[Side effects]
  multiple sclerosis, 217, 220, 229, 251-252, 256, 260
  neurologic, 25, 123, 136, 138-139, 193, 268
  neurophysiological, 139
  neuropsychiatric, 137
  recombinant IFN, 24, 220
  reversal of, 139
  serotonin, 323
  systemic, 135-137, 153
Smith, R. A., 116, 193, 321
Species specifity, 5, 109
Steady-state concentrations, 105
Strander, H., 6
Subacute Sclerosing Panencephalitis (SSPE):
  blood-brain barrier, 188
  clinical features, 187-192, 198
  CSF findings, 188
  epidemiology, 190
  IFN titers, 192
  isolation of measles, 189
  matrix protein, 189
  measles antibody, 188-189
  NK activity, 192
  treatment, 191-192, 194, 198-200, 210
  vaccination, 190
Surface antigens, 83
Synergism, axillary cells, 70
Synergy, 71, 76
Systemic interferon, 214

Takakura, K., 321
Talas, M., 295
Target cells, 78
T cells: 66, 68, 70, 73, 174, 209, 211-212, 219, 221, 295

[T cells]
  cytotoxic, 18, 20, 75
  differentiation, 83
  dosage effects, 71
  HLA, 73
  interleukins, 69
  ratios in MS, 219, 221, 255
  PHA stimulation, 66
  production of IFN, 67
  self recognition, 73
  suppression, 70
  T suppressor cells, 70, 74, 211-212, 221
Therapeutic application, 22-24 (see Disease and Virus)
Therapeutic response, 279
Therapy: 83, 149, 152
  monitoring, 53
  selection, 320
Thymosin b4, 46
Thyrotropin, 139
Tilorone hydrochloride, 159, 267
Tissue distribution, 114, 116, 122
Tomila, E., 146
Toxicity, 135, 241-243, 245-246, 252, 268, 298, 322
Transfer factor:
  MS, 226-227
  SSPE, 191
Transferrin receptors, 71
Transformed cell, tumorgenicity, 48
Transmembrane signals, 45
Treatment:
  brain tumor, 277-280, 290, 293, 310
  follow-up, 219-220
  herpes, 151
  MS, 214, 220, 223-227, 230-231, 241-251, 253, 257-260, 320
  rabies, 161, 171, 175-177

[Treatment]
  SSPE, 194, 198-200, 210
  trial design, 229, 246, 257
  trials, 81, 219, 221, 227-228, 230, 242-243, 256-257, 267, 269-271
  trial, side effects, 251, 260
  varicella, 152
Trigeminal rhizotomy, 147-148
Trincheri, G., 65
Tryptophan, metabolism, 322-323
Tumor necrosis factor, 74
Tumors: 23
  activity, 75
  mammary carcinoma, 17
  mice, lymphoma, 17
  necrosis factor, 321
  transplantable, 18

U937 cells, 72

Vaccination: 190
  rabies, 160
Vaccinia, protein kinase, 54
Ververken, D., 213
Vervliet, G., 80
Viral:
  etiology;
    ALS, 264-265
    MS, 209, 240
  genome, 266
  latency, 145, 147, 151
  replication, 145

Virus:
  canine distemper, 209
  cytomegalovirus, 149
  encephalomyocarditis, 51
  Epstein-Barr, 22, 71
  hepatitis B, 22, 318-319
  herpes, 67, 145-154
  HIV, 54
  influenza, 14, 22, 50, 65
  measles, 81, 187, 190, 209, 265
  myxovirus, 67
  paramyxovirus, 67
  polio, 265, 267
  rabies, 157-179, 318
  retrovirus, 209
  rhinovirus, 22
  Sendai, 66, 217
  Theiler's, 265
  vaccinia, 54
  varicella, 152-154
Virus-induced demyelination, 210

Warts, 23
Wiktor, T. J., 160
Winkler, K., 296
Winston, D. J., 153

Yoshikawa, H., 109

Zoumbas, N. C., 70

About the Editor

RICHARD ALAN SMITH is Director of the Center for Neurologic Study in San Diego, California, and he also serves on the neurology staffs of Scripps Memorial Hospital in La Jolla and Harbor View Medical Center in San Diego. He is the author or coauthor of numerous articles, book chapters, and proceedings papers which focus on research and clinical aspects of presently incurable neurologic disorders, including amyotrophic lateral sclerosis and multiple sclerosis. His pioneering studies on interferon have greatly expanded our knowledge of the pharmacokinetic behavior of interferons and their application to neurologic disease. In 1968 the San Francisco Neurologic Society honored Dr. Smith with its Henry Newman Award. An associate member of the American Academy of Neurology, he is a member of the International Society for Interferon Research and the American Association for the Advancement of Science. Dr. Smith received the M.D. degree (1965) from the University of Miami School of Medicine and completed his internship (1965-1966) at Jackson Memorial Hospital in Miami, Florida, and residency in neurology (1966-1969) at Stanford University Hospital in Palo Alto, California.